THE
CHRONIC MIASMS

PSORA AND PSUEDO-PSORA

BY

J. HENRY ALLEN, M.D.

VOLUME I & II

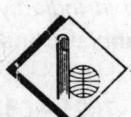

B. JAIN PUBLISHERS PVT. LTD.
NEW DELHI - 110 055

NOTE FROM THE PUBLISHERS

Any information given in this book is not intended to be taken as a replacement for medical advice. Any person with a condition requiring medical attention should consult a qualified practitioner or therapist.

© All rights are reserved. No part of this publication may be reproduced, stored in a retrieval system or transmitted, in any form or by any means, mechanical, photocopying, recording or otherwise, without prior written permission of the publishers.

Price. Rs. 129.00

Reprint Edition: 2006

© Copyright with the Publisher

Published by
KULDEEP JAIN

for

B. Jain Publishers (P) Ltd.

1921, Chuna Mandi, St. 10th, Paharganj,
New Delhi-110 055
Phones: 2358 0800, 2358 1100, 2358 1300, 2358 3100
Fax: 011-2358 0471
Website: www.bjainindia.com, Email: bjain@vsnl.com

Printed in India by
Unisons Techno Financial Consultants (P) Ltd.
522, FIE, Patpar Ganj, Delhi-110 092

ISBN 81—7021—082—8
BOOK CODE B-2006

DEDICATION

THIS BOOK IS DEDICATED TO ONE WHO, THROUGH ALL TIMES
AND THROUGH ALL TRIALS AND DISCOURAGEMENTS,
IN ALL DIFFICULTIES AND PERPLEXITIES, HAS
BATTLED FOR THE TRUTH OF HOMOEO-
PATHY LIKE A VALIANT
KNIGHT OF OLD ;
TO THE AUTHOR'S PHYSICIAN,
PRECEPTOR, TEACHER AND FRIEND, TO
THE ONE WHO FIRST TURNED HIS MIND TOWARD
THE LIGHT AND TO THE LAW OF CURE ; TO THE NESTOR OF
HOMOEOPATHY IN THE WEST, DR. H. C. ALLEN.

THE AUTHOR.

PREFACE

"As our institutions are, so are our people."

As the teacher is, so are our schools and our students. We see these truths demonstrated every day, as we study the internal workings of our medical institutions, and we meet with the finished product of their teaching, in the form of the yearly out-put of graduates. In a brief period of time we see the effect of the Alma Mater upon the people with whom our graduates come in contact—"as our institutions are, so are our people."

We can only teach the people that which we are taught. We heal our patients as we are taught to heal them. The fount and source is our sea-level—we seldom rise higher.

It was these and like thoughts which prompted the author to write this book. The younger men of our profession stand greatly in need of such a work; they must become acquainted with Hahnemann's teachings and precepts, so wonderfully laid down in his Organon of Medicine (yet so difficult for many to understand), in order to apply the law of cure. The busy practitioner has no time, and perhaps no one to help him to work out the vital problems given us by the great teacher, Hahnemann. The demands of my students, and requests from the profession at large, have induced me to put my knowledge of these subjects into book form.

Like many others of the professors, we have patiently waited for years, hoping that some zealous student of the Organon might come forward and write such a work, but no one came, so, the author has humbly taken up the work, hoping that it may in some degree meet the demand, if not the approval, of the profession.

*The second volume, *Sycosis*, which is to follow soon, will give, not only a full and exhaustive description of the action of this malignant miasm in all its forms, but the diseases and complications that arise in the primary, secondary and tertiary stages, besides a complete therapeutics of Gonorrhoea, the Kidneys, Bladder and Urinary organs in general, together with the treatment of Dysmenorrhoea in its multiple presentations, that of itself will be of great value to the profession.

A short description of how to use this work will be given at the back of the book.

THE AUTHOR.

*Chronic Miasms, Sycosis Vol. II, see Part II.

INDEX

	PAGES.
Abdomen	226–229
Bacteria and Their Relationship to Pathology	77–83
Basic Symptoms of Psora	164–269
Bowels and Intestinal Tract	230–238
Cavity of the Mouth and Teeth	195–197
Chest, Heart and Lungs	212–221
Closing Remarks	269–277
Desires and Aversions	201–205
Disease States	148–149
Ears, Hearing	186–189
Eyes and Vision	183–186
Face	192–195
Head, Outer	180–181
Heart	222–226
History and Philosophy of Psora and Pseudo Psora	9–73
Hunger	200–201
Idiosyncrasy	149–159
Mental Sphere	44–50
Miasms and Relation to Abnormal Growths	84–102
Miasms, Suppression of	103–109
Miasms, Their Relationship to Pathology	51–73
Miasms, Ways in Which Suppression Takes Place	109–139
Nose and Smell	189–191

INDEX.

	PAGES.
Predisposition	154–159
Psora	139–148
Rubrics	164–269
Scalp	182–183
Scrofula and Its Miasmatic Basis	159–164
Secondary Diseases	73– 76
Sensorium	176–180
Sexual Sphere	241–250
Skin	257–269
Stomach Symptoms of Psora and Pseudo-Psora	205–212
Suppression of Miasms	103–109
Taste	197–200
Upper and Lower Extremities	250–257
Urinary Organs	239–241

THE CHRONIC MIASMS

PSORA AND PSEUDO-PSORA

The discovery of the chronic miasms by Hahnemann was a deathblow to the erroneous conceptions of the etiology of disease, in his day, and it is none the less true in our day, although a century of years lies between, and an army of thinkers, and investigators, along these lines have arisen, and many of them departed this life since Hahnemann said that Psora was the parent, or the basic element, of all that is known as disease. Since his day many an etiological structure has arisen, but to fall with its own weight, or to be torn down and its debris removed to make room for other structures no less endurable. Probably one of the greatest and most endurable of these structures, or in other words, one of the greatest attempts at formulating a theory, or basic principle of philosophy for the present so-called regular system of medicine, was Virchow's cellular pathology theory. So numerous were the followers of this high-class leader of that school that he has been styled the *high priest of cellular pathology*, which for more than twenty years formed the basis of orthodox medicine, but which has been largely displaced and abandoned for other theories of no greater therapeutic value. Klebs has declared Virchow's theories to be undemonstrable and, indeed, extremely improbable. But in his doctrine of independent activity of the cell there lay concealed *vitalism*, a thing untenable by any materialistic school of medicine. He came up to the very doorway of the truth. His cell, the unit of life, was vivified or deified, as the case might be, by chemical processes, or by chemical change. But the great Hahnemann had conceived of a life force that was before the chemical or mechanical; hence, his theory of the vital force, without which there would be no organic chemistry. Thus arose chemical medicine or chemical therapeutics, with all its multiplicity of chemical compounds and formulas, as seen in the prescription writing of today. It has ended, as we might expect, in empiricism, which is governed only by the seeming necessity of the case and the judgment of the individual in charge.

Hahnemann had gone all through this, had weighted and measured it, analyzed it from every standpoint, but found it wanting. No one can read carefully the sixty-eight pages of the introduction to his *Organon* without coming, positively, to that conclusion. He not only understood fully the unscientific workings of all the systems of medicine of his day, but he went farther; he was able to prophesy the outcome and the progress and path of these systems. Why? Because he understood so well their unscientific basis, that he knew that their development could not be otherwise. "The spring could not reach a higher level than its source." How true this is. The systems have not changed materially; their modes and methods of procedure are unaltered. While they have abandoned some of their grosser and more objectionable methods, they have adopted others which are no less objectionable and no less harmful, and fully as detrimental to the good of the race. In this I refer, of course, only to their therapeutic methods. Nor can it be otherwise where "no other law save man's reason regulates events," when no law dictates, or where there are no divine principles to which to conform; where nothing is stable or fixed in the entire system, be it therapeutic, etiological or pathological, even; all are subjects of change and uncertainty. But Hahnemann has brought order from confusion; having formulated substantial laws and principles, he has removed uncertainty, and all his true followers are of one mind and one accord because of these facts.

Some one may ask, why it is necessary for a true homœopath to know about these chronic miasms. As long as he prescribes according to the law of similia he cures his cases. There are many reasons why he should be able to distinguish their presence in the organism, whether it be psora, latent syphilis, especially the tubercular form, or whether it be sycosis. Dr. Hering, however, in his introductory remarks in the *Organon* (3d

American edition), thinks it not of vital importance: "What important influence can it exert whether a homœopath adopt the theoretical opinions of Hahnemann or not, so long as he holds the principal tools of the master and the materia medica of our schools? What influence can it have, whether a physician adopt or reject the psoric theory, so long as he always selects the most similar medicine possible?" The last line is well timed: "*So long as he selects the most similar medicine possible.*" The fact is, we can not select the most similar remedy possible unless we understand the phenomena of the acting and basic miasms; for the true similia is always based upon the existing basic miasms, whether we be conscious or unconscious of the fact. The curative remedy is but the pathopoesis of a certain pathogenesis of an existing miasm. The proving of a remedy would be very indefinite to us if the name were withheld from us. Suppose that you were making a proving of sulphur or aconite. Why, the first thing you would do, would be to ask for their names, you would say, I shall not attempt to use these remedies without knowing their names. So it should be with the disease-producing agent. We should know, not only the name of that underlying principle that fathers that phenomena with which we are so diligently and earnestly contending and combating. It is the difference between an intelligent warfare and fighting in the dark, it is no longer a battle in the mist. Again, suppose that we prescribe the similar remedy and have no

THE CHRONIC MIASMS. 13

knowledge of the laws of action and reaction (or primary and secondary action), how can we watch the progress of a case without a definite knowledge of these disease forces (miasms), with their mysterious, but persistent, progressions, pauses, rests, forward movements, retreats and attacks along unfamiliar lines, and of whose multiplied modes of action we have taken no cognizance? In fact, if we know nothing about the traits and characteristics of our enemy, is it possible to wage an equal warfare? Suppose that one would say that disease was due to bacteria, to a certain germ, to atmospheric conditions, to taking cold—facts to which the majority of diseases are attributed, would those facts assist us in the selection of the similar remedy? Would they help us to understand the phenomena of germ development, of taking cold? Why should he take a cold? Why should one have germs or be subject to atmospheric changes? are thoughts that come to the reasoning mind. Why should disease return in the same form or some diverse form? These are the things that disturbed the mind of Hahnemann, and in the end, led him to discover the psoric theory of disease. I say to Dr. Hering, NO, the men who select the similar remedy and who are ignorant of causes and effects are not true healers of the sick and have not the mind of the master. His is a true system of medicine, but there are thousands of men and women who become familiar with but a few remedies or a few pages of our materia medica, and who go out to fight against the complexity of disease, which are due to the combinations of psora, syphilis and sycosis, and have no knowledge of the character and habits of the enemy. Their work is often hidden for years, so latent and pent-up are these forces in the organism. How many times have we based our prescription upon the totality of the symptoms that were entirely nervous or reflex, when, really, in the totality, values were not considered. But values *must* be considered, for reflexes are always secondary, and primary or basic symptoms directly of miasmatic origin. The nervous phenomena may be palliated by such a procedure; but it returns, and time is lost in the experiment; while the physician skilled in anti-miasmatic prescribing overlooks the foamings upon the surface, and dips deeper into the case, looking for *prima causa morbi*, and applies a remedial agent that has a deeper and closer relationship with perverted life force. The results were always better, and thus he soon learns to familiarize himself with these basic groupings that lie beneath all that may be called disease "simply because of their more tedious and burdensome operation (as psora, syphilis and sycosis), can not be overcome or extinguished by the unaided vital energies until these are more thoroughly aroused by the physician, through the medium of a *very similar*, yet more powerful, morbific agent,' (a homoepathic remedy.) (A footnote from See. 107, Organon.) You see it must be a very similar remedy suited to the nature and action of one of these chronic miasms. In this way we get at the natural disease itself whose existing dynamis lies in the peculiar dynamis of the miasm, Hahnemann has said (paragraph 13, *Organon*) that all the antipathic schools consider disease to be something separate from the organism, and the vivifying principle that animates or vitalizes the organism to be some obscure or hidden thing stored away somewhere internally. They could not discern, it seems that invisible something, called life, that suffers from these miasmatic influences. Continuing the thought in paragraph 15 : "The suffering of the immaterial vital principle which animates the interior of our bodies, when it is morbidly disturbed, produces symptoms in the organism that are manifest" etc.; and it is these morbidly produced symptoms that constitute what is known as disease in all its multiplied forms, whether functional or structural.

A knowledge of all miasmatic phenomena would be, in toto, a complete knowledge of all that is known as disease, and beyond these symptoms there is nothing discoverable or recognizable as disease.

Paragraph 19 : "Disease is nothing more than changes in the general state of the human economy, which declare themselves as symptoms;" or, in other words; disease is but the influence of some subversive force, acting in conjunction with the life force, subverting the action and changing the physiological momentum. Thus we can safely say that disease is but a modified mode of motion, a vibratory change. Hemple's definition of disease covers this ground, to my mind, more fully than any other philosophical definition: "*Disease is the totality of the effects, by which we recognize or perceive the action of a peculiar order of subversive forces upon an organism which has been exceptionally or specially adapted to, or prepared for their reception.*" We might draw a little closer if we say disease is the vicarious embodiment of some miasmatic influence that has bonded itself with the life force, producing disease according to the type, as is seen in psora or any other of the chronic miasms, just as we see in a piece of lime or charcoal an external, visible type or embodiment of an internal dynamis that through the process of potentization develops the artificial subversive force. The difference is that one has an existing natural bond (that is the miasm) with the life force; while the other (drug) can be introduced into the organism and, by its bond with the life force, produce the artificial disease phenomena, a fact that is undemonstrable to science save through the action of the life-force's dynamis.

It might be well to recall some of the simple reasons given by Hahnemann as proof of the existence of a chronic miasm, lying beneath all these multiplied outward expressions of disease. The first to be mentioned was the persistency of chronic ailments, seen when the diet, hygiene and general health of those patients were carefully considered. Even then the life force was unable to disengage itself from certain recurrent expressions of disease, conditions which were constantly repeating themselves ; although the apparently well-selected remedy was given with what appeared to be success, as the symptoms were, for a time, removed ; removed but to return with all their former energy, or with a new expression of symptoms, having to all appearances the same root or origin.

With no external etiological reason they seem to come from within the organism itself, developing from some peculiar dynamis within. Hahnemann also observed that they accompanied some physiological process, or were in some way connected with the functions of the organism. Was it possible that disease was perverted function and, too, that function governing the life processes was deranged ? Again he saw, under the action of the homœopathic remedy (curative action) disease disappear suddenly by the use of the higher potencies, often changing its expression, a sort of retro-metamorphosis, or a receding of disease in the reverse order that it came, going back through all the changes and processes that it came up through, finally disappearing altogether, leaving no trace of its prior existence. These thoughts came to him, when did it begin ? what was the source of its existence ? It must be that some latent, inherent, internal, pre-existing cause, having its habitat in the organism, yet not connected in a material way with that organism, but, with that dynamis, the life force itself, becoming a part of it or co-existent with it, and having a similar dynamis, which arose and fell as it was disturbed by other causes from without, known in our nomenclature as secondary, or exciting, causes. Thus he noticed that the skin never produced an eruption upon itself (outside of traumatic or chemical causes) ; never assuming a morbid state unless obliged to do so by some previous perverted change or abnormal activity in the organism itself. Again the eruptive disease would, as a rule, cause the disappearance of the whole of the original trouble. Not only was this true of an eruptive disease, but it was equally true of all the eliminative processes of all organs of the body. This was equally true when diseased processes were suppressed. For a time the disease forces assumed a latent condition, but sooner or later new diseased processes set up that were deeper and profounder in their ultimate actions, assuming often malignant states or acute processes, dangerous to life. It, therefore, could not be possible that external causes, alone, did lie at the bottom of all this. In suppressions, whether by local means or by the use of strong drugs internally, secondary manifestations of these *chronic affections* appeared sooner or later. He further noticed that when the organism, either by its own action or by the use of some powerful remedial agent (such as sulphur) threw an eruption upon the skin, that the original disturbance disappeared or became quiescent so long as the secondary process (eruption) was left undisturbed. Hahnemann further noticed that the use of crude drugs not only produced dangerous medicinal effects, but that they greatly embarrassed the life forces, complicated the diseased processes and undermined the whole organism in all directions. Especially was this true when there was present a marked psoric or miasmatic state, which proved to him that some one specific cause (outside of venereal diseases) lay at the bottom of all chronic, as well as acute, expressions of disease; and this unknown, devitalizing principle he named PSORA.

Hahnemann began to trace the history of this miasm, psora (*Greek which means to itch*), and found it to be of ancient origin, its history running back through the history of all nations, even to the most ancient oriental.

Hahnemann in a footnote (page 25, vol. I, Chronic Diseases, old edition) refers us to the third book of Moses (Leviticus), where the priest differentiates the eruption in its earliest stages from the plague of leprosy. It is evident, however, that the name psora has been given to various, if not numerous, eruptive diseases appearing in the human family in all the nations of the earth. Today we understand psora to be a basic miasm, not confined to any special form of eruption upon the skin of the individual, but that it is the parent of a multitude of functional and pathological changes that take place in the human organism. True it frequently presents itself in some form of an eruptive disease, and, undoubtedly, it originally began as a vesicular eruption accompanied with an itching or itchy sensation, a *pruritus* being, probably not only a primary factor in the acute form of the miasm, but a persistent, if not a constant, symptom throughout the whole history of its existence. No other symptom is so pathognomonic of psora as a *pruritus*. In syphilis and sycosis it is absent, and when we find it present in these miasms we can assure ourselves that they are closely intermarried with the psoric miasm.

The pure life of the Israelites up to near the time of Christ left them comparatively free from the severe internal inroads of this miasm. Their simple lives, good habits, freedom from over-indulgence in wines or spiritous liquors, meats, rich foods, etc., kept the disease largely confined to the surface of the body. The physical training and physical culture of the early Greeks also greatly mitigated its action. Not until men began to locate or congregate in cities, and their habits began to be corrupt do we see it breaking forth in its true vigor and virulency. Outside of a study of the disease in Europe, Hahnemann could say but little of its ravages in the earlier periods of the human race. There is no doubt, however, that its action became greatly intensified, and the diseases that it brought forth became more numerous and more complex as the orthodox schools became more acquainted with chemical therapeutics and the minerals came more commonly into use, especially those of arsenic, quinine and the mercuries. In the use of mineral medicines and local medicants, suppressions became of more frequent occurrence, and soon new and more malignant manifestations presented themselves, in the form of severe epidemics that broke out during and before Hahnemann's time. Today these suppressive methods still flourish. Though not confined to the same methods, yet many of them are still in vogue, and new ones added, such as the extensive use of electricity—the X-ray being the most modern, and probably the most positive—means of suppressing the deeper and more profound pathological expressions of these chronic miasms. Even such malignancies as cancer, lupus, tumers, enlarged glands, even psoriasis, eczema and other eruptive diseases have been suppressed by the persistent use of this most powerful of the yet known forces ever discovered by man, and to have been palmed off for genuine removals of the cause, and bona fide cures. Of the other modern methods used to suppress these chronic miasms and which might be mentioned, are mineral baths of all kinds, medicated douches, actual cautery, surgical operations, especially the removal of organs, curettements, etc.

Hahnemann mentions the excessive indulgence in such drinks as coffee, tea, also the use of tobacco, which is more or less drugged with arsenic, strychnine, opium, tonka beans, and other nostrums, besides the general use of spirituous liquors, stimulating and highly seasoned foods, as having a very marked effect in stirring up these latent miasms and rendering their actions more complex and difficult to cure.

As has been already mentioned, psora originally came as a form of itch of a contagious nature, of so contagious a nature that a shake of the hand or even a touch of the garments of the affected one would carry the disease to another. This can not be said of the other chronic miasms, syphilis and sycosis. That psora first made its appearance as a pruritis of some form, followed by a fine vesicular eruption, is no doubt true, as has been the testimony of Hahnemann, as well as that of many of his followers. It could not appear primarily in any form of eruption in such diseases as eczema, psoriasis, etc., as they are all secondary processes of psora or some other miasm (psoriasis being of a gouty or sycotic origin). It was only through the unscientific and suppressive methods of treatment that psora has assumed such diversity of character, and, as a natural consequence, through the natural law of progression, its future manifestations would be greatly magnified in their distinctive action, until structural changes in the organism took place. These outward expressions of the latent power of psora could not forever contend against or contest the epidemic field with the therapeutist who saw nothing in disease but the local expression, therefore attacked it with such powerful local measures as the ancient, as well as the modern, orthodox healers of the sick were wont to use. Frequently psora took in its flag, and then a contest took place within the inner tabernacles of the organism itself, and was continued until the life forces were baffled and had to give up the fight by a rendering up of the life to their prolonged influences ; and all, too, because the ignorant therapeutist misguided the life forces that, under favourable circumstances, would have kept their enemy *psora* upon the surface of the organism, or upon the skin. When a suppression took place in an organism where two or more miasms were present, all the conditions above mentioned were magnified and intensified, as is frequently seen when psora and syphilis are perfectly combined by hereditary transmission. I say "perfectly combined," for there can be no other such perfection of bond of the miasms with the life forces as is produced through heredity. The tubercular diathesis is the result of such a union, which is one of the profoundest in its depth of action of any diseased state or condition that can be named. So we see that pseudo-psora is worse than psora by itself, and the same thing may be said when psora and sycosis are combined; but they do not compare in their destructive action as when the tubercular element is present. Specific and malignant, acute, febrile or inflammatory states, as pneumonia, diphtheria, maligna, syphilis, erysipelas phlegmonous; inflammation of the brain, heart, kidney, or destructive appendicitis, as a rule, always have the two miasms present. I always look out for them in every case of the above-mentioned diseases.

Again, when we meet stubborn and determined pathological states or diseased conditions of an apparently simple nature, such as pain, neuralgia, headaches, epistaxis, nausea, vomiting, rheumatism, piles, ulcers, boils, or any simple localized condition not easily amenable to treatment, we may expect two or more miasms present. I would like to illustrate this fact more clearly by a simple case of rectal trouble: Mrs. M., aet. 24; dark complexion; small in stature; mother of one child and one of a family of twelve children, all of which are dead except two (herself and a sister) from tubercular diseases. I was called to treat her for a rectal trouble, a fissure in the rectum extending to the edge of anus. So severe was her suffering that I was compelled to operate or lose the case, as she had no faith in homœopathy. I did so, but on the sixth day a little tit-like process came down close by where the fissure opened externally. New symptoms developed quite generally, which were as follows: Hot, burning hands and feet, wants window open, wants fresh air, can't bear any covering over her, although quite often she will have hot waterbags about her; weak, hungry feelings between meals; all her symptoms worse in the evening; tosses about the bed all night and can not sleep as she is too warm, then falls asleep near morning and rests well most of the forenoon. She is cross, irritable, scolds and finds fault. Skin dry, harsh, red, itching, pimples on different parts of the body. Sulphur 50m was given, and within forty-eight hours all the above grouping of symptoms began to disappear, and in their place came a profuse greenish yellow leucorrhœa, excoriating and acrid in its nature, biting and burning the pudendum. The rectum began to heal rapidly and was soon well, after which the leucorrhœa disappeared. While I was treating this case her husband was taken down with acute rheumatism which followed a severe wetting he had received, having been exposed to a drenching rain for several hours. This, of course, only strengthened my diagnosis of acquired gonorrhœal sycosis by her husband and that my patient had also contracted the disease from him and later on suppressed the disease, thus the rectal trouble as a result. This case was cured with sulphur c. m., although the operative procedure was condemned as a wrong thing to do.

We must always be on the lookout for the basic miasm in these cases that is so unwilling to yield to treatment. Nature always sets up, if possible, peripheral inhibitory points of disease, pathological often, but sometimes functional; and if they are interfered with locally, whether operative or not, the life force, according to the law of progression and through the law of reaction, sets up another inhibitory center of reaction, within the organism and nearer the deeper centers of life. A peripheral inhibition can no longer eliminate the effects of the degenerative process in the life forces set up by the more profound hold the miasm has taken on the organism. Then, again, the vitalism of the organism is often so lowered that it has not that reactive power or resistive force to set up another peripheral inhibition; therefore it yields readily to the new order of things, and at once accommodates itself to the new order of change, for the new condition was induced by new modes of action or of motion, and the stress of the miasmatic force was centered upon new areas of the organism, and the perverted physiological process became more complex in their derangements or functions, and the retrograde metamorphosis more difficult to analyze, until the therapeutist and the pathologist are so lost in a maze or tangle of symptomatology that they can not systematically arrange or classify. It is in this way that cachexias come, through a prolonged intoxication of the whole system, even to the remotest cell and fibre of our being, due to a damming up in the organism, of some active miasms that ought to be eleminating these toxics from the body, through some eleminative process peculiar to itself, and which, if not remedied, will continue into a chronic form until every feature and outline of our being expresses malignant manifestations of their presence, until the whole house in which we live, becomes an unhabitable place for the in-dwelling of the life.

So universal is the action of psora and so generally does it affect all organized life, that there is scarcely any creature that exists unaffected by it or which does not show some sign or manifestation of its destructive processes. This is true of the lower forms of life ; even vegetable life is not free from it ; for in the deformed, decaying and dying leaf, we see it. Yea, psora is the primary manifestation of primeval sin, of the primary curse, the prophetic fulfillment of "thou shalt surely die." In order to understand these things, we must understand some of those fundamental principles governing homœopathy—the dynamic origin of disease, the dynamitization of the drug or remedy, and the application of similia. It was the application of similia that led Hahnemann to see the miasmatic cause of disease ; he saw that it was a contest between the dynamics of the drug and the dynamics of life, a battle waged by dynamitized, subversive influence upon the living organism which was a constant thing, an unceasing thing, because it resided ever in the organism and was in bond with the life ; and although the life forces might at times apparently free themselves from that influence, it invariably returned, often changed in its expressions of action and its character, but invariably it was the same old psora, though in a new garment or in a new disguise. How generally we see the landmarks of one of these chronic miasms stamped upon the organism. We see it in every feature and every physiological process; in the shape and contour of the body; upon visual expression, the face, nose, lips, ears, mouth, upon the hair, its growth, luster and general beauty or lack of it. We see it upon the skin in its colour or shadings, its local temperature, yes, we can tell the miasm often by a touch, by that response in our very inner being, the mental, the moral, even the spiritual, give us responses of its presence and of its influence.

For thousands of years psora has disfigured and tortured mankind. The business of the miasms is to kill, to destroy, to tear down, to murder life through their multiplied processes. They kill by sepsis, by devitalizing the blood, by anemic states, so reducing the red blood corpuscles that there is no means left whereby the organism can be fed. Not alone are these patients deprived of food, but of that life-giving and sustaining principle, oxygen. If they build, they build false structures, such as tumors, nodes, enlarged glands, fibrous growths, cancers, etc. These we call abnormal growths or pathological states, which simply means another way of life. These false or abnormal growths are constructed out of false material, because all the processes of life are false or perverted, so that a physiological truth becomes a physiological lie, or a death-dealing element working, or attempting to work, with a life-giving principle.

The action of the miasms is to make gaps and breaches in nature that the debilitated life forces can not repair. They deform the body, dull the intellect and destroy reason. They destroy men's wills, hope, courage, and drive the sunshine out of life, bringing all under shadow, making him down-hearted, low spirited, hypochondriacal, even to suicide. They are co-workers with sin and with death. They smile when men go mad, and laugh when he agonizes. Their instruments of torture are pain, neuralgia, rheumatism. They hate life and health and strength, and glory in death, in weakness and in feebleness. Their febrile fires burn, scorch, dry up the tissues to a crisp, and exhaust us even to death. The ever-vigilant life forces are forever contending with them. When their presence is felt in the organism every process, every organ is up in arms, every reserve is brought into action, and every nerve impulse into play, to oppose their inroads and to arrest their progress ; secretion, excretion, even the whole circulatory system becomes exaggerated and intensified to accommodate itself to the new order of things. The miasms are like enemies entrenched. They attack us at all our weak points, recede and advance, advance and recede. They never seem to tire or grow less. When we are asleep they break in upon us ; when we become tired or exhausted they come upon us unawares and take us by surprise. So, like sentinels, we must be ever on our guard ; we must be ever watchful, ever ready to oppose their advances ; to understand their tactics, both when they are active and when they are passive, when they give forth their acute, chronic or latent expressions.

To the follower of Hahnemann the word *Psora* convey a most important meaning. It means that disease is more than it seems to be on the surface. It means that no external expression can exist (that is outside of some mechanical or chemical cause) but that has the pre-existing internal dynamis, and however slight and trifling the external latent expression may appear, nevertheless the internal psora affects the whole organism, and any part or portion of the organism may sooner or later manifest it upon its surface. Often the psoric fire may be so latent and so inactive that one may deem himself healthy, or, others may think that he is healthy until he receives some injury, or until something unusual happens. Joy, grief, fear, overwork or some trifling cause arouses the sleeping monster, and the patient, to his astonishment, finds himself ill. True, we may live a comparatively healthy normal life for an indefinite period, especially if we are endowed with a strong, robust constitution, a cheerful disposition and a contented mind; but overfatigue, either mental or physical, or some trifling irregularity of life may develop some acute disease, which means that the miasm is aroused from its slumber. A slight mental shock, a fall, a slight injury, a broken bone, an injury to a ligament or muscle may become the disturbing element that develops the sleeping miasm and brings it into action. The nature of the disturbance may be varied, often depending on the original constitution or previous life of the patient, his character, vocation, education, temperament, predisposition, latitude, altitude, season of the year, circumstances of life, and many other conditions that might be mentioned. These are only a few of the causes to be considered that may arouse the internal miasm. Often a simple error in diet, an excess in eating or drinking, a cold drink, a hot bath, a mineral bath, over heat of the sun, wetting the body or the feet, a too long walk, carrying a heavy burden, an undue excitement or overjoy, continued grief, disappointment, failures in business or in life generally, may be the starting-point whereby psora is aroused from its slumber, when, without mercy, it assails the whole or a part of the organism.

and nothing can save it but the removal or cure of the psora.

When psora develops some local disease, or, perhaps, some positive local symptom that relieves the internal stress of the disease, then the old phenomena of the internal disease or psora is hushed, or, for the time, is calmed down or is quiescent as long as the local trouble upon the skin is not interfered with locally by the attending physician. The local manifestation assists the physician very much in his cure of the psoric state, for if similia is applied the external disease will disappear in proportion to the annihilation of the internal psora. This is the most simple method of procedure in the cure of psora. Of course, it is impossible to get such splendid results when cases are mismanaged, as a perfect similia may not present itself again for a long period of time, owing probably, to a misdirected, if not suppressed condition. Hahnemann says that the sensitive and irritable fibre is so disturbed by massive doses of medicine, frequently repeated by the allopathic physician, that the vital principle soon modifies the action of the organism so that, for a time at least, it is protected, or, in a manner, shielded from their assaults. But it will soon be seen that this irritability and sensitivity is soon diminished. This condition of things may be carried even to the mental, as is frequently seen in hospitals for the insane, from the overuse of nerve sedatives, such as the bromides, opium, and the coal tar preparations now in common use. These conditions are the ones of which Hahnemann speaks as being incurable, or the most difficult of all to reach by the aid of the homœopathic remedy. Generally, however, those dealing in this kind of treatment usually attribute the cause to the malignant working of the primary disease. These cases are the ones in which the homœopathic physician does not consider well the extent of the wreckage or the length to which the destructive processes have been carried before promising a cure in a stated period of time. Often the patient, for a time, sinks down under the sudden removal of strong tonics or stimulants given by the opposite school, and their effects have to be counteracted before the similia for the original disease can be selected. The healer now has not simple psora to deal with, as in the first place, but a drug miasm, if I may be allowed to use the term, plus a disease miasm or psora. Sometimes, in cases of recent drugging, this can be accomplished by simply giving no medicine, making a careful arrangement of the diet and the hygienic condition of the patient, and then the life force will of itself throw off the bad effects of the crude drug, and the primary disease presents itself in a clear and concise manner.

From what has already been said, the true physician should not base his prescription on pathological names which he finds so clearly set forth in the numerous works on pathology, but should go deeper down into his cases and gather together the bedrock symptoms of psora or of the present acting miasm, and around this diseased grouping arrest and the disease process at its, and in its, dynamic origin; and, further, when he has found the similia he should guard against interfering with its action in any way, such as prescribing for some simple intercurrent disease, as headache, cough, diarrhœa, offensive perspiration, leucorrhœa or any new development, unless dangerous to life; for we can have but a very faint conception of the manner in which the life force may eliminate the original disease upon which our prescription is based. In the majority of cases the new developments, or new symptoms, have appeared some time before in the history of the case, that were probably suppressed; therefore, their reappearance is only a necessary step in the progress of the recovery of the case. In sycosis such symptoms may arise as irritability of the bladder, frequent, and often painful urination, the same being often of a strongly ammoniacal odor or highly loaded with urates.

In my earlier experiences with homœopathy I would frequently give an intercurrent remedy, and, as a rule, the true similimum would never present itself again, and what should have been a success was turned into a failure. We can not emphasize this truth too much, as it means failure every time we yield to the wishes of the patient. The very fact that the first well chosen remedy called out the new symptoms or new phenomena was sufficient proof that the remedy had laid hold of the existing miasm at its innermost center of existence. Hence, the first remedy should not be disturbed in its action, not until it has ceased to work completely, and further progress can be discerned in any direction recognizable either to the patient or physician. Many of these troublesome symptoms, says Hahnemann, disappear of themselves, and in the natural order in which they came ; but if they are persistant and a constant annoyance, they are to be taken into consideration and a new prescription made, as the original prescription has not been well chosen. Often, however, the giving of a higher potency will do the necessary work without a change of remedy.

There are three errors, says Hahnemann, that we are all liable to make : "1st the selection of the improper remedy ; 2d, the improper potency ; and, 3d, not letting the remedy act a sufficient length of time." The trouble with most of us is we do not study the Organon sufficiently to become well enough acquainted with the principles and laws governing the action of disease or of drugs. For that matter, we are too apt to center all our efforts upon the study of our remedies and their provings, and thus neglect the other vital part, the knowledge of the way to use them, which comprises, among other principles, the third law of motion brought forth by Newton, *"that action and reaction are equal, but opposite."* In the study of optics we see a similar law revealed, and that is "the angle of incidence is equal to the angle of refraction." If you deflect the life forces in any way, whether in disease or health, the law of reaction, or the law of deflection, will surely assert itself sooner or later in the history of that life, and the results are, new and more profound expressions of disease or disease processes. If, after giving a deep-acting antipsoric, a diarrhœa or some acute process is set up and we arrest it either, by antipathic or homœopathic means, especially if the remedy selected does not cover the totality of the symptoms, but is directed to the one symptom of which you wish to dispose, the result is : the curative action of the antipsoric is, as a rule, at once arrested. Again, if the latent symptoms of psora, upon which the antipsoric remedy is based, should develop more prominently or of a more intense nature we need not feel alarmed, for more often than not, they soon subside, and the undue disturbance is often an assurance of a cure rather than a discouragement. When psora, or any of the miasms for that matter, have existed in an organism for years, and during that time have manifested themselves in both latent and acute manifestations of a various nature, and we come to treat them homœopathically with the antipsoric remedy we may, through the workings of its curative action, have in some order or degree, a part, if not all, of these manifestations again presented. This is one of the strong reasons why we should not interfere with the action of the well selected anti-miasmatic remedy, as it has so much to do in evolving and working out these different series or expressions of the miasm's own workings. This is especially true when the highest potencies are used. No one can conceive of the hidden secrets and infinite depth of action of similia, which reaches from profundity to profundity in the different potentials now in use today.

"*The fundamental rule,*" says Hahnemann, "*in treating chronic diseases is this* : *to let the carefully selected homœopathic antipsoric remedy act as long as it is capable of exercising a curative influence,* and there is a visible improvement going on in the system." This is the secret of success: to be able to watch with patience the wonderful workings of the well selected remedy upon the natural disease and the artificial disease disappears with the curing of the natural disease.

There is scarcely a day passes that we do not see some new manifestation of psora. It presents itself in a diversity of forms and characters.

There are certain conditions or states of the organism due wholly to the action of the miasms and recognized in our works on pathology under special names, as cachexia, dyscrasia diathesis, scrofula, struma, idiosyncrasy, predisposition, hereditary predisposition and hereditary states, all of which are due, directly or indirectly, to the workings of, or they are expressions of, miasmatic action. When we speak of cachexia we mean a depraved condition of the whole system, we mean blood changes often due to toxic causes, whether they be due to drugs such as arsenic, quinine, plumbum, mercury or to animal poisons, vaccination, or to malarial poisons ; diseased states as smallpox, diphtheria, syphilis, typhoid fever, etc., it is an advanced chronic, active miasmatic state, often a disintegrative process taking place usually in the fluids of the body, especially in the blood, an involvement of every cell and fibre, a dissolution of chemical constituents and biological elements, a stasis often in the elimination of waste products from the organism. Cachexias may be acute, subacute or chronic. Sometimes they depend on a single miasm, and again all the chronic miasms may be present. If sycosis or syphilis is specifically combined with psora the cachexia usually assumes semi-malignant, if not malignant forms, even to the destruction of life, ending in toxic states, specific anemias or general exhaustion and collapse. To cure a cachexia, we must select our remedies with care, basing our prescriptions upon the true symptomatology of the active miasm, when often the most discouraging and complex conditions disappear.

In our study of miasmatics we are brought into a closer relation with the nature and cause of the disease, than we can possibly be drawn through the study of disease, under any other system yet conceived or taught in our schools and colleges. Indeed diseases become no longer a mystery, but a clear problem, which is to be solved by a careful study of the phenomena that each case presents; each case being a distinct and separate study in itself. Our cures are not made through the application of our therapeutics to a nomenclature, but to a classical grouping of all the phenomena therein presented and that which we see often, is invisible to the physician who has no knowledge of miasmatics; but these things are made clear to those who have investigated carefully Hahnemann's anti-miasmatic theory of disease, which reveals its true nature and origin : for lying behind his theory, we see *sin to be the parent of all the chronic miasms, therefore the parent of disease.* It never was intended, nor can it be possible, that disease could have any other origin. Man was the disobedient one, and through his disobedience came disease. "The wages of sin is death." Nature may, in some ways, assist in bringing about disease in man, but nature did not become his enemy until after his fall. Yea, even all nature, too, is perverted, for all has come under the curse of man's fall. Therefore, why should we blame the climate or the elements or bacteria or micro-organisms, when the Creator tells us plainly that sin is behind all the ills to which man is heir?

Thus it is: "and even as they did not like to take God in *their* knowledge, God gave them over to a reprobate mind," or a mind "void of judgment," as the new version gives it; his mind is "void of judgment," Rom. 1: 28. He wanders about the earth looking for the truth and cannot find it. By not believing His word, he leaves out his Creator, Who is the Source of all true knowledge. So, it is no wonder that man is ever bringing forth new cause for disease, and ever changing his etiology and his therapeutics. As disease is the result of sin, so are micro-organisms, and all physical expressions of disease whether they be physiological, pathological or micrological. This leaving God out of his knowledge can be seen in his theory of creation, of evolution, whether it be of living organisms or the formation of the earth and the planetary systems, he will have it *his* way and not the *Creator's* way. Thus is he given over to a mind "void of judgment." It is the natural course of things, for in his studies of life or of creation he has made God's word a lie, and he assumes to know and teach the truth; but how can he with a mind "void of judgment?" Hahnemann saw this great truth in his day, as his mind was illuminated by the light of his new discoveries, or the light of law. It is only through a law or by a principle that we can see the Creator's plans and work out His hidden mysteries.

The antipathic schools today can no longer be said to be governed by this old formula, *contraria contrariis*, as it no longer expresses the exclusive character of these schools, since they have thrown out physiology and the vital idea of a life force and adopted the physio-chemical methods now in vogue. This makes the practitioner a physio-chemical physician, who bears all relationship to chemistry and none to dynamics. Disease, according to this latter theory, becomes often a chemical accident—a dietetic error; there is no primary vital principle, no separate and supreme cause of life. They would have us believe the physical, mental and moral expressions of life are dependent upon chemistry; function of organ, muscular contraction, idea, thought, loss or repair of tissue, physiological growth and pathological change—yea, the whole superstructure, etiology, pathology, physiology, therapeutics, all must conform to this far-reaching chemical formula converting every organism into a laboratory for chemical purposes and for chemical debauch.

In the study of *psora* we must look at it not from the chemical side, but from the potential side; for it is a potential, and a potential that bonds itself with that great potential, the life force, that vital energy which not only vivifies the whole organism, every cell, every fibre of our being, but sustains and controls all cell life and every physiological expression of life. Psora is the potential when it becomes well bonded with the life force; this same life force has no power, within itself, to disengage itself from that bond. It is a potential, bonded and co-operative with a potential, which through its co-operation with this life force, together with other miasms, causes all physiological deflection, functional disturbances and physiological change, always in the beginning functional, and later structural or pathological.

As we become more familiar with these subversive forces in their action upon the life force, or as we see their character expressed upon the normal vitality and function of the organism, how much more easy is it for us to follow their tracings or prophesy their probable developments in any given case. If we become acquainted with the character of psora, whether expending its force upon the organism, simply, alone or in combination with some other miasm, we are more able to give a prognosis as to the probable outcome in a given case of disease ; *for the character of the miasm gives us the character of the affection or the disease formula.* If in some severe acute trouble, as gonorrhœal arthritis, we first look for sycosis, suppressed by douches or injections of some drug, or drugs, capable of producing such results ; then back of that we look for a deep psoric or tubercular taint. Why ? Because we know we cannot have this particular form of arthritis without gonorrhœa, and further we can not have it without a suppression. The character or the expression gives us its history, and its history gives us its character. It can be nothing else. In this kind of a case how foolish it would be for us to prognose a speedy cure knowing the nature of the acute miasm and with a history of chronic psora, born into the world with hereditary changes whose physiological and histiological elements are a false expression of true biologics, whose whole physical, mental, moral and spiritual nature is a deflection of the truth. It is here we must test our knowledge of miasmatic action, and we must not limit it to our knowledge of the primary action of sycosis, but it must extend into the secondary and tertiary history of that disease. We see disease here to be the expression of these great potentials (psora, sycosis, syphilis) ; the life force in the grasp of two other potentials, sycosis and psora, each a powerful subversive force striving with all their power to destroy the life. But he who has become acquainted with the higher homœopathics of Hahnemann, which comprises not only these disease potentials, but the drug action, he has familiarized himself with the higher, and even the highest, potentials now at his command, whereby he can combat these fearful miasmatic combinations through law, *even the law of similia*.

The absolute in disease, then, we see to be miasmatic action. There is no other cause behind it, save a broken law (*the Decalogue*), which was given that we might follow its teachings and have life, even life in the larger sense. As we study these miasms, we see they express themselves in these degrees of action, acute, chronic, and latent; this fact we all recognize in their secondary or tertiary expression, or that which comes under what is known as pathology, for all pathology originates from the secondary and tertiary manifestations of the miasms. *Primary action has no pathology ; it is functional*. It is only reaction that gives expression, physical form or genesis of any kind. What we are in the habit of calling primary is really secondary. A miasm is only made visible in proportion as we have these stages and degrees of action presented in the organism. I have heretofore called them modes of motion.

The bond of the subversive force with the life force we saw was an invisible thing to be recognized only in its workings with the life force, or in the new and strange phenomena it presents as it hinders life action. The nature and character of the disease depends wholly on the form of the miasm and the character of the bond with the life ; therefore, the study of disease becomes a study into the nature of the miasm present in the organism and the degree of its activity.

When a miasm enters the organism it immediately bonds itself with the life force, and the life force immediately takes on its subversive nature, and its actions from henceforth are in accordance with its nature. If it be syphilis the phenomena of that disease are at once presented in the usual order of their appearance in cycles of action, or stages, as seen in its primary, secondary and tertiary manifestations. We see the new perversion gathering strength and power at each new setting of the disease, until the whole organism is involved, becoming subservient to the potentiality of its power as it becomes bonded with the life force, until every expression of life, physical, mental, moral, even spiritual, begins to show false processes and alterations from the true standard of life or health, which means whole or holey. Thus its wholeness or *holeyness* is interfered with from the moment it bonded itself, or intermarried, with the miasm syphilis.

From this we can readily see where cometh our subversion in idiosyncracy, dyscrasia, predisposition, and even certain forms of temperament. They are all climaxes of perversion or change, and stand forth as the finished work within the organism of the action of chronic miasm.

THE MENTAL SPHERE

Frequently we hear the remark among physicians "I have better success, or have greater success, when I base my prescription upon the mental symptoms." Thus you see any expression of life may be affected by the action of these miasms, and the nature of the mental perversion, if carefully studied and compared, can be traced to the prevailing active one. If the syphilitic miasm is present the symptomatology will revolve about some anti-syphilitic grouping, such as syphilinum, mercury, nitric acid, kali iod, etc. ; and if of a sycotic or psoric nature we will undoubtedly find the mental grouping in such remedies whose provings meet the sycotic or psoric taint. It is an immutable law of physiologics ; it is also a therapeutic law that governs any toxic element. The majority of us can see this fact to be a truth of great value when we study the action of the miasms upon the mental sphere in their acute stages, when all the phenomena are clear and positive, in fact they stand out so prominently that even the lay mind might, with little difficulty, diagnose the condition present. But it is when they present themselves in their chronic and latent forms that the difficulty arises ; when we can see but faint tracings of their presence, faint outlines in the shape of single isolated symptoms, when the groupings are imperfect and the local or physical signs are absent, or nearly so, or when we have mental phenomena due to a mixed miasm, or in fact all the chronic miasms and, perhaps, added some mental worry of long standing, some distress of mind which magnifies the prevailing condition and confuses the mind as we attempt to analyze the mixed phenomena. It is then that we feel our great weakness in our knowledge of miasmatic action, we fail to select the true basic remedy, because we first fail to understand the miasmatic phenomena, and the relation they bear to each other, and also, to the life force. If the miasmatic grouping is located about some one organ, as the liver, heart or lungs, the task, usually, is a simple one; first, because the functions of those organs are limited, simple, and their expressions physical; and, secondly, because the patient recognizes the physical pain, perhaps, or tenderness, soreness, pressure and such phenomena. Then we can oscultate, palpate and in many other ways secure the symptoms that are necessary in our pathological or therapeutic groupings. This, however, is not always the case when mental phenomena are to be studied, as in the brain, where more than one organ or the faculties may be, and is apt to be, disturbed; for then we come to a complex organ, that not only gives forth physical expressions, but mental; and when we come to the mental we are mystified to some degree, for we do not clearly see the relation between the mental and the physical. In the morbid phenomena seen in the heart, lungs or liver we seem to understand, for we are more familiar with their offices and their functions. We know their anatomy and their functions, but those strange and multiple expressions emanating from the brain confuse us. We see in the other groupings the relations between the secretion of bile, of blood, or of air, the relation between the bile and the processes of digestion, the relation between the air of the lungs and the blood or the circulation as a whole ; but we can not understand in like manner the organs which secrete (if I may be allowed to use the term) thought, or all the mental phenomena of that life, whether they be normal or abnormal, whether they be from a conscious or an unconscious mind. I say it is here that we must become familiar with the action of the chronic miasms upon the mental sphere if we hope for success in curing our patients, or ridding their systems of those miasms.

In sycosis the mental symptoms that make their appearance, such as the anxiety, the consciousness, the fear, the patient is constantly examining the organs, looking for signs of the disease. In psora the mental symptoms develop after a long illness or at the close of severe acute expressions of that miasm, as in typhoid fever, etc. This is also true of syphilis, the mental phenomena appearing, usually, at the beginning or during some period of the secondary stage. Often in syphilis or sycosis they are due to lesions such as congestion of the meninges. Many of us have seen the symptoms of failure of the memory following the suppression of a gonorrhoeal discharge, which increased as the basiler meninges became more and more congested, until the symptoms of mania or true insanity were fully developed. Often, however, years are consumed in this slow process, the memory failing by degrees, this condition first showing itself in the failure to remember recent events, the things of the present, while events long past are vividly recalled. This can readily be seen under the provings of Medorrhinum.

I recite these facts to show to you the importance of the mental phenomena in disease. It is through the mind that man sins, therefore it is frequently through it that he becomes diseased. This is true in most cases of the diseases emanating from lust. *He thinks, he wills, he acts*, and out of that triune cometh the visible physical manifestations of the venereal disease. The mind is the vice-regent of the body, the government, the ruling power. The body is subject to it in many ways, therefore subservient to it; but if, with the mind, we violate a law or a principle of life, the body can not shield it, for it, too, is under the same law; therefore we see it witness against itself. A syphilitic eruption is not only witness against the body that it has sinned, but a witness against the mind and against the spirit of that human being. "That which is born in darkness must be revealed in light." We can hide nothing from law, *for law is a revelation*. A broken precept crieth out throughout eternity until it is made right. Oh! would that men whose business it is to deal with and study human life continually could but see these things in their *true* light, especially the physical law. We must ever remember that all things are under law.

There is not a thing in existence but is governed by law. It could not be in existence a moment without it. Law is the very existence of things. Therefore, in our dealings with life, let us ever keep this thought before us, that all normal life is governed by law and is in harmony with it, but that all sickness is a perversion of law; or, the symptomatology of all disease is the symptomatology of broken law. The vibrations of the life forces in true biological action are numbered and fixed, as capable of measurement as are the vibrations produced in a perfect note or tune; but the vibrations in a sick man are changed, as is seen in perverted physiological action; they have no perfect rythm; the notes, even the whole scale of movement, are interfered with, and the action of the sickness depends upon the perverted vibratory changes. Thus it is in the case of the remedies we use, each has its own peculiar mode of motion, of action, of vibration. No two are alike, and when their modes of motion, of action, rythm and character are concomitants of each other we call that *similia*, and the result of their action is a cure; then law is again restored and harmony is again established in that perverted life force. We see that grace came to our aid through another law, even a law of life, known as the law of *similia*. In our study of these laws governing the philosophy of function of the body, we must not lose sight of the fact that these same laws govern, to a great degree, the mental sphere also. Therefore our study of these laws must not cease with the physical.

Indeed, as we study these physiological laws, we enter into a closer relation with the life and all its purposes. As we study the faculties of the brain and become familiar with their office we enter into a closer relationship with their mental phenomena. When a patient enters our office and we see fear, caution, combativeness or any of the leading faculties very prominent, we can assure ourselves that much of the mental phenomena will evolve about these centers. This we often see to be specified as fear of death, of being incurable, of falling, as seen under the remedy borax ; fear of dogs, as under lyssin ; fear of darkness, night, a storm, etc. (phos.) We can well say with Nicodemus of old : "how can these things be ?" There is no pathology behind them, no disease process that he can detect, and yet there exists in that brain a morbid phenomenon that is as persistent as any pathological state. Speaking of a similar phenomenon in a patient, said a prominent old school physician to me, "there is something behind that grouping of symptoms that I do not understand ; it is there, nevertheless. Your miasmatic theory is true, but I am not well enough acquainted with it to make the analysis." When I showed him that sycosis of a tertiary nature lay beneath that mental grouping, he was greatly surprised and at once readily called to memory its history of suppression and the sudden rise of the mental symptoms. Of course, all the miasms are capable of producing mental symptoms, and many of them are due to a combination of miasms. A mental miasmatic symptom is like a miasmatic symptom anywhere in the organism. It is often known by its persistency, by its positiveness and by its constancy. Quite often mental symptoms rise and fall with the general state of the health or through the influence of the moon, or other planetary changes, by atmospheric or barometric risings and fallings. Why? Because the centers that govern these things are not acting normally; the powers that control are out of tune; thus the discord, and that discord being within ourselves, causes our disharmony with all nature. We have lost our dominion over all the earth and earthly creations; we are subservient even to the elements, and the mental sphere bears no exception to this rule. Our calmness, our self-government, too, is often disturbed by the action of the miasm upon these centers of the brain. The mind, or the mental, works through the physical; thus, when the physical is out of tune, the mental is often disturbed. This may take place directly in the brain itself, or indirectly from a disturbance, remote from the brain, as is seen in reflexes, known as reflex disturbances. Now as the mental, to a great degree, rules over the body, so can we lay great prominence upon a mental miasmatic symptom. This is the reason Hahnemann gave them such great value, as they were primary or basic, and when a remedy was carefully selected, basing it upon the mental phenomena, the cures were prompt and quite often permanent.

THE MIASMS AND THEIR RELATION TO PATHOLOGY

We all recognize that there are two distinct schools of homœopathy, yet very few of us are willing to admit the fact; most of us being desirous that the name *homœopathy* should cover every phase of that school and every conception of the different teachings in vogue today. But this can not be so; for, if there are two distinct schools, there must necessarily be two distinct doctrines or teachings. These are sometimes designated as the false and the true, the pathological and the symptomatological, the materialistic and the non-materialistic, the chemical and the dynamic, the scientific and the non-scientific, the high potency and the low potency. Other terms are sometimes used, as the "pure,' the "straight," the mixed, the Eclectic, the school of Hughes, the Hahnemannian school, etc.

The fact of the matter is this, when Hahnemann promulgated the science of homœopathy and made it public to the world it was then a very complete science; and, although he had not brought out all the minor details as clearly as we see them today, it was nevertheless a comparatively perfect science, for he had formulated it all under law, and that law stands today the same—just as sound and as scientific as any law ever discovered by man. Now, a law can not be set aside, can not be compromised with ; it can not be tampered with without spoiling the whole science. This is just what a part of our school has done, or has tried to do. They have attempted to conform this wonderful law, or set of laws (for there is more than one physical law involved in the science of homœopathy, as we will see further on, but all co-operate in one law, even the law of similia) to their own meaning and to their own way of thinking. Hahnemann teaches that the remedy given in each case should be the one that has been proven in each particular case to be able to produce symptoms as like as possible in the healthy individual. We are to understand by "symptoms" that all the deviations from health, all morbid phenomena, found in the organism, with their conditions of change and concomitants, circumstances which we perceive or conceive with our senses of those of the patient ; or, in other words, the totality of the symptoms is all that there is to disease when considered from a therapeutic standpoint. Now herein lies the departure which draws a distinctive line between the false and the true, sometimes called the physiological and symptomatic. But there can be no physiological school, for "physiology is the science or theory of function and change in healthy bodies," while pathology has reference to the diseased body. Therefore, it must be called the pathological school.

Dr. Richard Hughes, who is high authority in this school of pathological homœopathy, defines the true school when he says, "I quite admit that there is many a *terra incognita* as yet in disease, and many a case which, as yet, we can treat only symptomatically. I am thankful that the law of similars enables us to fit drugs to disease, even when we are unable to say what the phenomena of either mean. But none the less do I reckon the other mode (the pathological) of applying the law as the more satisfactory, and, in most hands, successful; and believe that a scientific pharmaco-dynamics, linked to a scientific pathology by the bond of the homœopathic method, will constitute the therapeutics of the future." Thus the adherents of his school departed from the teachings of Hahnemann by making the pathology of the disease and the remedy the basis of the treatment, the modalities and the minute symptomatology being rejected as of only secondary importance; whereas the followers of the Hahnemannian school make the minute symptomatology the basis of their treatment, pathology and all else being subservient to it.

Now there are three points to which we would take exception in Dr. Hughes' teachings, specially waiving all the others that might be considered :

First.—Dr. Hughes was thankful that the law enabled him to fit drugs to a given case, even when he can not give the disease a pathological or man made name ; or, in other words, before the miasmatic disease has given us any physical expression of itself, or, when they are yet functional. Now, if the law can be applied in any one case it can be in all cases, and if it comes to our rescue when we do not understand the phenomena, is it not a greater test for the law than when we claim to understand its phenomena? Nevertheless we do not understand the phenomena any better after the pathological expression has been made manifest than before.

The second point is, has pathology any more relation to causes than symptomatology? Do not all arise from the same fountain head, and why resort to the other when the former fails?

Thirdly. Diagnosis is not always a positive thing, while symptomatology is always positive and they mean the same to all men, making the law a universal and harmonious thing. Pathology must be as complete and as positive a thing as symptomatology before we can arrive at a universal acceptance of it as a system of medicine. There can be no security in pathological prescribing *per se*, as each case depends upon the judgment and knowledge of the individual. Therefore it can not be in accordance with Hahnemann's teachings, and, from the very fact that Dr. Hughes is thankful that the law has provided another way, shows the weak place in the system, for in his distress he flies to the law—that law which every true homœopath learns of and loves every day of his life, and that in which he trusts and to which he pins his faith in time of trouble.

But let us always remember these facts, that *post-mortem changes and pathology are not always the end of miasmatic action or the end of disease, although they may be the end, or death, of the patient.* Hahnemann never rejected pathology, and there was probably none more expert in making a diagnosis; but when he was through with pathology, for the sake of knowledge, he put it where it belonged, as a part of the great whole in the pyramid of symptomatology.

It is to this minute symptomatology that I wish, in particular, to call your attention in our investigation and study of the miasms, for a single symptom often in miasmatics may guide you to the discovery of some one of the chronic miasms that you have overlooked for an indefinite time in your treatment of the case—a single persistent symptom is often quite a positive sign of a suppression, and if suppressed, compels the life forces to set up another symptom no less positive and no less persistent, taking a deeper hold on the organism, therefore more difficult to eradicate.

Another departure of the pathological school from Hahnemann's teaching is found in the prominence they give to morbid anatomy or post-mortem changes. They attempt to base the relation of the remedy on these changes or on the analogy existing between the disease processes and the morbid appearances found after death. At first sight this would seem plausible; yet, on careful examination of the subject, we find these hopes to be illusive; first, for reasons already mentioned, that our knowledge of pathology or morbid anatomy is uncertain and by no means complete, as its history has been and is ever being presented to us as a succession of changes of beliefs and theories. Besides, these post-mortem changes are neither the beginning nor the end of these disease processes, although often the end or death of the patient. We might illustrate this by two cases of pneumonia : One begins in the right lung and travels to the left, and the other in the opposite direction. On examination of the morbid anatomy we might find no distinguishable difference, yet the phenomena might have been quite similar, that is, the symptoms covering the pathological groupings. Again, they may be entirely different. The pain in one may be sharp, shooting, stabbing, while in the other there may be a comparative freedom from pain, or if any were present it was of a dull character. No doubt there exists some minute distinction in the pathological change, but we can not detect that difference. So you can readily see the impracticability of using these changes as a standard of therapeutics, while on the other hand we can always take the totality of the symptoms as a perfect standard and as a constant thing, which, if carefully taken, is found to be an agreement with the therapeutic agent and in correspondence with law. This, you see, makes Hahnemann's theory the more simple and the more positive of the two. In this way, the symptomatology is not a local thing, but a general one, and we no longer confine our study of the case to local manifestations, but we are free to make our therapeutic application from every visible or discernible change from the standard of health in the whole organism, whether it be physical, mental or moral ; for they all become partakers of the sufferings of the offended organism or member and deserve the same attention from the true healer. The oneness must not be lost sight of, for they are inseparable in sickness or in health, a biotic whole, and it is only the pathological eye that does separate them and not the physiological or the pathogenetic one. It is the sick person that is to be treated, not the pathological name. It is the disturbance of the inner processes of life to which we are to look, and not alone to the outer processes ; for the inner processes govern the outer, as the outer manifestation is but an outward expression of the inward process. As this is true of one pathological expression so it holds good in all. The miasm, psora, will give us psoric expressions, and so on through syphilis and sycosis. If we have a mixed miasmatic action, a pseudo-psoric or pseudo-syphilitic manifestation is the result. And it is here that a simple cause becomes a complex thing, difficult to understand or analyze, as new coloring is given to the symptomatology, as well as to the pathological groupings, as they partake in part of the nature of the combined miasms. This fact can be clearly demonstrated in the syphilo-psoric blendings of scrofula, and in the tubercular diathesis. We see clearly, especially in the physiological developments of the whole organism, the tracings of psora underlying the gross and exaggerated workings of syphilis as seen in the thick protruding lips and mouth, the irregular and imperfect dental arch, the serrated incisors, the high cheek bone, the large head and a thousand and one other changes not to be found in a case of simple psoric taint. Again as has been said we see pathology to be ever changing in its character and why should this be so? Can the Pathologists of today give any positive reason for this thing? Why should the pathology of today differ from the pathology of ten years ago? It differs because of the increase of sycotic diseases which we know to be greatly on the increase, by the constant suppression of these disease processes, by the present modern powerful suppressive agents in use today, by the imperfect life, diet, hygiene, etc. Have we not vast heaps of literature on the subject? Are we not confused and overwhelmed by facts that are inharmonious, and are they not continually accumulating? And even today would we not all be hopelessly bewildered, had it not been for Hahnemann's wisdom and foresight in recognizing the fact that *disease* lies not in the pathology alone, but in the totality of the symptoms in each individual case? The pathological symptoms are not first causes in any case. There is something behind pathology, something a little deeper down in each case. Pathology may be a death process, but it was first a perverted life process, first a perverted physiology, a perverted function, and functional change preceded, and does precede, all pathology. Pathology is the finished work of the perverted life action—the ripened fruit, the lie made manifest, the truth verified that good and evil produce death and degeneracy when associated with each other.

In pathology the term pathognomonic symptoms is intended to express the keynote of a disease, just as we use keynote in drug proving. But it does not express that disease in its fulness or designate the distinctive features that characterize one disease from another. So, likewise, we say of pathology that it does not represent fully the expression of the disease in a given case. *The true pathognomonic symptoms of a given case are those that cover the existing active miasm.* In this way our therapeutic grouping becomes a miasmatic one and not a pathological one. The chief feature in pathology is a constant factor in all persons attacked by the same malady, which has furnished the name of said malady. Yet we must all admit, with whatever school we may be associated, that we are able to detect by some sign, symptom and all-pervading condition that there is a characteristic difference in each individual case that gives it its individuality, causing it to differ from all other cases. We are not (I care not to what school we may belong) quite satisfied with pathology, although it seems to have a sort of monopoly over us, a sort of controlling influence, that to some degree deflects and biases our judgment, and the first thing, we know, we have selected a remedy on the pathological grouping which does not fully cover the case, any more than do the pathological symptoms of a proving of a drug bring out the whole character of that drug. We selected that which groups these patients into families, and not that which individualizes each. The one is based upon a pathological law and the other upon a physiological one, and the perverted physiological law is behind all pathology, that is, the pathological plus the existing miasm. How freely we express ourselves to our patients in pathological language : "You have a tumor" or "you have an infiltrated lung," "a valvular heart lesion," "a retroverted womb ;" and the anxious patient replies, "Is that what is the matter, Doctor ?" "Is it dangerous ?" the next question. "No," you say "Is that *all* that is the matter with me, Doctor ?" Now, such answers may satisfy the patient and quiet a disturbed mind ; but do they satisfy you, my good reader ? Do you not feel somewhat guilty ? Have you told all the truth ? Would you not like to tell *all* the truth sometimes ? Would it not satisfy us much more to be able to say, "you are psoric," or "you are sycotic" or "tubercular" as the case may be ? Does pathology count for much with any of us when we see a hypetrophied cervical gland or a tubercular osseous process in a joint ? Does it amount to much when we see a tubercular infiltration ? I am speaking therapeutically now and I leave you, my reader, to answer the question. The tumor, the infiltrated lung, the pathological condition as manifested anywhere is not all that there is to disease, and you know it. But you have lost the finer tracings in symptomatology that lead to cause, or that lie between cause and effect. "Remove the cause of this effect" said the great revealer of nature, Shakespeare. So, what we thought was disease was but the effect of disease, and that which we named as disease to the patient we only gave them the name of a physical effect, or a disease ending a miasmatic centralization or correlation. Shall we look upon this correlation, this fencing or walling-in process, as that with which we are to combat or contend against, or shall we look further and deeper? We may ask ourselves such questions as these: How did this pathological manifestation make its first appearance? What was the mode and manner of its evolution? Did it develop a local thing as a fungus does, or were the fungoid properties in the system itself?

We know that behind every expression of life or matter there is a dynamis. If this be true why not look to the dynamis for the cause of the pathological expression? This is just what we *should* do. The life force *is* that dynamis, and the life force in a normal condition could not do other than give to that organism true physiological impulses and health and life giving qualities. But it is no longer a true dynamis, for it is now under the power of another dynamis, even the miasm that knows no law and has no life giving qualities in it—yea, all its dealings with the life are death-dealing and destructive to that life. It at once turns the life force about and, as it were, endeavors to conform all its movements to its own will and nature.

In the study of the causes of disease in the human

family we notice first the distinguishing features of the race, then the distinctive markings of the nationality, the characteristics of the family, and, last of all, the lineaments, positively or faintly traced, that characterize the individual. The provings of a miasm upon him—as that is what disease is—gives us a picture of a setting quite distinctive from an individual of some other type. We might use the remedy belladonna as an illustration of this. Many of its symptoms are identical with the proving of other drugs, but there is something pervading throughout its every effect that bespeaks of belladonna, something that we say is *pathogenetic* of the remedy. It is this principle that enables us to differentiate between remedies. Thus it is in the miasms; there is that in the phenomena of each that points distinctively to the action of some miasm or a group of miasms. By this means pathology becomes a servant and not a master of our art, and in this way it is brought into greater use instead of being a hindrance to our system of prescribing. In this way we have not only diagnosis, but we have the true picture of similia, which proves to be a better help and a greater power in the hands of the true healer than pathology can ever be to us.

The logical man, in his attempt at establishing any art or science, knows full well that it can only be established with any standard of surety by founding it upon some one of nature's laws. There must be some fixed principle, some standard of value, or the thing becomes an uncertainty and leads to confusion. The first principles are those which establish the professional harmony, the union of purpose and the mutual co-operation among men. The man who firmly believes in homœopathy and its principles can under no circumstances or under any shading of sophistry embrace other principles than those in harmony with the law.

The pain-killer doctor is another type of the pathological therapeutist, with his pain-killing reagents, knowing full well that the pain that is lulled and deadened is not cured, and, indeed, he knows that as soon as the action of his pain-killer has ceased the patient is in a worse condition than before. When men make the claim that they do not desire to be governed by any fixed set of principles then we know that they are not men of law, and that law has no dominion over them. The question then arises; should we employ these men to treat our families who not only ignore law, but who are, in every scientific sense of the word, lawless men? If medicine is a science we know that it must be governed by law. And in order to advance it, we must be guided by law, and in time we will be asked to prove our advancement by demonstrating our *modus operandi*. Yes, we must have law as the foundation upon which to erect any great structure, or we fail; we can not build upon man's multiplicity of opinions, for if we do the whole edifice will become Babylonic and end in confusion and disaster.

We can not apply the law of similia in any degree of

perfection through pathological similarities, for the simple reason that they never cover all the case. There are symptoms behind pathology, symptoms that lie at the cause to which pathology is due, that fathers' and mothers' pathology. Therefore we have not the *tota-causa* in any pathological grouping ; we must go back to the fountain head in order to find out that which taints the rivers of life, for pathology is not fed and nourished by pathology, and we, as men of science, must acknowledge its miasmatic fatherhood and birthright ; that symptom similia does not begin nor end in pathology, although we do not, by any means, ignore pathology. "Cancer," says Dr. Ostrom, "is primarily a dyscrasia." If that be true, then let us ask this question : What is behind dyscrasia ; or, in other words, what is the first cause of dyscrasia ? Here investigation ceases in all schools of medicine except the school of Hahnemann, and it is here he has opened secret, doors both in science and philosophy, and he invites all to enter therein and behold the secrets of disease and disease changes or if you please, pathology.

Let us read a few paragraphs from Hahnemann's writings, Chronic Diseases, Vol. I, p. 18-19.

"*Ever since the years 1816 and 1817 I have been employed day and night to discover the reason why the homœopathic remedies which were then known, did not effect a cure of the above named chronic diseases. I tried to obtain a more correct, and if possible, a completely correct idea of the true nature of these thousands of chronic ailments which remained uncured in spite of the incontrovertible truth of the homœopathic doctrines: when, behold! the Giver of all good permitted me, about that time, to solve the sublime problem for the benefit of mankind, after unceasing meditations and research, careful observations and most accurate experiments. I observed that non-venereal chronic diseases, after having been repeatedly and successfully removed by the then known homœopathic remedies, constantly reappeared in a more or less modified form and with a yearly increase of disagreeable symptoms.* This proved to me that the phenomena which appeared to constitute the ostensible disease ought not to be regarded as the whole boundaries of the disease; otherwise the disease would have been completely and permanently cured by the homœopathic drugs, which was not the case—*but that this ostensible disease was a mere fragment of a much more deep-seated, primitive evil, the great extent of which might be inferred from the new symptoms which continued to appear from time to time.* This showed me that the homœopathic practitioner ought not to treat diseases of this kind as separate and completely developed maladies, not that he ought to expect such a permanent cure of these diseases as would prevent them from appearing again in the system, either in their original or a modified form."

"I became convinced," said Hahnemann, "that to discover one or more remedies which would cover all the symptoms characterizing the whole of the disturbance *was to discover all the ailments and symptoms inherent in the unknown primitive malady.* The medicines so found would be able to conquer or extinguish the whole disease, with its successive groups of symptoms and its endless change of phenomena."

Now in an analysis of this most precious page of homœopathic literature we find the following revelation: Hahnemann had been prescribing for a certain group of symptoms that to him seemed prominent and important. No doubt, many times, these symptoms were either pathological groupings or reflex phenomena. However, they were not basic or miasmatic in his arrangement of them, hence the return of the symptoms in a modified form or in new groupings. But when he found remedies which covered the whole of the phenomena the disease did not return, but the patient remained cured. A little farther on he says, "*This primitive disease evidently owed its existence to some chronic miasm.*" Now this wonderful revelation, and it *is* wonderful, for no man, before nor since, has seen such a *revelation* of disease, nor had such a flood of light thrown upon the *phenomena* of disease. The prescribing of a true antipsoric remedy covered all the phenomena of disease, both its pathological and symptomatic expression, even the *inherent primitive unknown malady*. That being removed, there could arise no new phenomena nor any expression or manifestation of what might be called disease. Why? Because the principle of *vitus-morbi* had been removed, yea, annihilated, and it no

3 F.B.

longer existed, and the organism was free from the first cause of its disturbance. Thus the cure and the preventive of its reappearance must follow as a law of cure. Hahnemann's recognition of this *primitive existence in a chronic miasm is the only true conception of disease*. The new phenomena, or that which is supposed to be new disease, is nothing more than the daily workings of the miasm, or the further development of miasmatic action, the forward movement of a perverted life action, a miasmatic revelation of that unknown dynamis, *psora*, or some other miasm, as seen in its pathological changes in the organism. Hahnemann's experience with his remedies is often ours; we give a remedy based upon a few of the more prominent symptoms in a given case, and what results do we get? Simply nothing more than palliative effects or a reduction of the miasm back to its latent condition, and when the least exciting cause makes its appearance, such as taking cold, undue exposure to the elements, injury, climatic change, errors in diet, or any of the many exciting causes that are apt to come in our way, we have a fresh outbreak of the miasm, either of similar nature or in a modified form. In that way the general health of the patient is switched back and forth with no permanent good result in the end. But when we come to understand the miasm well enough we can select the basic miasmatic symptoms in each given case and, basing our prescription on them, we reach *prima causa*, and not only are the secondary or tertiary manifestations of the miasm removed, but the effects of the miasm as a whole, or the sum total of all that is known as disease.

There comes a time when we can not do this or, at least, it would not be wise to do so, as is seen in cases of incurable disease or when the miasmatic action has progressed so far that no permanent reaction can be solicited and any attempt to make a positive cure results in injury to the patient and often shortens life. This is frequently seen in such diseases as diabetes melitus, in the last stages of cancer, tuberculosis in its third stage. Here it is well not to base our prescriptions upon the basic miasmatic symptoms ; as the attempt made by nature under the basic remedy causes overaction and death follows sooner than if we left the patient alone. Here it is better to palliate the disease by remedies not based fully upon miasmatic symptoms.

When we undertake to treat pathological miasmatic formations we get no permanent results from our potentized remedies unless we *do* base our prescription upon the true miasmatic symptoms in the case. And, naturally, we may see that this might be true, for the growth, formation or whatever it may be depends upon the miasmatic principle in the life force ; or, in other words, the life force is in the pathological business and is prepared to manufacture any pathological formation depending upon the nature of the internal existing or acting miasm. If the miasm be psoric we have psoric manifestations. If it be sycotic, we have sycotic pathology ; and if syphilitic, we have the polymorphic pathological presentations of that other great lust miasm ; or, if we have the miasm syphilis and psora combined, we have the multiplied changes and infinite destructive processes known as tubercular pathology. In order to magnify the tubercular pathology we have but to add the sycotic miasm, when there at once develops the malignant types of tubercular disease. This is not to say that a malignancy could *not* develop without the sycotic, but that it greatly increases the possibility. We often see this fact demonstrated in patients who are infected with sycosis that has been suddenly suppressed by injections or medicated douches, when suddenly new, acute and persistent symptoms develop, such as stasis to lungs, heart, kidneys, brain, or to any internal organ or part. Some secondary processes may arise, like la grippe, to develop this stasis, but it comes, sooner or later, often unexpectedly. Tubercular infiltration in these cases is said to be due to la grippe. But is it due to la grippe? No, it is due to the newly acquired miasmatic disease (sycosis), and the new or acute miasm la grippe—(it, too, being of a sycotic origin) stirs up, as do all the acute miasms, the chronic suppressed or latent miasm or miasms, as the case may be. They again become active and set up a stasis of that disease which, in time, is converted into a new or secondary point of elimination which is destructive, of course, to the organism, as it attacks a vital center of life. The frequency with which we meet this condition of things is amazing if you will look carefully into the history of each case, as fully eighty per cent. of the cases we treat today, especially in men, are sycotic in some degree ; they are suffering either from the acquired form of from hereditary transmission.

It is dreadful to contemplate such a condition of things as is present on the earth today. Almost every man you meet is polluted with this disease ; and it is ten times more difficult to cure diseases at the present time than it was fifteen or twenty years ago. The difficulty increases every year, and that is one reason why many of our physicians of today resort to palliatives and suppressive measures. The study of these cases is difficult, and the connection between the disease processes harder to understand and more difficult to analyze ; but it is greatly simplified by a thorough knowledge and understanding of the miasms. When we become acquainted with the phenomena of the chronic miasms, psora, syphilis, and sycosis, or their blendings, it is then we begin to understand their pathology, for their pathological manifestations are peculiar to themselves. It is only when they are suppressed, or in a latent condition due to a suppression that the pathological readings become at all difficult. Quite often the well indicated homœopathic remedy will in a very short time develop such cases, bringing them to the surface in the nature of an eruption, or by some special lesion or discharge peculiar to the existing miasm, thereby revealing it. Of course, no miasm will give us tertiary pathology if it has been properly treated through the homœopathic law, especially when the higher potencies have been used—and what I mean by higher potencies is the 1 m and upwards. I have never seen tertiary symptoms develop even in syphilis when the 1 m, 50m, cm and potencies of this power were used. The law of cure will arrest their progress before they have reached the tertiary stage. The cure does not take place while a disease process is advancing. It is possible for us to have suppressed symptoms reappear, or latent ones develop, but we can have neither a new setting nor a progressive advancement of any disease in the presence of the law of cure unless it be of a malignant or incurable nature. The chronic miasms, syphilis and sycosis, ought to be cured in the primary and secondary stages, before they have formed such a perfect bond with psora as to induce tertiary manifestations. Tertiary manifestations are in these diseases permitted to develop, principally because we have neglected psoric manifestations that were latent before the new bond (with syphilis or sycosis, as the case may be), but now aroused by them into new activity by the new stimulii and the bond with the venereal miasm. Here often arises one of our greatest mistakes, an almost inexcusable one. On general principles we are giving mercury sol. for the syphilis, the ulcers or the mucous pathes; continuing it on and on for an indefinite period, while at the same time it is acting only as a suppressive and not in any sense as a curative measure. No; the miasmatic similia now lies largely in the psoric bond and in the psoric phenomena, and a remedy may have to be selected whose provings cover the present phenomena of both miasms, which would be, of course, more homœopathic, indeed, it is the only thing that is homœopathic. Should we continue the mercury we may suppress the syphilitic phenomena entirely; but then new developments of psora appear which are often difficult to deal with, if not incurable. And we have thereafter a true case of persistent chronic disease to treat.

The true internal nature of disease is made manifest wholly in the study of the chronic miasms. Pathology can do nothing more for us today than it did in Hahnemann's time, and it can never do any better, for the simple reason that pathology is not at the bottom of that *mysterious process* by which morbid changes and alterations take place in the organism. What is said of disease may be said of potency. Although we see no material in potency, it still has the power to disturb the healthy organism in its own peculiar way. And thus it is with the miasmatic potential, it is an invisible and unseen thing, yet we see the effects of its presence in the organism long before any change of tissue takes place. We see it first, as a rule, manifest in the mental sphere, then in the physiological or functional, then, finally, in the pathological, the pathological, of course, coming last. To many of us it is in this intervening space that the mystery of disease lies, the culminating act or the pathological formation. It is in this stage of the disease that the dynamis of the organism (the life force) is undergoing change or perversion—the intermingling of the false with the true, or the miasm with the life force, and *the disturbances are in accordance with the existing active miasm, modified by previous heredity or miasmatic states of the organism.*

SECONDARY DISEASES, OR SEQUELAE

Where latent chronic miasms have been aroused from their slumberings by the violent action of some acute miasm such as typhoid fever, la grippe, scarlet fever, etc., often at their close we have left what are known as sequelæ or secondary processes, supposed to be due to the acute malady. But this is not so. They are secondary or tertiary processes of the chronic miasms that have been overlooked in the treatment of the acute miasm. The acute miasm, we know, is self limiting in its action, for in a certain fixed period it should disappear. Therefore its non-disappearance and the appearance of the secondary disease is due to the chronic miasmatic bases that previously had its existence in the organism. "The vital forces," says Hahnemann, "were (previous to the appearance of the acute miasm) able to keep down the psoric or chronic miasm which always strives to get the upper hand." Now, by the aid of the acute miasm, it is assisted into prominence as the resistive power of the life forces are overcome, or overwhelmed by the combined power of the two subversive forces. This fact can be clearly seen through the failure of the homœopathic remedy to any longer arrest the disease process that has now assumed a pathological proportion or state. We are now compelled to select a remedy covering the chronic miasm in order to arrest this process which, up to this time, has been overlooked or neglected, and which could have been avoided had we, in the first place, or earlier in the case, based our prescription upon the symptomatology of the underlying basic principle or chronic miasm. This thought might be illustrated by a case of scarlet fever where belladonna was indicated and which was given far beyond the period of usefulness, and the result was an abscess of the middle ear. Had we looked deeper we might have seen sulphur, silica, psorinum or some other deep acting miasmatic which would have headed off this secondary or tertiary process and at the same time greatly mitigated, if not aborted, the acute disease. By this method of prescribing scarlet fever has lost its terrors and its danger to life has fallen to a minimum; the fever diappearing usually about the eight day and convalescence following rapidly. Of course, I give these patients no solid food, and the usual caution and care is taken to prevent the possibility of taking cold or chilling the body where such a large area is affected as in this disease and where such an important organ as the skin, with its multiple processes of elimination, is involved. These acute epidemic or sporadic miasmatic diseases must not be allowed or permitted to complete their course, for the longer they are allowed to exist in the organism the greater danger there is to the life from their rapid destructive processes as they combine their action with the chronic miasms, psora or either of the others that may be present.

"They, in the first place," says Hahnemann, "could not exist except in the presence of the chronic miasms, syphilis, sycosis and psora." That is, the acute miasm, such as la grippe, malaria, exanthematous fevers and all infective and contagious diseases can not and do not bond themselves with the life force independent of the miasms. There must be a basic miasm, there must be a *sin process*, already present in the organism. The inner *vitus potens* must have in some degree failed, and prepared the soil for the acute miasmatic toxus. Then again we see that in order to arrest pathological developments or processes we must search for the basic miasmatic symptoms in each case, for even after we have dispelled the effects of the acute miasm by the use of our acute anti-miasmatic agents (remedies), the psoric or chronic miasmatic process has been forced to set up a stasis or a new central point of elimination for its own pathologic *debris*. This was, of course, unnecessary, and had we carefully taken into consideration the chronic miasmatic process that was co-operative with the acute disease we would not only have arrested the whole process but would have shortened the disease period and the sufferings of the patient.

This is one of the strong distinguishing points between the true homœopathy and the false, between that which corresponds to a *true science* and that which might be called a *pseudo-science* or an imperfect science. It is the point of gradation or of valves in the homœopathic doctor; it is the difference between palliation and cure; between a true knowledge of disease processes and an imperfect knowledge.

If we have some understanding of the nature of the miasms, their history and action upon the life of the organism, we are able to follow these processes, liking them together into an unbroken chain, and our knowledge is not confined alone to the present, but it becomes prophetic and we can prognose their possible developments, even to their intricate processes and mysterious movements, in that way we are able to head off the new developments and new processes that come upon us unexpectedly.

BACTERIA AND THEIR RELATION TO PATHOLOGY

Another doctrine that has come to our knowledge in the past quarter of a century, and which has become a sort of appendage to the pathological schools of medicine in general is the doctrine of micro-organisms, which, for a time, threatened to swallow up the dynamical doctrines of Hahnemann, *that, disease is nothing more than the disturbance of the life force.* But law, in time, always resumes its equilibrium, for they too (that is these many forms of *bacillus*) have come under the same law, even the law of similia and under the law of potentiality. The homœopathic remedy covers all the phenomena of disease of whatever origin it may be, even to the micro-organisms. The life principle restored, or when the perverted life force resumes its normal, it puts an end to their existence. Thus we know that their existence is but an expression of that perversion. True, they exist in a latent state, even as their parents, the miasms, exist in a latent state. True, often of themselves, they are able to convey disease, even as they partake of the same toxic elements as the miasms ; as like produces like. Even their medium is a miasmatic production ; therefore their medium has the same disease-producing power and is of the same potential, and what is true of the chronic miasms is also true of the acute miasms, or what may be said of one may be said of the other so far as their power to produce disease is concerned.

The Physico-chemical schools freely accepted the teachings of Dr. Koch and others, receiving them with great enthusiasm, sincerely hoping that the medical profession had at last arrived at a means or found a method whereby the true remedial agent could be found and applied to the diseased condition. But in this they have failed as did those before them and as will their followers, because there is but one way to study disease and that is the way mapped out by Hahnemann, that disease is but the varying conditions of the life principle which not only *creates but controls the organism.* Do not the scientists of this present time deny that there is a living vital force which animates and dominates the human organism as a whole? "Yes," they say, "it is a chemical entirely; there is nothing we can find beside that." But they can find what they see in the chemical, even when the spark of life has fled. We can not demonstrate life in the chemical any more than we can gravitation. It is not demonstrable, because it is *behind* chemistry and was *before* chemistry, and organic chemistry came into existence by virtue of the dynamic. When we first begin the study of any science we should first look for the law which governs it and must not strive to make the application independent of it. This is true whether we study bacteria in their relation to disease processes or whether it be in our application of *them* to disease. Behold the bold, daring

THE CHRONIC MIASMS.

experimenter who attempts to apply these toxic elements such as tuberculinum, vaccinninum, diphtherinum or any of the viruses of commerce in use by the serotherapeutists of today to combat diseased states and processes with no law or no principle behind their application. Instead of pursuing a course of investigation based on natural laws and inductive reasoning, a theory is first propounded and then every effort is made to substantiate it empirically. Thus, when a bacillus is newly discovered they immediately *declare caus morbi ; ergo,* to cure, the bacillus must be destroyed. *This is but an epitome of what has been done throughout the world for the past twenty years anp in no instance has the mortality been lessened nor the prevalence of any disease decreased.* Smallpox increases, becoming even epidemic ; tuberculosis multiplies and day after day the public press publishes announcements of the deaths of the unfortunate victims coming under this unscientific and unjustifiable empiricism, saying nothing about the thousands of organisms ruined and weakened by these toxic elements, these degenerate, degrading animal poisons which weaken the race and multiply disease processes without name and without number. Some of the fearful conditions that follow are skin eruptions of all forms, malignant diseases, heart failures and even death may follow their use ; post-diphtheretic paralysis, malnutrition, non-assimilation, tuberculosis and a host of conditions which are frequently overlooked by many of us.

But there *is* a law governing the *life* and *health*, a law governing *disease* and a law governing *cure*. Why will our scientists not seek and find these laws and these principles and strive to make the application of them for the safety and for the benefit of their fellow men? Should they do so, they would upset all their fine spun theories of the present and of past centuries, and would reveal to the world the fact that they are neither men of science nor men of law. Satan is up in arms when men attempt to either keep law or any attempt he makes to apply law. They do not look deep enough to see the sin process or the miasmatic dynamis that has ever been a mystery and a secret of all, except to those who have become followers of Hahnemann. This invisible potentiality (*the miasm*) in some form is imposed upon the life of every unborn child in some degree, often to such an extent as to destroy the new life or drive it from its living house by its invisible expelling powers. These are the influences that break down the resisting power of the organism, that force the organism under false laws, thus bringing in all perversion, even to cell perversion and cell change. It gives to the unformed and imperfect creation in utero that principle of cell perversion which after birth, generates the false processes, even the tubercular processes in all its forms, whether marked or unmarked, whether functional or structural: it is all the same. The cause is found in the blendings of the two chronic miasms, *psora* and *syphilis*. This is also the reason why the disease should attack one

THE CHRONIC MIASMS. 81

person and not another, one family and not another. It resolves itself into the fact that the only and supreme influence which determines its action and its development in any human being is an inheritance of the above mentioned chronic miasms. They alone can produce what is known as tubercular processes and tubercular taints. They do not only furnish the soil for germs, as we often hear said, but they *father* the germ. They are the propogators of the tubercular processes and the tubercular bacilla *in toto*. The perverted cell of Virchow in any disease is not at first a pathological one, but a functionally changed cell, only cognizable by symptoms that are not normal or that are below the standard of life or what is known as true function. So, it can readily be seen, that cell perversion which in time becomes pathological must first be functional, and that there may be *any* intervening time between that functional change and the appearance of the pathological. The question may arise in your mind, why is it that one person in a family becomes afflicted with the disease and another should escape? The answer is: they all have the taint, for they were all conceived under that law of perversion due to the presence of the miasms in one or both parents; if in *one* parent *only*, then the danger is lessened or minimized to a great extent. Thus we often see the boys in a family free from tubercular affections while the girls are affected early in life, but the disease is held back often by that natural physiological resistance that each organism is endowed with and other conditions favorable to the development of health and strength such as physical training, climate, diet, fresh air, etc.

It is only when the miasm has created something that the pathologist recognizes it as *true* disease, and if the miasm be psora or sycosis in a tertiary stage he either sees no relationship whatever, or he can not understand that relationship. Every man sees the potentiality of life in the heart, and in the respiratory movements, the circulatory phenomena, cell construction, but they do not discern it clearly in disease before the pathological appears.

Professor Virchow, the father of cellular pathology, advanced the theory that structural change (the pathological) began in the cell. This, no doubt, is true as far as it goes, for the cell is the unit of the body; the body is made up of these cells or these units. But as men of science we will ask this man of science, for the sake of bringing forth our point (although he has departed this life), what disturbed this little unit, the cell; how do the cells become diseased when, often, there is no external apparent cause? Why should the blood cells die or decrease or multiply either locally or generally? Why should they pile up in heaps and form tumors and abnormal growths; or, in other words, what is that power that is behind the cell change, behind the cell disturbance, or the life perversion in that affected part or portion of the body? *Bacteria*, is the answer. Shall we carry the question further and ask from what source do these bacteria emanate; from whence is their parentage, their origin, their existence? Shall we wait an answer or is the question unanswerable? Are they a product of inheritance; are they prehistoric? Professor Virchow says not, for in an address before the Tubercular Congress held in Berlin on May 27, 1899, he declared before that body "that there is no evidence that tuberculosis is inherited, as I have never, in the course of my microscopic investigations, found any trace of its presence in the unborn babe," although he admitted that it could acquire the disease one day after its birth.

I would like to ask my readers if this bears out the experience of any of us? Is it any guaranty of its absence or of the future possibility? Does it bear out Hahnemann's theory, or is it in accord with the history of our experience or with the history of tuberculosis in the race? That potentiality that is behind the cell is the thing that Dr. Virchow did not see, nor yet has any materialist seen. Their eyes are veiled to all such light. This is where Dr. Virchow turned about, and where the immortal Hahnemann went on and *on* and *on*, until he found his life force. Hahnemann, by his remarkable and comprehensible philosophy, by his keen analysis, his wonderful research, enables us to make a clear generalization, taking a mountain-top view of things, and brings about an orderly arrangement of the different phenomena presented in disease, which, without his instruction, would be incomprehensible.

THE RELATIONSHIP OF THE MIASMS TO ABNORMAL GROWTHS

We have seen the relationship which the miasms bear to acute diseases, and to all diseases as a whole. We also saw their relation to functional disturbances and to pathology in general. We have seen that all disease was first disturbed function and that later on, as the functional disturbance increased and became more intensified, it became pathological. Indeed it is the perverted function or physiological stress that produced the pathological. It is the multiplied impulses that have not life giving power or life giving principal in them that changes the physiological, and from these continuous perverted impulses the false creations develop, but separated from all sin process, the life forces act in all harmony and its resistive, sustaining and creative powers are magnified.

Thus all life is magnified by continuous normal impulses from the great nerve centers of life such as the brain. We see this great potential dynamic in the power of speech, the action of the mind, yet after all overlook the potentiality of disease. Yet all these energies, all these potentials, are invisible, and when they have finished their work we saw not the workmen. It is the same stupendous potentiality that gives us these wonderful manifestations in life, so in disease, the life potential combines with the miasmatic potential.

THE CHRONIC MIASMS.

Herbert Spencer says, "We have no state of consciousness by which potential existence becomes actual." But we see in nature innumerable manifestations of these ever present and ever acting potential forces, working out and through the material and bringing forth and developing the actual or material as is seen in the action of growth by sunlight, heat and moisture upon all life, stimulating, nourishing, developing, and showing that the actual is latent, dead, lifeless and undeveloped without the potential; therefore they are inseparable. *Then we say all actual existence was first potential existence.* If there were no potential existence there would be no life nor no motion, therefore it is the genesis.

Again, without life or motion there were no action existence. Medicinal and chemical action are not directly potential; they, it is true, have a crude potentiality of their own which, as in the case of the chemical, can be, by potentiation, changed back to their original potential.

Then we base the theory of all pathological formation and of every expression of pathology upon the grand truth that in all our dealings with matter, or the material whether it be an organism imbued with the highest form of potentiality or be it some inert medical substance, any therapeutic agent, *we must deal with them from the potential side wholly.* To deal with them otherwise is to ignore the potential, its power over all, and its dealings with matter. Indeed, to ignore the potential means even more, it means to catalogue life with the material, with the chemical, and to raise it no higher than the chemical plane. In the actual it is the consciousness of form, of size, of color, etc. In the potential it is the consciousness of action, of change of position and motion. In medicine it is more than that : it is the power of their action (the miasms) upon the life forces. It is this power that the miasms wield over the life that we have constantly to deal with. It is through their influences that all disease change takes place from the slightest functional disturbance to the most exaggerated pathological creation. There is no other builder in pathologics but the life force and there is no provision made in a healthy organism for such creations. But let us infect a healthy organism with the miasm of syphilis and then, knowing of the possibility of its presence, let us watch the action of its constructive and destructive forces at work. At first only slight tracings, faint outlines of its presence are detected ; gradually, however, it gathers strength from day to day as the system becomes more and more intoxicated with its presence. Soon we begin to see the beginning of false processes and multiple false expressions both within and without the body. We see the false structures built up and again torn down, we see the *neoplasm* arise apparently out of healthy tissue or with healthy structures all about it, pushed up or through by that miasmatic power that is co-operative with the life. How easy it is for us to combat visible enemies, but when such an invisible dynamis gifted with such power as is manifest in syphilis confronts us, no wonder we are often at a loss to understand its multiple manifestations and its multiple processes. If any where we should become acquainted with this dynamis of the miasm, it is syphilis, where the phenomena is *so regular* and *so constant*, while in psora no such uniformity of phenomena exists. We might also say that if there be anywhere where we might set aside the chemical and accept the dynamic, it is in this disease syphilis. Let us watch its pauses of weeks duration, its progressions, its strange presentations, its specific *aura*, its destructive cell infiltration, its concrete lesions and its vicious ulcers with their necrotic *debris*. When we study carefully all its strange and progressive phenomena, we ought to be fully convinced of its potence in dealing forth its death principle and we may also have some conception of the seeming unlimited end of power of its sin process, more especially knowing that a violated principle of the *decalogue* is behind that power. Again when we consider what a positive bond it has with the life force, and how it never expresses itself until it has fully made that bond, even should there be a pause in its preparation, extending from 17 to 50 days before that preparation is fully made, and before it may express itself upon the organism in what is known as syphilis as it demonstrates this power throughout the organism. The first potential is seen in the intoxication of the system long before the pathological appears. The second potential manifests itself in the glandular involvement and the secondary external or skin eruption and the mucous ulcers. The third potential is seen to partake not only of the syphilitic miasm but of the latent psora which is aroused from its lethargy and intensifies and magnifies the action of both miasms. Indeed, the syphilitic miasm gathers strength and power at each new setting of the disease, for such is the law of progression. "The wages of sin is death," and the death process becomes more manifest as the sin process develops and proceeds in the natural order of its development. The life force yields more fully to the influence of the miasm (syphilis) as the latent process (psora) comes to the assistance of the syphilitic miasm, thus weakening its resistence until the false process overrules the life process, and the organism succumbs to its fate.

The real object or office of the pathological is to relieve the organism of this dual action of the miasm with the life force. The pathologic is necessary, as false, eliminative centers; indeed lesions of whatever nature or in whatever form they may appear are eliminative points of disease products. They all bring relief to the organism threatened by the internal workings of the miasms. The truth is that an *internal* disease process, when it becomes *active*, must in the general course of events and through the natural evolutive process, *soon* become an *external* disease process. Yea, not infrequently, some of the natural eliminative processes, like those of the kidneys or of the skin, become accelerated in their action. This may increase even to an incipient diabetes or hyperhidrosis, or a diarrhœa may intervene and in that way, for a time, relieve the internal disease process, thus preventing some pathological lesion or stasis of disease. Should the natural eliminative process take on such action it must soon become an overworked process, or what is known as an overactive one, which is followed by reaction, which means some form of paralysis or paresis. It is safer, then for the organism to be relieved by some superficial pathological lesion rather than through a physiological eliminative process that in time must become pathological. If we do not understand the laws governing the dynamis of life we are soon deceived, as we are apt to take the results of action for their cause; or, in other words, we take the finished or completed work of the miasm, the lesion or the pathological for the real disease. For instance, we say the tumor is the cause of pain or pressure or some reflex condition, which is true, perhaps but the tumor is never the first cause of the disease. No lesion or pathological condition is the first cause of any disease, for the disease process precedes them all, and the *true* cause always lies (outside the mechanical) in the disturbed or distressed life force itself. We must go back to the life force for all action and all change in the structures of the organism itself. A tumor is but an inhibitory point due to perverted life action. It is a miasmatic correlating process. The difference often between an abscess and a tumor is that one is an inward process, while the other is an outward process, although they both may be either an inward or an outward process. The abscess throws off or out the disease, while the tumor correlates it. One is destructive, the other constructive, both of which, up to a certain degree, become, as it were, safety valves to the organism. The life force of itself is a true potential and all its processes should be creative, and it can not be deflected from its true action save for the presence of some miasm within itself. The life as begun in man must have forever moved forward in the same unchanged and unchangeable state, never to grow old nor to be in any way related to environment to death or to time.

The father, then, we say, of all sickness of whatever nature it may be, is, directly or indirectly, a subversive force whose action is co-existent with the life force. Therefore, through this co-existent action we may have any conceivable anatomical, physiological or histological imperfection—yea, more: we may have a mental, moral or even spiritual imperfection.

To us, as homoeopaths, a tumor or any abnormal growth, in fact, any pathological formation, is but a landmark of miasmatic action or change, for these manifestations present in themselves the prehistoric history of such change and such action and a recognition of the real, the miasm, the subversive force as distinguished through the phenomena of disease action. They are simply ripening or ripened fruit of that prolonged perverted life action. As the action of physical forces for ages has changed the whole face of nature, so has the action of the miasms changed the whole physical, mental, moral and spiritual nature of man. He is a wreck of his former self, all due to this subtle nonentity, as mentioned by Hahnemann in paragraph 13 of the Organon. It is a subtle nonentity as compared with the pathological.

Let us now notice more closely this dual action of the life force. The life force itself, in a normal state, is endowed with a creative power; but when we add to it the destructive action of some one or more of the miasms then we have a dual action set up. "All vital action," to again quote Spencer, "considered not separately but in their ensemble, have for their purpose the balancing of certain outer processes by certain inner processes." This balancing of the effects of force we call equilibrium, and as soon as this standard barometer falls we have disease, and this prolonged dual action must sooner or later set up a counteraction, which gives us the inhibitory point heretofore mentioned and which becomes anew and fixed center of disease action or a wheel within a wheel. Here is where the pathological begins in this inhibitory point, and therein is set up by this new and false action the new and false creation. In this way we can establish some true relation between what is seen,—the *real, the pathological*—and what is *producing* the *pathological*, a connection of subjective states and objective agencies or actions.

We see then in abnormal growths two things: the

pathological condition and the phenomena of that condition; and in the phenomena of that condition lies the cause of the pathological, while the *real* (pathological) represents only a portion of that truth, as it is the finished work or last cause; but for the first cause or first action we must study the remainder of the phenomena, and as we analyze perverted vital action as a whole it conducts us back to cause and to a true conclusion of the unknown.

Then we conclude the thought that what we see in the real, is not only impressed upon consciousness as a mental impression, but it is substantiated by our senses of sight, touch, hearing, feeling and taste ; while, on that other hand, we can, by the extension of the same mental process, prove that the real came out through the action of the potential, and the pathologics are buildings or creations of a life force perverted by miasmatic action, and that the phenomenon of appearance is not *prima causa*—rather is it the phenomenon of that invisible *potens*, psora, or some other miasmatic influence upon the life force.

Even when we can not always locate or name the existing miasm we can, from our knowledge of its action, locate cause through our study of the phenomenon, for we know that the disposition of cause is the disposition of that phenomenon; or, to be more definite in our statement, we say the application of the law of similia to the active miasm is the only true method of curing the disease even when it has reached the pathological state. We must always look upon all disease, whether of a functional or a pathological nature, from the potential side, and regard all phenomena, whether produced directly or indirectly, as manifestations of some power within the organism itself. The science of homœopathy is the correct grouping of all the relations existing in the pathogenic phenomena of the life force, applying it to law, which is the shortest and most direct route back to cause.

In our study of this retrograde process of disease many complex groupings of symptoms may present themselves for consideration and analysis, until perhaps along history of perverted life action has disappeared in the reverse order in which it came. In the end we are able to establish and locate cause, and the unknown becomes manifest when a clear light is thrown upon both the actual and potential.

The truth of the matter is that what we call real as seen in pathology is only the appearance of the real, the true real being potential or dynamic. If we, on the other hand, would say the real (the pathological) had always existed, there would be some truth in the statement that disease was pathological. But knowing that the pathological did not always exist, that it belongs not to the perfected organism, it becomes an objective reality, and the true real is now seen to exist only in the potential which may have always existed in the organism, although in a latent state. This study of the potential as seen in the action of the chronic miasms becomes the ultimatum of all ultimates, and the whole science of homœopathy, so far as therapeutics is concerned, becomes a study of the science of the forces and the laws governing them, taking the true biological action of the life forces as a basis. On the other hand, as the real or visible (pathological) came through the medium of the potential, or the perverted life action due to the miasms, so, in like manner, it disappears through the potential by virtue of the power of the potential and by the assistance of the *other* potential, the remedy. This is *true* healing and is embraced in the teachings of the first paragraph of the Organon.

This conflict between the life force and the miasms furnishes us, as healers of the sick, with material for a life study, and the suffering one, with all the ills life is heir to, with all the phenomena, subjective and objective, visible and invisible, that fill our works on practice and our volumes on therapeutics, with data of the phenomena of disturbed vital force. In the beginning of this miasmatic conflict, or when the miasms are in a latent condition, we see only signal flags of distress, only threatenings of greater future action, as seen in flying pains or the mild sensation of heat and cold, peripheral irritation; and then we may see great centers profoundly disturbed, as in epilepsy, spasm, convulsions, until we get any degree of perversion.

All movement ought to be governed by fixed laws, and when motion is interfered with we know that law is interfered with, or the law governing that movement. Every force in the universe should be under law. The life force is not exempt from this rule, hence in any disturbance of it, it must be admitted that the laws which govern it have been disturbed by the interference of some other force.

A nebulus of disease is but a nebulus of perverted motion, and a climax of disease is a climax of action in the perverted life force. We live or exist on a higher plane of action, even as the life forces act upon a higher or lower plane. It is the momentum that kills or makes alive; force must be multiplied or diminished before lines of action are changed or destroyed.

How do we know that we have uniformity of law in the forces, even in the life force? By uniformity of action. And how do we know that we have uniformity of action? By the constancy of the same phenomena we know to be present in the normal life action, which becomes a standard from which we judge all perverted life action.

In the study of the miasm we see that there is a something in disease, in fact in every case, which is beyond consciousness and which persists, and *it is this persistence that premeditates causes other than that which we now see in the pathological*. We are compelled to confine ourselves to the study of the phenomena, the nature of which confirms the kind of bond the subversive force has made with the life force. When it proves to be an inseparable one we call the disease malignant, and when it can be separated, a benign one. The positiveness or the persistency of the bond establishes the relationship between the life forces and the subversive forces. If the balance of power be on the side of the life force the subversive force is latent. But if the balance of power be on the side of the subversive force, then we look for any degree of intensity and persistence of disease, and the *real* or the *actual* becomes magnified as the *potential* becomes magnified. Then the history of disease is a history of something coming out of the imperceptible, out of the invisible or potential, and in the course of time through similia it disappears in like manner. This is as true of the functional as it is of a simple pathological state, and the phenomena that has passed must, in some degree, become the phenomena of the future in the correlative action of true similia until the whole past is expressed and the history of all the disturbances of the sick one is complete through the law of similia. Thus we have found that the real, the actual, is but the creation of the potential ; that the real has no existence but through the potential ; that the correlation of the forces is behind all things, and if we wish to know or to see what disease is we must know and see it through the potential ; also if we would remove disease from the suffering organism we must remove it in like manner—that is, by and through the potence of medicine. We may be wanting in knowledge, but we are not wanting in law or principle. We may lack knowledge or thorough conception of these principles governing disease and cure, but we are not lacking in the resources of power.

A recognition of the results of the dynamic action of the life force is one of the points of departure of homœopathy from the old school. Then, having the previous reasoning in our mind, we at once look for cause, and the cause is found only in the miasmatic phenomena.

But to return again to our study of abnormal growths: after this philosophical discussion of the subject, we will now consider the manner in which such growths are formed. In the first place we must all admit that no abnormal growth can be formed without it be the work of the life force. We will further admit that a normal or healthy life force *could* not and *does* not construct one, as it has no power, outside of its normal physiologic action. Then how was it formed? There are many ways by which the life force might be disturbed that would bring forth an abnormal growth, such as a suppression of a discharge, injury to a part, suppression of disease states, such as eruptive diseases, pain, ulcerations or any marked disease process. *Any stasis of disease or miasmatic suppression may produce an abnormal growth*. Even should it be an hereditary expression the law holds good, for all abnormal growths are *inhibitory* points or inhibitory centers, and an inhibitory center is usually a tertiary expression of a miasm, although in acute diseases it may be a secondary process. When a miasm is acting along certain lines, say in a chronic or subacute state, producing simple external expressions, as papular eruptions, warts and such like, the system is through these simple mediums eliminating from itself all that is necessary of the effects of miasmatic poison. Should the unskilled physician who is not acquainted with this law governing miasmatics, suppress these conditions, some other eliminating avenues or points must be created, as the miasm is still in that organism with the same strength and power of action. *The same stress is there*, the same dynamis; therefore, when we suppress its manifestations do we simply change its nature? No, its action or its manner of working in the organism, and the same miasmatic force is directed along other lines and against other points or parts in that organism, which is along lines of heredity. New phenomena, therefore, or new symptomatology develop. The more profound the suppression the greater and deeper the new manifestation or new process. Each succeeding suppression involves more vital centers or organs, so that if we hit a single persistent symptom in disease we are like the Irishman at Donnybrook fair whose rule was to hit every head he saw. So the physician without this knowledge hits with some specific remedy, or some suppressive measure every inhibitory point that manifests itself, and in that way *he is constantly forcing every external manifestation of miasmatic action upon the organism itself*, thus cutting off all avenues of elimination of the disease whose true nature he does not understand. It is in this way abnormal growths develop, or that any new disease process develops which is classified by pathologists as a new disease, independent, probably, of any former disease or state of the system.

We will now admit that abnormal growths come by or through this process of compelling the life forces along certain lines, due to combating a part of the phenomena of disease and not taking into consideration the totality of the symptoms ; we will now suppose that after we have done this thing we come to the true knowledge of disease and desire to undo the work we have performed. How shall we do it ? There is but one way, and that is by taking carefully the present existing totality, which uncovers cause, and by taking carefully these new totality groupings in the order of their appearance we are led back to the primary simple miasmatic state and in the meantime we have removed pathology and uncovered cause, and, as we uncovered cause we removed all suffering and what is known as disease. In the first place, as we study this totality our knowledge of its grouping tells us to what miasm or miasms it belongs. And in this way we get at the basic principle of our abnormal growth. If we happen to be a physician of the old school our first anxiety is to know whether it (the growth) be of tubercular origin or not ; knowing *that* greatly modifies our prognosis or possibility of a cure. And yet to know this does not lead us back fully to cause, as a tubercular process is not *prima causa*, for we know that certain miasms originally produced this condition. So then, in order to get at the basic principles of a tubercular process we must investigate its miasmatic origin. But, you say, how do you know that a miasm is behind or at the root of all abnormal growths? We know, in the first place, that this subject received a careful study from Hahnemann himself for twelve years, and after the most earnest thought, careful analysis and experiments he saw that the miasm lay not only at the basis of abnormal growths but that they fathered all disease outside of chemical and mechanical irritation. In the second place, when the law of cure was applied, basing the prescription on the totality of the prominent and most dependent miasmatic symptoms, the abnormal growth no longer developed and immediately began to diminish and finally disappeared. This occurred when the highest potencies were given and when all chemical action was lost, or destroyed, in preparing the remedy by the process of potentization. Usually the local symptoms or the pathological phenomena were either not taken into consideration or were only given their due place in anamnesis of the case; that the tumor or abnormal growth lost its power to increase in size and began to diminish, and furthermore that the general health of the patient began to improve immediately with the arrest of the growth, was sufficient proof of the basic principle lying at the bottom of the disease had been reached; besides, no new disease process developed. On the other hand, when the growth was removed by surgical measures, it often became recurrent, or some new development succeeded it, frequently of a nervous or mental nature, that was difficult to remove, if not incurable. So we see that this same physiological stress or functional perversion clearly demonstrated the presence of a something in the organism that maintained a ruling or governing influence over that life, and the removal of the tumor by surgical measures was simply the removal of this inhibitory center, this correlative point, which the life forces were compelled to set up, owing to some former interference or some deflection of its action by unscientific procedure, either by the patient himself or by the attendant physician. What further verification do we need to prove that the basic principle of disease is potential, than that of the removal of abnormal growths or any profound pathological condition by the highest potentials we employ and which are to be found in our remedies? The process of absorption taking place in any abnormal growth, under the law of similia, through the influence of a potency, is nothing more than a cessation of miasmatic action and the retrograde metamorphosis of the life force resumimg its normal again, and as we analyze perverted life action as a whole it leads us back not only to cause but to a true conclusion of the unknown—it finds the secret power, the miasm, that is behind the perversion and which neutralizes its action and annuls its power over the organism.

In looking upon disease from this standpoint we readily see that reality underlies appearances as the law of similia unfolds the mystery of *prima causa*; "and the disposition of cause is the disposition of miasmatic phenomena, and the true real is now seen to be the potential. It is also true that law unfolds like mysteries in the physical universe, as seen in Newton's discovery of gravitation by which the mystery of the great inhibitory forces and the complex movements of the planets were made known.

"The philosophy of today does not tear down, does not destroy, but constructs for us magnificent temples of truth where he can store and securely keep its archives." Our conception of cause is becoming more cosmic, more positive, more polar and less anthropomorphic. Being heirs to the files of ages we are able to compare, classify and to weigh in the balance of truth the many grand, though oft conflicting, theories of our forefathers, until today we have a new philosophy, discovered by Hahnemann, clothed with *dynamics*; it is not a mere Organon of scientific methods that are man-made, but a true synthesis of truth concerning the unknown. We have the requisite basis of a distinct science—one that is capable of a progressive development—which can not be ignored or set aside; one that is not amenable to the opinion or beliefs of men, because it is founded upon laws and principles which are unchangeable and invariable. The laws governing the life and disease corresponding to our therapeutic laws and thus altogether they work out in harmony, each having an agreement with another.

SUPPRESSION OF THE MIASMS

Hahnemann, speaking of the treatment of psora in his Chronic Diseases, Vol. I, says: "The older physicians were much more conscientious than modern doctors, they were much more enlightened observers. Their practice was based upon experience, which showed them that the removal of psoric eruption from the skin was followed by innumerable ailments and grievous maladies." However true this may be, today we have reason to believe that they saw in the psoric eruption an internal constitutional disease and attempted, in their weak and very imperfect way, to treat it constitutionally, and not locally. It is true that thousands of practitioners today recognize psora, and all the chronic miasms, for that matter, as internal constitutional affections. But, not knowing the methods which Hahnemann employed, or not being acquainted with a law of cure, they can not apply internal medicines in a way that will remove their effects from the organism; therefore, not knowing what else to do, they resort to expedients of all kinds, not as a matter of choice, but from that of necessity. The majority of men are honest in these things, and would gladly adopt our methods if they understood them; but they are so diverse and so different from the teachings of the scientists of today that in order to change their methods of treatment they would, to a great degree, have to abandon or cast aside their present teachings and knowledge of physiology and pathology in general; even their conception of life, as well as therapeutics, must be changed. They would have to put a dynamic life force behind their physiology and abandon their theory of chemical action as governing the growth and repair of the organism, for Hahnemann's dynamic theory of both disease and life. Thus you see some of the reasons why men use expedients and all sorts of methods in the treatment of the sick. And what are they contending against? *Disease* they call it.

But the truth is: that against which they are contending has as yet no name in their nomenclature. It is true that secondary and tertiary expressions of that which they are really contending against have been given innumerable names and with them are coupled conditions without number. They have endeavoured to tabulate and give a special name to each miasmatic expression present in the organism, but often the name itself is confusing and misleading; old names are retained such as *rheumatism* and many others we might mention which were conceived in ignorance and framed from a misconception not only of life, but of disease. New names are today coined with almost as poor a conception of their origin or their nature. Often the organ or part affected is coupled with changes that are apparent or which really take place in the circulation. Again the character of the lesion is coupled with the organ or affected part and thus the disease manifestation receives its permanent name; with this name they are compelled to place a pathological or etiological explanation, in order that it may be understood. Again, their so-named diseases have their primary, secondary and tertiary expressions of values; even then we do not get at cause or do they reach back at the true etiology or the nature of the contending forces which have their habitat within. When these acute expressions pass by they think that the disease has disappeared from the organization, save for the predisposition to a relapse or a return. You see such a state of things exist because men do not understand the *causus morbii*, the miasms, which are the true etiological factors in disease, which are to be studied carefully in order to understand the relationship to disease, whether functional or pathological. These multiple expressons of disease, known by certain specified names, are but the fruits of the miasmatic action and its power over function and over life. In our study of disease we may lose sight of the miasm itself for a time, as it becomes more or less latent in the organism or is presented in new forms and as new phenomena, but we can never lose sight of that force, that unknown quantity, which is constantly perverting the life and bringing changes in the organism, and although we may not recognize it as one of the chronic miasms, it nevertheless is, and if we bring the life forces under law we at the same time bring *it* under law, "that is the miasm." Now if we bring the life force under law we have brought *all* under law, and we can have no suppression. Should we, however, not recognize either law, life force, or miasm, we are forced to go back to chemical medicine, and to our empiric measures, and the life force must suffer the consequences and become more and more deflected until pathological states and conditions arise without name and without number.

We can only understand the forces of nature by and through law; because law is the relator of all things, as it is only through it that this unknown principle (the miasm) is clearly revealed to us with all its attending phenomena. It is also true that we can only see through law the mystery of a suppression, for suppression itself is a retrograde process or a deflection of law, or it is physiological law opposed. The physician who suppresses any miasmatic state, or disease process, if you wish, is an enemy of law, or at least there is no mutual understanding between him and law. We must first know that law rules not alone the visible things, but all invisible as well. It stops not at potency, but governs even that—yea, all the forces are subservient to law, and in disease there is no exception. You may ask the question, shall we under any consideration apply our therapeutics locally? No. I say most emphatically—*no*, as that is not according to any law of life, or disease for that matter. Why? Because both the life and the disease—(and you know disease is perverted life)—work from within outward, and from above downward, and not from without inward; even the very unit of life (the cell) works from within outward or from its nucleus. The life is within, not without; the disease is within, not upon the surface. It is only an expression of it that you see. You can never see disease, any more than you can see the life itself. If it were possible for it to be visible it could not bond with the life force, and this fact is true in every expression and every phase of homœopathy; to withdraw from this is to withdraw from homœopathy, as thousands have done, leaving only the name behind them as a memorial, although that name is by no means represented in its true light. "*Life*," says Hahnemann, "*is a vital principle, a self-moving force, a vital power which, if acting in harmony, preserves our bodies a harmonious whole; a disturbance of which is disease; a lack of which is death.*" Herbert Spencer says, "Life is a continuous adjustment of internal relations to external." It is by virtue of this fact we are entitled to be called alive. True, we are constantly adjusting ourselves to changes, so that any altered condition in our life force throws us out of correspondence. If we correspond not with a part, a part is affected; and, with the whole, the whole is affected. The adjustment is always imperfect in the presence of the miasm, and it is this imperfect adjustment with which we are constantly dealing. The external adjustment is imperfect only when the internal is imperfect. It is the internal, the life, that rules the organism. When it is perfect the organism is perfect, and when it is imperfect the organism is more or less imperfect. So, we see that the life correspondence dwells in the law. If it is the internal, the life that rules, we can not assist it from without otherwise than by protecting it from its environments. Therapeutically speaking, then, we must enter into correspondence with it, we must deal with that which animates the organism and gives it its being, the life. Nature is the complement of the life ; but we must assist nature through its right channels and by the way of law. *Disease appears through the medium of the same law that governs life, and we must work with it along these lines.*

The miasm is the opposing force to the life force ; *therefore, the forces we bring against it must be in true opposition to the miasm*, and not alone against the life itself or we disturb it more. It must go with the life and work through the life and be in co-operation with the life. Any other procedure endangers a suppression or a greater deflection of the perverted life force.

The life force often relieves itself from the possibility of a suppression due to our treatment by presenting the existing miasmatic action in some new form or by an external expression, for instance, in an eruptive disease, in a diarrhœa, in a neuralgia. I now recall a case wherein a uterine hemorrhage, suppressed by viburnum oppulus, was followed by a facial neuralgia. The secondary process, as we can readily see, was an indirect one, forced process, and it must be equally as prominent a process as the former or it could not relieve or represent the physiological stress. Thus the outward expression must relieve the inward expression. Death follows when these conditions are not equalized. And that is what is meant by equilibrium, which is the balancing of the effects of force or the effects of the miasm upon the perverted life force.

SOME OF THE WAYS IN WHICH A SUPPRESSION MAY TAKE PLACE

Hahnemann in his Chronic Diseases, Vol. I, devotes seventeen or eighteen pages of that small work to the subject of suppression, wherein he gives special cases illustrating almost every form of suppression and the means whereby they are produced. He puts particular stress upon the suppression of skin eruptions, such as itch (scabies), tenia, eczema and other such eruptive diseases, out of which arise some of the most fatal results, or which may be the means of establishing new disease processes which are even more dangerous to life or are more difficult to eradicate. The most frequent methods used were local applications, such as itch ointments, salves, medicated lotions, mineral baths, applications of cold and heat, also the persistent use of crude drugs internally. The same author says that the removal of the local expression of the disease only gave the miasm an opportunity to become centralized upon some organ of the body and that while the local expressions were removed the internal conditions were unchanged, and the internal disease increased in the progress of time. He recognized the local symptoms as secondary expressions, or vicarious expressions, of the internal disorder. He also noticed that the suffering of the organism was greatly relieved when the patient broke out with an eruption or when any external manifestations of disease presented themselves, whether they were skin eruptions, catarrhal discharges, diarrhœa, dysuria, hemorrhoids, abnormal growths or any other local manifestations. He further noticed that with these sufferings and attended with these comings and goings of the disease or these inward and outward miasmatic manifestations, the internal suffering either ceased entirely or was greatly relieved as the local expressions presented themselves, such as eruptions, perspirations, abscesses, discharges and so on. It was such expressions that enabled him to see the true nature and character of disease, which he followed to its bond with the life force itself and from which all disease emanated.

While the local methods of treating skin eruptions, ulcers and local lesions is still in vogue they are not so generally used at the present time as they have been heretofore. However, still more powerful agents are now in use which not only accomplish the same purpose but do it more effectively and with more certainty. A few of these I will mention, such as the actual cautery, so large in use to destroy chancroid ulcerations and other ulcerations where bacteria are supposed to be abundantly present. The X-ray is one of the more modern, and probably one of the most powerful, suppressive agents yet discovered. Under its prolonged application and use such fixed lesions as lupus, psoriasis, eczema and other kindred lesions have disappeared. And, strange to say, these removals have been palmed off upon the public and also upon the profession as *bona fide* cures, and that, too, before a reasonable time had elapsed to give any assurance of the fact. It is true that the X-ray will cure some of the above mentioned lesions, but it must be done according to the principles of homœopathy and according to the law of cure. A proving of this wonderful and yet almost unknown dynamic has been made from the sixth to the c. m. potency, and since its proving a number of cures have been made and recorded in our journals. The law of homœopathy is so broad and so sweeping that we do not have to go outside of its bounds or away from it one iota, for it is applicable to all diseases, states and conditions. So when any new thing is brought forth let us prove it as we always have done and catalogue it with our great therapeutic list and bring it under the banner of law.

No, we can not remove local or external expressions of disease by the use of the X-ray and call it a cure, as there is but one law of cure, that one promulgated by Hahnemann : that disease is cured from within outward, and from above downward.

We have in skin diseases and all external manifestations of disease peripheral expressions through nerve transmission. It is taken up from within and transferred outwardly as a relief process. This is nature's provisional safety valve. This is as much a biological law and a physiological process as the elimination of the urine or sweat is a physiological process. When we suppress any local disease we overcome that process or we annul it, and we are then enemies of biologics or physiological law. This is the secret of all suppression—we have deflected, if not destroyed, nature's eliminative process, which is a life process, and have forced nature and its processes back upon itself. We must not lose sight of the fact that while we are dealing with disease we are dealing with life, "for all disease processes are perverted life processes," and all must be brought under the laws of life in order to restore that disturbed harmony. If we study closely we will see that it is the same law that governs all life. It is *biological law* governing; not chemistry, but biological dynamics. What do we see? Motion active—the keystone of all organized life; motion sensible and motion insensible; motion visible and invisible; motion voluntary and involuntary, giving us redistribution of matter and the external transposition of disease processes, and while not always visible, can in time be easily proven to exist by its change of arrangement that becomes clearly manifest. This is not chemical or mechanical, as some would have us believe, but life motion (plus some miasmatic force), living energy which is influenced by all motion or by external or internal influences. I say: "by external and internal influences," for the law that governs its absorption and the external transmission of disease is the law that governs all life.

As we rise in the scale of life and begin to deal with multicellular forms and biotic life as a whole, when organs and life processes are multiplied, then we get that multiplicity of phenomena which makes it the more difficult to analyze and harder to understand. We might illustrate this, in a way, by taking into account the child at puberty, when the reproductive processes are developing. Previous to this we had not this sphere to deal with, and if at all, only to a very slight degree. But now we have a very complex process that is subject to numberless changes and disease processes. So we see, as organs are added, the life process becomes more complete, therefore the disease processes are more numerous and complex. Again, as the miasms are multiplied the disease processes become still more complex and multiplied, so that the effects of a suppression is then more complex in its phenomena, therefore more dangerous to life. If we suppress psora we are aware of the profound changes which take place in that organism from a simple pruritis to pain, spasm, convulsions, coma, and death. But when we suppress a mixed miasm, like psora and sycosis, what can we expect? We certainly must expect multiple processes and fearful conditions to follow; for the character of each subversive force, each miasm will be characterized and, to some degree, expressed in that organism. Here are two sin processes, the sin of disobedience and the sin of lust, both having their own peculiar lines of action in the organism, one along one line or against certain organs or tissues, while the other is against others. So it can readily be understood how necessary it is to be able to discern the presence of those latent miasms in the system, and we should deal with them according to the principles and science of homœopathy. If we deal with disease from any other standpoint, we can not give it the positive assistance we would like in each disease state and prevent all danger of suppression or deflexion of the miasms action. The suppressed action of a chronic miasm means much to the patient, to the family and to the race in general, for it not only weakens the race, but it means (as a rule) hereditary transmission of either that perverted state, or that deeper and more profound envolvment, by these newly developed processes, coming out of such suppressions.

There is another point to be considered in our study of the suppression of the miasms and that is the resistive power of the life force. One person is gifted with more power than another; different persons resist to a greater or less degree the action of drugs. One patient is sensitive to a certain drug or remedy; another one is comparatively insensitive. A local application of a certain crude drug applied to certain eruptive diseases readily dissipates it in one patient, while it has comparatively no effect upon another, and vice versa. This may be due to some idiosyncrasy in the patient or it may be due to some natural protective or resistive force in the organism. I have often noticed that when many crude drugs, now in use for the supression of some local manifestation of disease, fail to accomplish the result, some other means has to be used to accomplish the work. Again, often when disease is suppressed, it will not remain so, but will be forever breaking forth, either in the same form and in the same locality, or in similar form and in different localities. In this way the life force largely protects itself against the inroads of this unscientific and incurative method of combating disease. Again the organism may be gifted with that inherent power to set up other local manifestations of miasmatic action, such as pain, neuralgia, rheumatism and such kindred diseases, which will largely take the place of primary eruptive diseases, and in that way prevent an internal miasmatic stasis. If we attempt to suppress the disease locally by local measures, in a patient with very little resistive force, or where the resistive power of the life force is below par, or where they have been under the effects for a long time of some mixed miasm, such as tuberculosis, the suppression is often an easy matter ; but where we attempt to suppress disease in some strong, vigorous constitution the life force rebels and the contest becomes a marked one between the therapeutic agent and the life force. All the principles of life governing the organism are principles of truth, and when any of them are interfered with nature rebels. This protective principle is an inherent principle in the organism and is governed by law, knows no other way of action, therefore is in opposition to any false methods or false processes that may be introduced.

The life force previous to the attempt at suppression was either eliminating, or endeavoring to eliminate all miasmatic products, or that produced by the disease process, which is in agreement with physiological law; it could do nothing else, for the good of the organism is dependent upon it; but the false physician, the violator of law comes in and opposes it, turning it about, and thus magnifies the disease process, by forcing a change of action, or some new process of disease upon the organism. In that way, not only is the disease changed, but the symptomatology is changed and as we attempt now to take the case, we get an imperfect picture of the true internal change due to the deflection, and besides only a part of the symptomatology is presented and that is in an imperfect light, and the rest is veiled or covered from our sight. Herein is the beginning often of malignancy as well as the turning point where disease is made incurable. This great truth can not be better illustrated than by giving a few cases to demonstrate the fact.

CASE 1.—Mrs. B., age 32, was infected with sycosis soon after the birth of her child; it was a vicious form, the vaginal discharge being dark yellowish green and quite offensive, it was also corrosive and irritating. This was suppressed at an early stage by medicated douches and was followed for a short time by a period of good health, and this is where the deception often comes in that leads us to believe that we have done no harm, but if we will follow the history of every case we will see this is not true; two years later uterine displacement (retroflection) with rectal adhesions (a marked subinvolution, and, by the way, this is the cause of the majority of our cases of subinvolution) things grew from bad to worse with a history of change of physicians and much suffering until cancer developed and death relieved her of her sufferings.

Case 2.—Mr. L., age 53. History of a tibial ulcer that he has been combating locally all his life with all kinds of ointments and local washes. Suddenly it healed under the use of a mercurial ointment and within a year interstitial Bright's disease developed which has gradually grown worse, and now he is a complete invalid.

Case 3.—Alice B., age 24, suffered with hay fever every spring, suppressed by local treatment which was followed by a chronic bronchial cough, that has since proved incurable. But every physician can give us many instances of such cases that have come under his observation for treatment. If there, seemingly, proves to be an exception, it is only a matter of time and endurance, gifted to the organism. We then fail to see the connecting link between the first and the last process of disease. A young woman came to me about a year ago suffering with a cystic ovary, the trouble was of long standing and incurable by remedies and therefore was removed. She regained her health and for six months or during the summer was apparently well but as soon as the weather became cold she developed a severe case of pneumonia of the right lung. She was thin in flesh and in no way would you suspect pneumonia or any congestive disease, the miasms present were psora and sycosis, a combination that gives us marked congestions and local inflammations followed with a cystic degeneration or abscesses. The abscesses, however, are more painful than the tubercular or syphilitic and have very little pus as compared with the tubercular. The pus or expectoration is scanty and a dirty, brownish yellow, while the tubercular is thick, copious and yellowish, or yellowish green in the later stages. In sycotic diseases, rheumatism is usually present while the psoric is often accompanied with neuralgic pains. The subject of suppression is such an extensive one that books might be written on it, giving the numerous forms that present themselves for consideration. Of course the manifestations following suppression are usually in proportion to the stage of the existing miasms. If the miasm is suppressed in the acute stage we will, of course, get acute expressions ; and if subacute, subacute expressions, and so on as the case may be. This is often found to be a cause of our many mistakes in diagnosis ; we to a great degree lose sight of the miasm in

THE CHRONIC MIASMS. 119

this way as the phenomena differs so in the different stages, or is modified as it verges into the subacute and chronic forms, besides it becomes a mixed miasm as it recedes from the acute and as it blends with psora, it is here where psora and pseudo psora begin. Chronic miasmatic expressions of disease are known as latent miasms. Often we have but faint tracings of their action upon the organism, quite often functional, although it is not uncommon to find some one persistent symptom present, occasionally of an annoying or distressing nature. It may be limited to one symptom or condition, as is seen in the profuse perspiration about the head, of calcaria children. Again it may be pain, pruritis or some simple expression and located in any part of the organism, or found in any anatomical region, part or system, in the bones, muscles, lymphatics, circulatory system, again it may be found in moral or mental spheres. As a rule the symptoms of the miasm can not be long suppressed or forced into a perfect latent state, for sooner or later, the life force is bound to give us some expression of it, and that expression will depend of course upon the nature of the suppression, the stage of miasmatic action and the blending of the miasms. Occasionally we meet with some form of cachexia which develops, in time, into some well defined disease or pathological state or condition. We have seen cases in which the first sign of a suppression, or of a miasm being suppressed, was in a spasm, convulsions, epilepsy, or in some form of chorea, hysteria or spasmodic disease of some kind or other. Asthma, one of the spasmodic diseases of the respiratory tract, is decidedly a disease induced by suppression; in fact it never comes from any other cause. I have given each case that has come before me a careful historical study and without any exception I could trace it back to where some suppressive measure had been used. Many of these cases were induced by quinine given in overdoses, or where the treatment was prolonged some time. I now recall one case that was due to suppression of an acute muscular rheumatism by quinine, given internally with local medication to the parts. Under treatment the asthma disappeared and the rheumatism returned. Another case, a very severe form of bronchial asthma (where the patient, a man of 40 years of age with a tubercular family history), came on soon after suppression of hemorrhoids (the itching and bleeding form, which are usually sycotic). The asthma disappeared in the first case under psorinum c. m. and in the second case under the use of arsenicum c. m. In the second case the hemorrhoids returned before the disappearance of the asthma. In another, or third case, ague had been suppressed by powerful doses of quinine, also cured by arsenicum 1 m after having suffered from the disease for ten or twelve years. In that case the old chill returned, followed by high fever and sweating, which lasted for several days. He also had marked symptoms of arsenicum poisoning following the giving of the potency, which was due to his taking Smith's specific, a patent medicine containing arsenic, that he had been in the habit of taking for years to palliate his difficult breathing. I recall still another case, that was of a nervous or hysterical nature, which came on from the suppression of hay fever due to local treatment; a woman forty years of age, a ballet singer, was confined to her bed for two years with nervous prostration and asthma; this was a severe form of asthma cured with a few doses of sabadilla. So sensitive was she to this remedy that I could not give her more than one dose of the c. m. potency, as each dose was followed with a severe numbness all over the body, copious perspiration, with a feeling about the heart as if she would surely die. The second and third dose was given her by strategy, but she nevertheless suffered more severely each time and was fully aware of the fact that the remedy had been given. No more was given, but the asthma soon disappeared and she has remained well ever since. Many cases of asthma in tubercular patients who came to me for treatment were induced by suppression of la grippe or bronchial cough induced by the use of cough mixtures. Tuberculosis develops in many of these cases or they become helpless invalids. There are three miasmatic conditions, which, as a rule, when suppressed, produce disastrous conditions; these are acute itch (scabeacris), gonorrhea in the first or second stage, and the malarial miasm often called intermittent fever. The first may give us any disease catalogued under psora and unless a secondary eruption should appear such as eczema, etc., stasis is sure to appear in some part of the organism, and which is often incurable unless the eruptive disease can again be produced. A gonorrhoeal suppression in my experience usually results in one of three processes—a gleety discharge or catarrhal condition of some mucus surface; a localized secondary inflammation of some form or other, such as metritis, salpingitis, appendicitis, or inflammation of the prostate, rectum or of some other organ. Not infrequently this form is manifest in congestion of the menninges, medulla or some other part of the brain, often inducing many aberrations of the mind such as acute or subacute mania, even to true insanity.

Moral insanity is of such common occurrence after a suppression of gonorrhoea, that the most casual observer can not fail to notice it. It does not always make its appearance at once, as you might suppose, often months or years pass, before we see the bad effects of a suppression; this depends upon conditions already mentioned.

I now recall a case of a healthy man 51 years old who had never been ill in his life until he contracted this disease. He was treated locally throughout the whole course of his treatment, still there remained a gleety discharge often with a marked irritation of the bladder and other annoying symptoms. At the age of 58, the gleety discharge was suppressed by local medication, while in a short time, his memory began to fail, forgetting trifling things at first and later on greater things, until finally discharged from his employment. It was not long until he was confined to his home where he has been closely watched for years by his family, owing to his insanity, which quickly developed. This is one of many cases that fill our insane hospitals and places of detention for these people. They are simply judged insane, and the cruel hand of the law takes hold of them, and many of them perish from that brain stasis, due to the suppression or live for years that lamentable life of one who has lost his reason.

In this treatment no thought is given to the probability of suppression, and often no research is made as to the history of their secondary disease. Indeed, cause is of no value to those who have not studied the history of the suppression of the disease or who are in the habit of giving brain sedatives to modify or quiet the mental phenomena.

The true physician and the true scientist will look deeper into the cause of the mental phenomena, for he knows that the royal centers of life are not disturbed by any trifling cause. No; it is only when some profound disturbance takes place in the life force itself. Generally a brain stasis is the last thing to appear, and yet it is about the great centre, the brain that all eruptive diseases (exanthematous especially) evolve, such as measles, scarlet fever, syphilis. And why not? Because a principle of biologics, a principle of physiology is involved in it, for from the great centers of life are evolved the great and profound expressions of life, therefore as disease is disturbed life force, it, too, is evolved from the great centers of the living organism. Then shall we turn back by false methods these forces upon themselves, so that they may correlate themselves upon the central organs—that they may destroy or disturb them more profoundly? We must not look to organs or to special localities for the cause of disease any more than we must look to pathology for cause, for cause is a deeper thing, a constitutional thing, a something co-operative with life; and from the fact that it does co-operate with life it gives us the phenomena of that co-operation, which is disease phenomena in all its shadings and in all its multiplicity of signs and symptoms. The dynamic must be looked for, no matter how it may manifest itself at any point or organ. We must not only look for it but we must study its nature and character and know its internal workings, its plan of attack and its developments and modes of action.

The last or third form of suppression mentioned, the malarial, is none the less important, although not met with so frequently as many others; yet we find that in the past it was frequently met with in all its grave forms and manifestations. It can not be overlooked by any practitioner who has had any experience in its treatment. The organism usually effected by this acute miasm (the malarial), is the psoric or pseudo-psoric, the latter more frequently; that is, we find the tubercular element often manifesting itself soon after the system becomes infected with this subtle poison. It matters not how this poison known as malaria, is propagated, whether it be by or through the old supposed process of heat, moisture and vegetable decay or whether it be that of more modern thought, insect bites or stings, we care not, the results are the same, whether it manifests itself in the usual phenomena of chills, fever and sweat, or in that peculiar and profound cachexia common to this poison. A suppression of this condition in its treatment by quinine, arsenic, or in the use of other similar suppressive means, often brings forth disastrous results, profound organic changes, and in the end death processes, even to the destruction of the life itself. No more unscientific thing could be performed, no more unjust or unprofessional act could be thought of from a therapeutic standpoint, than the producing of a stasis of this profoundly acting, acute miasmatic poison, that has blended and bonded itself with psora or pseudo-psora, giving us a disease producing element that is probably unequaled in our study of any sick-making process (nosansis). Some of the developments of suppressed malaria are asthma, chronic headaches, chronic liver and splenic difficulties, tubercular developments, bronchial coughs. Insanity, so frequently met with in farming communities, often has its origin in suppressed malaria of some form. Take it along river bottoms of such rivers as the Wabash, Ohio. Mississippi, and we find many of the chronic diseases that are not sycotic or syphilitic, depending on either suppressed itch or a suppressed malarial poison. How frequently we have seen the tubercular dyscrasia, especially in young girls, develop soon after a malarial suppression ; first the liver becomes involved, or the spleen, or both together, then we see that peculiar ashy complexion begin to show itself as the dyscrasia develops. Finally the tubercular element itself soon appears, and in a short period of time it has developed into a true case of tuberculosis.

Much could be written along this line of thought, and many revelations of the facts be made if space would permit, but we must take up other subjects, not less important to this work. Should you wish to get a clear revelation of these things, you can only get it by close study of similar suppressions. Hahnemann said "that without a knowledge of that *threefold origin* and the *homœopathic remedies*, the successful treatment of chronic diseases is absolutely impossible." In the threefold origin, he means the three chronic miasms, *psora, syphilis and sycosis*, as they are the first cause in every case of disease ; all other processes or means of disturbance in the life force, is secondary.

A few cases of suppressed malaria, given in brief, will not be out of place here and will serve as an illustration of the facts herein stated.

CASE 1.— Mr. John B., age 42, light brown hair, fair complexion, lymphatic temperament, contracted malaria in 1889 and was treated more or less for a year with quinine in large doses. He was suffering from the effects of that drug in many ways, when he came to me for help; indeed he was having a marked proving of its toxic effects upon his whole organism. He came to me in 1890 suffering from Bright's disease; he had a constant pain in the back, thirst, prostration and frequent urination. From these and other symptoms of kidney trouble, I made a careful urinary test and the test revealed Bright's disease of the right kidney. I put him on a suitable diet and gave him arsenicum 200, which relieved many of his symptoms. This was followed by silica c m, which cured the case in less than one year. This was twelve years ago. There has been no return of the disease. The pain in back and region of kidneys came soon after the suppression of the chills by quinine.

CASE 2.—Mrs. Ella Herman, age 32, mother of three children, the oldest 13 years, the youngest 7. The history of her case is as follows: Always well, never employed a physician until at the birth of her children. She contracted sycotic gonorrhea from her husband five years ago, suffered with pelvic inflammation and pelvic abscesses until she was compelled to have the uterus and its appendages removed. She made a good recovery from the operation, but soon after developed a severe form of nasal catarrh, large accumulations of pus, yellowish green in color and of a lumpy consistency, would form at night in the posterior nares. I gave her a number of remedies without any effect whatever. I was then treating her by correspondence. Some time later, however, I advised her to come to the city and see me, as she lived about one hundred miles away. On a careful analysis of her case the following symptoms were noted : Symptoms and feeling always changing, no two days alike, dreads cold weather, better by warmth in general. Before the removal of the uterus her menses were very offensive, she was always better when the flow was on. She was low-spirited and despondent. I gave psorinum c. m. and within a week a very decided leucorrheal discharge came on, which was attended with much burning and itching of the pudendum. At once the catarrhal symptoms disappeared and she quickly regained her health.

There are other conditions found in mixed miasms as well as in malaria, which bring forth even as dangerous results when suppressed, some of which might be mentioned here ; they are such diseases as tinea sycosis, tinea tonsurans, tinea vessicular, verruca in its many forms, the eruptions of vaccination and some of the vegetable parasites, such as alopecia circumscripti, and others, all of which are sycotic. These skin diseases are syco-psoric, as they are a combination of both miasms, although partaking largely of the former or of the sycotic nature. Any of these above mentioned diseases, if suppressed, may bring forth almost any nameable disease or expression of disease action in either the physical, mental or moral spheres ; thus a suppression of tinea sycosis or barbæ, may give us subacute or chronic rheumatism of some form, throat affections, ringworm in different parts of the body, etc.

"Suppress," says Dr. Burnett, of England, "any form of ringworm and there often follows it tubercular diseases," which lead him to think that ringworm was of a tubercular origin, but this is not so, for a careful study of these skin affections by one giving their time more fully up to the study of skin lesions, it will soon be clearly seen to what family they belong and to what miasmatic basis they depend upon. Of course, we often have to get at these things through the deductive method of reasoning, excluding them from syphilis, seeing that they have none of its characteristics and in the same way of psora. Again we can combine them with psora, by carefully noticing that they partake of the primary action of psora, such as pruritis and other peculiarities of psora. I have often noticed this in the treatment of gonorrhoea. After treating it for a week or longer with anti-sycotic remedies, the psoric element would develop in the form of an intense itching about the sexual organs or in some portion of the penis, or psoric eruptions such as furuncle, psoric papules or pustules appear in different parts of the body without any apparent cause, and in patients who heretofore had shown no signs of active psora. Again psoric aggravations of time, or of heat, and cold, would appear. Sometimes psoric manifestations in other organs are found, as in the liver and stomach, that would lead us to prescribe anti-psoric remedies which would complete the cure of the sycotic condition. Again, psoric lesions or expressions would vanish as sycotic lesions came to the surface. I now recall a case where sycotic moles, that dotted the body of a physician like polka dots on a piece of cotton, disappeared under the homoeopathic remedy after an eczematous eruption made its appearance upon the left tibia. This sycotic form of skin trouble is very difficult to cure, as it is a tertiary expression of sycosis.

Hahnemann says that "in the study of the chronic miasms and their suppression, three things ought to be considered, first, when the period of infection took place; second, when the whole organism is tainted; third, when external symptoms make their appearance." In the acute miasm, such as exanthematous eruptions of all kinds, as seen in scarlet fever or measles, or the eruptions of psora or syphilis in the chronic, the catarrhal discharge of sycosis. "The psoric infection," says Hahnemann, "is instantaneous." It is performed in a moment of time. No means can be employed to arrest this process of infection or contagion when it has come in contact with the blood flow or the nerve endings. While it is usually a material contact, it is not the material that infects; it is the dynamic; therefore how useless to cut out or to cauterize, to douche or to get at it in a material way. No, we must send a similar dynamic after it in the form of a potency, and by and through the way of law.

5 F.B.

A disease process must be set up in the infected organism before a local or constitutional disease manifests itself to the eye or senses of the observer. Why? Because it is the life force that is disturbed and the organism, by virtue of that disturbance, gives us a secondary or a tertiary process, a secondary or tertiary change in that life action from the normal standard of action. Often these secondary and tertiary processes are forced upon the organism, by virtue of the suppressing of the miasm. The suppressive measures do in a day or a week, or a month, what the natural disease process would take years to accomplish, and often, if left alone, would never take place. For instance, a gleety gonorrheal discharge has been known to have existed for years, with no bad effect whatever to the patient, but which, when suppressed by operative measures, or the use of strong medicated lotions, produced a stasis to internal organs, and death in a short period of time. This I have often noticed when itch was suppressed; only a year ago a boy of six years was affected with itch, which was suppressed with sulphur ointment, and was followed in a few days with convulsions, which ceased only when sulphur was antidoted, and the itch broke forth on the body again in a modified form. If syphilis suppressed in the primary stage develops a cachexia and tertiary as well as secondary symptoms, when there should only be secondary manifestations, we know that it was a forced process, and that that process was hastened as well as magnified by the suppressive measures. The regular school was forced to cease their method of cauterizing the hard chancre, on account of the fearful secondary processes that developed. They found that the secondary symptoms were less severe when the initial lesion was not interfered with and the tertiary stage was not so liable to develop, and they were less severe when the primary syphilis was treated constitutionally. What is true of the syphilitic process is true of all processes; they all came under the same nosantic law, all under the same perverted physiological process; there is no difference. Probably fifty per cent of all so-called cures are nothing more or less than suppressions of some form, or some deflection of the disease processes, and arrest of elimination in some part of the organisms, and a closure of the sluce-gates of relief to a diseased body. We so often find that through suppression, the internal disease is formed, and the external expression of disease (the pathological) is the natural evolution of miasmatic action; which is from above downward and from within outward, and the unnatural procedure is to hinder or arrest that process; in fact, it is an arrest of this process that constitutes a suppression or a stasis to organs or localities that were sound and well, before this backward movement of the disease took place; by these false methods of cure they soon become diseased and often show marked destructive processes within a very short period of time. When we think we have checked the process of an external disease which is a manifestation of an internal one, by local measures, we are greatly mistaken, for there really is no such a thing as an external disease; it is all the peculiar workings of an internal dynamis. The internal disease for a time becomes more latent or slows up, as it were, in its action for a time, but it soon assumes its former mode of action, though often changed in its direction and vibration. For a long period of time it is silently gathering strength in some other direction or preparing to undermine in new localities, and unobservently instilling itself into the innermost centers of life. Hahnemann compares the suppression of pain or acute disease, to the poor man, who to get rid of his poverty stole a large sum of money and in place of *obtaining* real wealth, he "goes to the dungeon or prison." Such chances and such procedures must be paid back in the same coin. *"Sin is the transgression of the law"* and the "wages of sin is death." *So any transgression of a physiological or therapeutic law brings forth a death process*, and its wages is more disease and deeper laid plans of destruction. There is no escape from the miasms' action or workings, but through the recognition of law. If we do not recognize law in all things, we are compelled to suffer from the results of no law, and that is therapeutic anarchy, for that is what no law leads to.

Those who have not studied the miasms, especially *psora*, are often ignorant of its presence in the organism. Therefore, when some new process develops, such as an eruptive disease, pain, or whatever it may be, they do not know to what to attribute it, so they endeavour to satisfy the curiosity of the patient by telling him that the new diseases have arisen, owing to the presence of bad humors in the blood. In a crude sense this is true, but the question arises, what are the humors? Where did they come from? Give us their origin and their history. Are not all humors the result of miasmatic action? Did anything else ever father a humor but a miasm? Could anything else create or form a humor? Why, of course not; humors are either syphilitic, psoric or sycotic, or a combine of two or more of these. We see clearly defined syphilitic humors or any one of the miasms. We see the tubercular humor in these patients who have an ancient history of psora and syphilis; humors enough in some of them to make us think, or reason out the cause for the sake of the existence of the human family. Often after an acute fever or some severe form of Lagrippe, some eruptive disease, like eczema, arises and we are at a loss to know where it came from, but if we will but look back into the history of the patient, we will discover psora or some other miasm which was latent, but by the new acute process was aroused, which explains all and makes plain the whole matter. *It also gives us such knowledge as to enable us to begin a plan of treatment in that patient which will, in the end, remove that which is behind humors.* The humors of the body as recognized by our ancient medical fathers were blood, black bile and phlegm. Yet foolish as seems this conception to us, it was about as clear as far as cause is concerned as many of us see today. Many of us have no better principle to work from.

It is our lack of knowledge of this latent or quiescent state that a miasm assumes in any organism that produces those multiple and mysterious processes known as Pathology, that deceive us. It is often very difficult to see the connecting link between the two or to trace out the lineage from one disease state to another. How shortsighted we are; these latent disease processes are slowly developing day by day, but we do not see the markings or tracings of perhaps psora or some other miasm all the way along. Here is a case of epilepsy, with no apparent cause, coming on in a boy at puberty. Why should this be? Look carefully and you will see a psoric or tubercular diathesis. Again here is a case of hysteria in a girl of twenty years. She is well developed and to all appearances healthy, but at each menstrual period she suffers in a way that is almost beyond description, violent dysmenorrhœa, extreme pain, spasms, mania with great mental agitation, dysentery and very strange symptoms, and what is the history of such a case? Tubercular, of course; an aunt and an uncle on the father's side died of that disease. It is only a mixed miasm that could give us such a combination of phenomena. Suppose we look over her latent miasmatic symptoms. She has light brown hair that is dry and lusterless, the dental arch is imperfect, the teeth club shaped and irregular, the incisors still show a slight serration, the face is pale, but becomes flushed easily from the least excitement, the eye-lashes are irregular and some of them are imperfectly curved, others stubby and broken, the edges of the lids scaly and red, the hands and feet are cold and clammy, the nails thin and imperfect, split or break easily. All of the above are tubercular or pseudo-psoric symptoms, her physical endurance is quite limited and she is forever complaining that she is tired; she has a history of suppressed menses from getting wet in a rainstorm, and all her sufferings have arisen since that time. She has been treated in both this country and also in Europe, but with only temporary relief. What are we to do in a case like this where so many have failed? Wherever climate is favorable to her she goes, to spots by the sea, to Europe, the mountains; all have failed. A careful analysis of her whole case revealed tuberculinium to be her remedy, which cured the case and she has remained well ever since. That was in 1896. Oh, how much there is in treating diseases from a miasmatic standpoint, which brings us at once down to bed rock, and in compliance with the law of cure. I feel that I have by no means covered the ground in my treatment of this subject, but space prevents my carrying it any farther, and yet it means so much to every honest hearted physician who has a desire to carry out the teachings of Hahnemann, in order to make perfect cures of the sick and not false cures;

for all know that suppression is not a cure, and that the result of suppression *is to throw back upon the inner life processes, that which the life has been ever pushing forward and outward to the surface, to the periphery, where it can keep it in abeyance and under its power.* Thus the inner centers are not in danger. The disease when thrown upon the surface not only frees the organism from that pathological stress, but it becomes quite accessible and amenable to treatment.

There is another form of suppression that has not yet been mentioned and it is probably as important for our contemplation as any yet considered, and that is the habit we have of suppressing certain symptoms that make their appearance from time to time, by the use of the homœopathic remedy. We become so over-anxious at times to please our patients and to carry out their requests, that we frequently prescribe remedies which will palliate or remove annoying symptoms; this we know is not in harmony with the law of cure or the teachings of Hahnemann.

The symptoms may appear either single or multiple, but quite often single. They may be any form or expression of disease or suffering and any part or organ may be affected. When these symptoms appear after the giving of a deep acting anti-miasmatic remedy, they should by no means be interfered with, as they are the reactionary workings of the life force, under the influence of the remedy that has been selected according to the law, unless, of course, the sufferings of the patient demand it. Sometimes the reaction becomes violent, and we have such an acute expression of the miasm coming up, as pain, neuralgia, inflammatory processes, such as inflammation, erysipelas, coming as a regenerative process, and it is true of all such conditions. In that case we often have to interfere with the anti-miasmatic remedy, giving an intercurrent until the violent secondary expressions of the miasms subside; then, if the symptoms are similar when the organism resumes again its quiescent state, give the same anti-miasmatic remedy. The curative process is a retrograde process, a stepping backwards, a going over the old trodden paths of life. Just as soon as we give a remedy, there is immediately set up a reaction in that life force, and that reaction is the process of cure that takes place through the law of cure, which is known as Homœopathy. Therefore the secret of our success is not wholly in the selection of the similar remedy, but in carefully and intelligently watching the retrograde process or the reactionary action of the life force in its efforts to throw off the disease in its own peculiar way. Now if we get in the habit of striking at every new symptom the life force works to the surface, we will sooner or later turn the tide of life action the other way or in the direction of some internal organ or part and the eliminative processes of the organism will cease, and a destructive process at once begin its development within the inner organism. This is an important part of the higher homœopathy, that we follow minutely the retrograde movements of the life force under the action or influence of similia, as long as it continues to act. When it ceases entirely, a new selection can be made, which will take up the miasm at that point and continue to neutralize its action upon that life and in the end drive every vestige and sign of its presence from the organism, and a perfect and complete cure is the result of our efforts.

PSORA

We now come to the study of psora from the standpoint of its symptomatology; it is only through the study of its special phenomena that we become acquainted with its action in general upon the organism. We have seen by our general view of it as far as we have gone, that its array of symptoms is very complex and that it was most persistent and profound in its action upon the organism, no part of which was free from its inroads or from its ravages. Like a mighty octopus, it takes in everything, both the physical and the mental, and in many cases largely influencing the spiritual. There is no life process free from it. Every zone or center may be involved and, besides, it readily combines with any other miasm, bonding itself with it in such a way that it would seem almost at times impossible to separate them. Indeed, only through the power of similia can the separation be accomplished. No other power yet conceived of by man has been able to make this separation. Another peculiar phase of psora is its power to assume a latent condition or state peculiar to itself. Neither syphilis nor sycosis seem to have this faculty of hiding themselves away in the recesses, as it were, of the organism, in such a manner as to be for a time hidden from our vision, only to appear again in some unexpected quarter or at some unlooked-for time. If syphilis or if sycosis ever becomes latent, it will again appear as a psoric expression or in combination with psora. These facts, above, make psora our greatest enemy. Hahnemann has said that "if it was not for the presence of psora in the organism, the organism could not become affected by any other disease, not even syphilis or sycosis." It is the basic principle of all expressions of disease. It is the bond of acceptance, that induces the life force to receive disease. It is the gateway of reception, the doorway wherein disease entereth. Disease can enter in no other way. It is the insignia of disobedience and the sin processes, therefore all disease processes must partake of it, or they can not enter therein. Seldom do we find psora, now an acute disease; universally, it now appears as a latent disease, affecting nearly every organism in some manner. Physicians of ancient times had recognized the fact that eruptions, when suppressed, were followed by direct consequences, and neither their modes of treatment nor any power then known could arrest or stay these processes, now known as internal disease. Conscientiously and faithfully they recorded their efforts and their failures to cure these multiple manifestations which we know to have been nothing more than *psora*.

Hahnemann spent many years in elucidating this subject, that we might know something of the mystery of psoric action upon the human organism. That wonderful image or picture which he gave to us has grown in its brightness as it has passed through the minds, and the experiences of such followers as Hering, Lippie, Wells, Fincke, H. C. Allen, Kent, and many others of his noted apostles and followers of the past and present. Many of his self-styled followers have drifted, not only away from his psoric theory, but away from the knowledge of the first principles of his law of cure.

Hahnemann was the first to classify *psora* as a chronic miasm and to give it the prominence it now holds as a disease-producing agent and as a parent or basic element of disease. Foster defines a miasm as a morbific emanation which affects individuals directly and not through the medium of another individual. This we do not understand to be always a condition of psora, for Hahnemann says it may exist with or without an eruption, or anything save itching or pruritis.

It is quite evident that he found that far back in the early history of the human race, there had sprung up this psora, or this self-producing miasmatic disease known by its progressive order or successive groupings of symptoms, and the apparent changing of its nature at each cycle of its appearance. This disease entity or ego, had through all ages presented itself in its multiple and varying forms, yet always with the same death-like grasp had held its countless victims. At one time it had presented itself in the form of a malignant itch, at another as a leprosy, again as "the plague," and so on through all time. To this disease *ego*, Hahnemann applied the name of *psora*. He discovered the law of *similia* in 1796 and published his *Organon* in 1810, but I believe it was not until 1827 that he made known to his followers that he had made a wonderful discovery, and it was then that his theory of chronic diseases was brought forth in which the doctrine of psora was inseparately and indissolubly incorporated. It was at this time that he discovered the true relationship between the *miasm, psora*, and all the subsequent sufferings of the patient. He arrived at this conclusion after years of constant study and thought, together with the repeated failures of the ordinary homœopathic remedies to cure the hosts of non-venereal diseases ; that the non-venereal diseases having been repeatedly and apparently successfully removed, continued to reappear in some modified form of the disease, proved to Hahnemann that each presentation of the disease did not constitute the disease *in toto*, but was simply an overflowing or a reaction produced in the life force by the presence of the psoric taint. "This ostensible disease was a mere fragment of a much more deep-seated, primitive evil, that had taken possession of the whole organism." This also was a positive proof to Hahnemann that we ought not to treat them as separate and completely developed maladies, that we find to be located in parts or portions of the body designated under special names known to our nomenclature, that like thunderstorms broke forth with violence, to be followed by calms, peace and temporary quiet at that point, only to break forth again at some other portion of the body. We ought not to expect to cure disease by assailing those points of the enemies attack when we know that there is something within the whole organism which is at variance with the life in general. As we attack these salient points therapeutically, we only drive back the foe temporarily. It recovers itself and repeats its attacks upon the same part, and in a similar manner presents similar phenomena, or at times involves new parts and processes under the false guise of new phenomena. This was the true secret of the basic miasm *psora* revealed, and so the totality of the symptoms came to the mind of Hahnemann as the therapeutic triumph as healer of the sick, and the perfection of therapeutic law.

Hahnemann found records of *psora* among the ancient Greeks, Romans, Arabians, and among the children of Israel, who were infected in one or another manner. The people of the middle ages were not less diseased, and the dreadful continental plagues that swept all before them at different periods and from varying causes, such as malignant syphilis, cholera, and leprosy, he attributes to the basic principle and far reaching miasm *psora*.

Studying psora from the light of our present day knowledge, just what conclusion are we to reach concerning the application of the true "*psora*"? It was a name that meant much to Hahnemann himself and to his earlier followers, and it means much to some of his followers of today, but to the rank and file of homœopathists it means nothing, as their lack of knowledge of its nature and character, gives it no significance. We believe, however, that the words conveyed a far broader meaning to the mind of Hahnemann and his early followers, than that it was not symbolic of *acarus* poisoning, as many of our friends would have us believe.

Hahnemann says, "at one time, the psoric eruptions which appeared after infection had taken place, was easily driven from the skin, by all sorts of lotions and contrivances." We believe from this that itch was not all there was to psora, but simply a form of or manifestation of psora, or in other language, itch was one of the secondary manifestations of psora. This we believe to be true that it has no fixed formula or symptomatology, but is made manifest in multiple forms, and in countless, yea, endless phenomena, varying often with the age, sex, nationality, zone, climate and other circumstances of a numerous order. Often the milder forms were more dangerous to the people, as they were not protected or isolated from it, as in the more malignant types of leprosy patients. The groupings of secondary ailments, that presented themselves after a suppression of the itch, was to him positive proof of the falsity of the treatment, as well as the ignorance of its true character among healers of the sick.

We do not understand, however, that the common itch of today is nearly as malignant as the itch mentioned by Hahnemann, although, perhaps, it still takes on largely the same nature and character, but in a modified form. We are not to understand that Hahnemann teaches us that all secondary or tertiary manifestations of disease are induced by suppressed itch. No, they are produced by supressing *psora* or any of the basic miasms. *Nothing can be suppressed but the chronic miasms or that which is in combination with them.* They are the only things that have that persistent and perfect bond with the life force.

Our great mistake is in not studying disease as a whole, as Hahnemann has so frequently pointed out. This separating of every manifestation into pathological groupings or segments, and losing sight of its dynamic origin, as well as its greater consecutive nature and successive development, is a mistake. If we attempt to cure these many manifestations known by pathological names, with no regard or with no scientific desire to look into the spiritual *ego*, we are sure to fail. *How foolish it is for us to try to bind together the vagaries of the life force.* We must first know and understand that disease originates in the life force itself, before we can treat it from the standpoint of Hahnemann's *psoric* theory. Disease does not originate in the life force or manifest itself through the life. Not because Hahnemann says so, but because when we stop to think, we know that everything in the universe of God is dynamic in its origin, and a dynamic law control every vibration of matter, from the smallest atom upward. What we need is to look into the action of these laws, so that we may see the miasms in their true light. So long as we neglect this internal disease (miasm), so long we neglect to attack the vital disturber of the patient's health. If this is not done, we will be forever having these psoric upheavals to deal with, and in the end accomplish nothing permanent. Today the psoric miasm is, to great degree, blended with sycosis; fully 80 percent, we are told, have sycosis in some form, therefore catarrh is now the prevailing expression we meet. Dr. Lippe noticed this fact, and I believe he speaks of toothache and neuralgia being so prevalent in early days and that now catarrhal troubles were the most common manifestations of psora to be met with, and today, fully 80 percent of them have in some degree the sycotic element present. But these miasmatic expressions of disease are ever changing, due to their multiple blendings, suppressions and unscientific methods of treatment, to say nothing of surgical and operative measures, intermarriages and hereditary transmission; all these tend to change the normal action of the life when the miasms are present and give us false or diseased physiological expressions, which sooner or later present almost any disease, either local or general. Unless we know something of the action of these chronic miasms, *psora*, *syphilis* and *sycosis* in their different stages of action and also their latent conditions, we can not follow disease in all its changes and mysterious presentations, but a thorough knowledge of the miasms makes all clear to us and we are prepared to meet them at any stage on therapeutic grounds, for they are no longer wrapped in mystery. We should also know something of the diseases and complications that present themselves in each stage of miasmic action, and in this way we are forewarned and we are always prepared to meet any emergency. A knowledge of suppression is another feature we must become familiar with. For instance, many cases of gonorrhœa are coming to us that are either suppressed fully or partially. Now we ought to know these symptoms that arise and are due to suppression. We get this by a study of all the symptoms of our patient, previous to taking treatment, and his present condition. Often a single symptom in the history of the case will call your attention to this fact. The patient may tell you that he has had a headache, backache or that he has felt badly since he began his treatment for gonorrhœa, or he has never had a well day since. You will find this in both sexes. Now the first thing to do is to re-establish that suppressed discharge, and the remedy based upon the totality of the present symptoms will do just that thing. Be patient and wait fore results, as a cure can come no other way. Of course, if sycosis has passed fully into the tertiary stage we can not as a rule re-establish the discharge, although we may be able to bring forth a warty eruption upon the skin either locally or general.

DISEASE STATES

There are many conditions to be found affecting the organisms, that we recognize as disease states of the system, which are due to the action of psora or its combination with other miasms. We have in the beginning of this work called your attention to these states, which are designated under the terms diathesis, dyscrasia, cachexia and idiosyncrasy, scrofula, struma and such states of the blood. These conditions have, strictly speaking, some degree of difference from each other, yet they all depend on similar causes. The difference in often only in the different proportion in which other miasms are combined with psora. Usually the tubercular taint is present and not infrequently the sycotic element is also present. In a study of the word cachexia, we will find it means a depraved condition of the system, and what is true of this word is also true of the others, they all express depravity in the organism and that which induces the depravity lies in that inherent power of the existing miasm to produce such changes in the organism. Indeed, it is the miasm that induces all these chronic, depraved states of the system. A diathesis may always have been present although it of course can be acquired, but it has within it that which at any time or period of life may induce a cachexia. Again we are told that a dyscrasia is a morbid state of the system, but that explains nothing or gives us no cause or reason for its presence; indeed, these names are so closely allied to each other that they mean the same thing, or modifications of it; they are simply degrees of miasmatic action going on in the organism for years, often from the birth of the individual. Even for generations these miasms have been doing their dreadful disintegrative work in the organism; like the fires that devastate a mine, slowly they are eating away, and gnawing at the vital forces of our being, and these expressions, cachexia, dyscrasia, diathesis, and idiosyncrasy, are but pictures of the ruinous workings of their presence in their organism.

IDIOSYNCRASY

This is a well-known state of the body or mind; in fact, we may have either a physical, mental or moral idiosyncrasy. It may enter into the desires, hopes, fears, cravings, longings, moods, and manners of life, or in any expression of life. It may show itself in any one or more of the faculties of the brain. For instance, we may see it in caution ; he is extremely cautious, painfully so ; or a patient may be over sensitive to the presence of odors, flowers, perfumes, gases, to light, noises, colors, animals, birds—that is, they faint easily when roses or violets are brought into the room ; when they are ill they can not endure a bright light, sunlight, or, may be, certain artificial lights, as lamp light or an electric light. Certain shades or colors are intolerant to them. They can not endure the presence of certain animals, as cats, dogs, and other animals. Often these peculiarities are a constant factor ; again, they may be only temporary, as one often witnesses during pregnancy, about or during puberty or in earlier childhood. Frequently these patients are born with these abnormal conditions, or they make their appearance during certain sicknesses, such as prolonged fevers, gastrointestinal diseases, in fact during any prolonged illness independent of pregnancy. We see it in the craving for salt. This I have frequently seen to be present in whole families from a remote date. These children not only desire an excess of salt in their food, but they will steal it from the cupboard or table and partake of excessive quantities of the crude article. You will find this in patients who have a tubercular diathesis or a latent syphilitic taint. They do not assimilate a sufficient amount of sodium chloride, for some reason, and when suffering from tuberculosis in an active state, they eliminate little if any, in the urine. I believe Professor Vaughan, of the

University of Michigan, speaks of this fact in his work on urinary analysis.

There are many ways in which idiosyncrasy is manifest in the organism besides those already stated. One person may be affected by a certain agent, another by some other. Certain kinds of foods or drinks affect one person and not another. We see this in the production of skin eruptions, as in urticaria after the eating of sea food, shell fish, or from eating certain vegetables or fruits, strawberries, asparagus, oatmeal; also animal products, as certain kinds of meats. Honey frequently disturbs the kidneys or the whole urinary tract. Again we see it clearly manifest in people who travel. They have nausea or vertigo while riding in a carriage or in a ship by sea. Others are affected by the approach of a storm, by the sudden fall of the barometer (as seen in sycotic or syphilitic patients), the wind blowing from certain points of the compass. They suffer from neuralgia, rheumatism, gouty conditions, depression of spirit, moody conditions arise, mental states are made manifest, even to temporary aberrations of the mind. One patient craves fresh air and must have the doors and windows open. And another desires warmth, so much so that the slightest draught causes suffering. Patients have been rendered unconscious by an approaching thunderstorm when suffering from prosopalgia or some other severe neuralgic or rheumatic pain. Certain kinds of foods or drinks have produced spasms, convulsions, gastric fevers, nausea, vomiting, and were repeated when such foods or drinks were given unknown to these patients. The idiosyncrasy seemed to be an inherent concomitant of the very life. Often what are known as aggravations and ameliorations are due to idiosyncrasies. Patients suffering from idiosyncrasy can not be said to be healthy human beings. They need antimiasmatic treatment; they need the similia that in their particular case removes or separates psora or the tubercular element, or whatever may lie behind the idiosyncrasy. Idiosyncrasy is, in a sense, a bad habit of the organism or the mind. We see these mental or physical peculiarities cropping out more particularly in the earlier years of life, that of childhood, and adolescence, when the organism is developing, as in the growing boy or girl. Often we see some process become tardy or completely arrested, as in the non-assimilation of bone making material, as is well known in hydrogenoid constitutions, seen in the proving of Calc. c., Calc.-phos. Sil., the limes, the phosphates, the silicates are not being furnished for the making of bone, and as a result there is a longing for such materials which the organism requires, and the patient is not satisfied until that physiological process is restored through the process of similia. We see it again, quite noticeable, in pregnant states, as the new physiological process is established in the productive function, which often disturbs these patients, even to the profoundest centers of life. Strange wishes, desires, longings, take possession of them. They desire or crave strange articles of food, such as salt, pickles, sweets, starches, acids, raw or uncooked foods and grains, such as wheat, barley, rice ; undigestible things, such as charcoal, earth, the limes. Again these perverted appetites may call for spices, such as cloves, nutmegs, mustard, peppers, etc. ; or they may desire wines, beers or stronger beverages. In fact, we may have any perversion of taste or desire. They long for travel, sight seeing, visiting, and they can not be kept at home Sometimes the sight of the sea or any considerable body of water satisfies them. Again they prefer solitude, to be alone, to be quiet. Music may solace them for a time, or it may make them sad. Often, however, nothing seems to satisfy or please, and their lives are made miserable. Their likes and dislikes become magnified and often exaggerated, all due to the looming up of some latent miasm, latent until the new or reproductive function began to manifest itself fully within the organism, when an extra demand is made upon the life force, upon the circulation, upon the nerve supply. In many ways this new process, or new function, draws from resources already taxed, perhaps, to their limit, in a weakened organism where it has been sapped for a whole lifetime by some deep-acting miasm, such as produces the tubercular element. It is then that dycrasias crop out, predispositions become manifest and idiosyncrasies show themselves in their fullest sense.

PREDISPOSITION

Another condition fully recognized, I think, by the majority of homœopaths, as well as many in other schools, and closely related to idiosyncrasy, is *predisposition*. They are so closely allied to each other that we can scarcely separate them—the one becomes the prefix, very often, of the other. To be predisposed to a thing is to have a weakness in that direction before-hand ; or, in other words, we have within us a sort of attribute (perverted, of course) or weakness that predisposes us to certain diseases or conditions of life. We might just here associate these two conditions mentioned, *idiosyncrasy* and *predisposition*, with another condition which, in the past few years, has grown into prominence with some of our modern teachers of therapeutics, and that is *temperament*. Temperament can not well be left out of any case in making up our anamnesis, for as we study temperament closely we see that peculiar temperament is predisposed to certain forms of disease. In this we see a fixed law, or principle, involved. As an illustration of this we might take for example the bilious temperament so characteristic of a nux vomica patient. We know, with a positive certainty, the diseases to which he is predisposed. Are they not hepatic, gastro-intestinal, directly or indirectly, the result of an abuse or excesses peculiar to his mental makeup, and moral weakness, peculiar to himself?

It is a difficult matter to say just where idiosyncrasy ends and predisposition begins. Quite often they are so intimately associated that we can not separate them, or they commingle and become a complement of each other. The removal of one is very apt to cause the disappearance of the other. For instance, a patient may be predisposed to orbital neuralgia, who has an intense craving for salt, the removal of which may take away the predisposition to the orbital pain and the desire for salt. The same may be said of gastritis. This we have often seen to disappear by a high potency of nat. mur.

Those patients who are so sensitively predisposed to every disease that comes along, that is, of a contagious nature, are usually of the tubercular type, or the miasm, psora, and syphilis (latent) is firmly implanted in that organism. Psora alone seldom predisposes us to any severe excesses or extremes in anything ; but the combination of psora and syphilis, which is the parent of the tubercular diathesis, gives us all kinds of excesses. These patients are either too large or too small, too thin or too fleshy, too tall or too short ; they develop too slowly or too fast, they are mentally too dull or too bright ; the teeth come slowly, are painful, and at long intervals, or they come in groups of half a dozen or more at a time, with spasms or convulsions often, or with febrile states, gastric disturbances, etc. These children are predisposed, of course, to all (if in a marked case) the sequences due to the combination of these two elements, syphilis and psora, which is one of the most destructive of all the miasmatic bonds with the life force.

Occasionally we see a patient who is not predisposed to natural disease states, but who is extremely sensitive and predisposed to artificial diseases, such as plant poisons, of which the rhus family is a fair example. Many cases have come to the writer almost blind from the effects of rhus tox. poisoning; with face and hands presenting that erysipelatous inflammation peculiar to that poison. The first thing these sufferers will tell you is that they are supersensitive to its influence, so much so that it might be called an idiosyncrasy. Thus we often have an idiosyncrasy behind the predisposition which intensifies the action of the poison. We know by experience and from careful observation of the history of a great number of cases that neither the idiosyncratic nor the predisposed patients are healthy human beings, by any means; all of them have either a deep psoric or some miasmatic taint from which these conditions arise, and that some special cause lies behind the effect, can be plainly seen. However latent these miasms may appear to be in the organism, we can always point quite directly to their presence by idiosyncrasy, or through predisposition. Here is an apparently healthy child, say of the age of nine years; she has many of the appearances of health and strength, but she is predisposed to every acute disease of a contagious or infectious nature that comes along, and within a few years she has gone through the whole catalogue of children's diseases which, if properly treated by the single homœopathic remedy, comes forth free from any sequelæ, and the general system is renovated greatly of its existing miasm ; but, if improperly treated, we may have any chronic miasmatic stasis which either remains with it permanently, or in time destroys the life.

It is right here that we would impress upon the mind of the practitioner this important fact, that we must have a wider knowledge of these latent miasms, in order that we may know when and how to select a deep-acting miasmatic remedy that will not only remove idiosyncrasy and predisposition, but cut short all of the history above presented with its sufferings, and dangers to the young life. As a rule, many of us only scratch upon the surface of this miasmatic soil, removing a few of the weeds of disease, when we ought to be preparing the soil so that it will bring forth only the fruit of health and strength, and magnify life and perpetuate youth. Idiosyncrasy and predisposition are the offspring of our failures to do this thing. Many times we do give the true antimiasmatic remedy according to the law of similia, but we give the potency too low to get the full breadth and depth of its action, and while it may abort the existing acute disease, it leaves, as a rule, the deeper pre-existing miasmatic symptoms ; therefore, the predisposition and idiosyncrasy are still there to threaten the patient with new disorders at every new cycle and turn of life ; while the highest potency could have removed or taken away all the phenomena that disturb that life. This is a great truth that can be substantiated by every physician who has given it a fair trial or who generally brings it into his practice.

An idiosyncrasy or a predisposition is then, as we have seen, a bad habit, and inhibitual condition formed in a life force, that has been under the promptings of some subversive force for years, yea, often through generations, of miasmatic action and the changes that are common to its subversion. We often see the effects of predisposition in climatic influences as in malarial districts, removed by the potentized remedy that cures the chills, never to return, although the patients may remain in the same location and under the same miasmatic influences and climatic conditions, simply because some anti-miasmatic remedy was given that either modified or removed the effects of the chronic miasm to which, not only the predisposition was due, but that which the acute (malaria) disturbed.

This phase of physiological perversion may be carried into the moral sphere, as we see manifested in the desire to steal, to the use of alcoholic or other stimulants, tobacco, etc., to many phases of degeneracy which can be traced back, quite often, to some miasmatic taint, such as sycosis, or to syphilis, or to both. They may be born with just the right kind of toxic element in their systems that will prompt the mind and propel everything in that direction.

Sometimes we see this condition of things fall upon some one child or member of a family, and a long history of hereditary perversions is the result.

SCROFULA AND ITS MIASMATIC BASIS

The world has known thee and has known thee well,
Thy age, no mortal man can tell,
Father of death, and Mother of poor health,
The grave is but the store-house of thy wealth.

We have from a remote period been taught that the miasmatic basis of scrofula was psoric in its origin, but I think we can readily see from what has already been said concerning the action of both psora and pseudo-psora that the disease scrofula owes its origin to that malignant combination of psora and syphilis. Indeed, from what we know from the study of these miasms, as far as we have gone, both individually and collectively, it is already apparent to us that from the complexity of phenomena of this disease (scrofula), it could not be wholly due to the action of psora, nor yet of syphilis, and while it partakes of many of the peculiarities and characteristics of psora, it has at the same time many of the more prominent features of syphilis.

We frequently use synonymously the words struma, scrofula and psora; we make no distinction whatever

It is a disease, we say, arising from a psoric constitution yet it is generally understood that in psora we have no involvement of the lymphatics, whatever, which is so characteristic of scrofula.

It is true that it has many features in common with psora, yet it has, in my estimation, a clear and unmistakable history of syphilis which is a miasm the action of which is more specific than that of psora.

The development of the scrofulous diathesis is largely due, not only to syphilis and psora combined, but to the suppressive measures and crude drugging used in the treatment of syphilis in the Allopathic School. The truth of the matter is, that these gentlemen of the Allopathic School who so distinguish themselves for their knowledge of the pathology of the numerous, yea almost nameless conditions, which arise from and have their sole origin in the miasms are totally ignorant of the nature of this poison (syphilis), save its mere toxic effects upon the different tissues it is prone to attack. A few powerful doses of Mercury, or Iodide of Potassium or some other equally powerful agent and this miasm is buried forever from our vision.

Such is the history of the treatment of the dominant school. No wonder, after all these years, with such treatment and taking into consideration hereditary transmission, it is so changed in its nature and so defaced that we mistake it for psora. We fail to see the stamp of psora with that of syphilis; we do not see the fine blending of these two powerful miasms ; and while anti-psoric treatment does often cure or modify the disease, it sometimes lets loose the reins of syphilis, as you have probably noticed. The cure of a number of cases of blepharitis with Syphilinum in scrofulous patients led me to think that scrofula does not depend on psora alone as a basis, as has been suggested by many leading authors, even of our own School, but principally upon syphilis or syphilis ingrafted upon a psoric basis. We might further prove the truth of this statement by comparative study of the two diseases, scrofula and syphilis. No close observer can have failed to have recognized their striking similarity. Both diseases in all stages concentrate their forces upon the glandular system and especially upon the lymphatics ; both have the same tendency to ulceration and to puriform, decomposition of their exudations ; also, both have the same preference to locate themselves upon the organs of special sense (showing a very marked anatomical relationship) in the form of an inflammation of the middle ear, of the eyes, conjunctive, ciliary apparatus, mucous membrane of the mouth, nose and lips ; also in the osseous tissues.

What other miasm would produce caries or destruction of the bones but syphilis ? None. What miasm would produce rickets or softening of the bone anywhere in the bony structure but syphilis ? Will psora do it ? No. Will sycosis do it ? No. Sycosis may produce gouty concretions, or amorphous deposits in the joints, but it never produces changes as we find in the scrofulous patient. The periosteal inflammations and changes that take place in those scrofulous patients are very similar to those produced by syphilis. Last of all, that most sensitive and extensive organ of sense, the skin—in both diseases it often becomes the seat of very similar deposits, syphilides and scrofulides. Both are generally multiform or polymorphic in character and are usually free from itching, except where the psoric features are prone to predominate.

The eruptions or skin manifestations in both diseases may come in the form of nodules, papula, litchen, prurigo, urticaria or hives.

Again in the involvement of the lymphatics, which is so characteristic of scrofula, we have as much if not more right to say that it partakes of syphilis as well as of psora, knowing that it so much resembles the syphilitic diathesis and has so many conditions in common with it. The primary action of syphilis is upon the lymphatic glands, that wonderful venis appendix, the great filtrator or renovator of the system.

As scrofula is the full-grown tree with all its luxuriant foliage, tuberculosis is the blossom, often the degenerative stage of scrofula. William Osler, in his pathological work, says "that scrofula is tubercle, and that the bacillus of Koch is the essential element." The virus which produces adenitis in scrofula produces in other parts tuberculosis. We know that whenever scrofula takes on a malignant nature, it usually ends in tuberculosis, either in the lungs or some other part of the body. In childhood it often assumes the form of tabes-mesenterica, and in no form can a syphilitic history be more plainly traced out than in this. Again, we see it in those forms of specific anemia found in scrofulous patients, and which so frequently ends fatally, and is almost facsimile of syphilis in its worst form.

Pathologists will tell you that scrofula is a disease that often affects the bones, producing rickets, and to be found in children who have imperfect nutrition, who are badly nourished, but we know this is only the reasoning of a materialist.

What, except syphilis or tuberculosis, makes the patients poor in bone, poor in flesh and blood, poor in the organic elements that go to make up a healthy bone? What difference is there between scrofulous ulceration and a hereditary form of tertiary syphilis? None to speak of. Both have the tendency to decomposition and to the formation of tubercle. Scrofulous opthalmia is only a modified form of syphilis: modified as I can imagine any form might be by mercurization, by suppression, by hereditary transmission, by the strong resistance of the life force, that one healthy parent might be endowed with, forcing it into a latent condition, probably for a generation and then suddenly aroused and fanned into flame by the intermarriage of some one of less resistance, or probably affected with some other miasm in a more active stage.

The more I study scrofula the more I see the stamp of syphilis on every feature of it, and to the practical eye of every true homœopath it never loses its identity. Look even unto the fourth generation and it is there, a standard bearer of sin, depravity is its companion, squalor and filth often its associates, although it is to be found everywhere—in the hovel, in the cottage, in the palace of the king.

BASIC SYMPTOMS OF PSORA
THE RUBRICS

Mind.—Mental activity, psora (dull syphilis), quick, active, psora (cross, irritable, sycosis), prostrated easily from mental exertion or impressions—heat of the whole body after mental impressions or exertions—anxious, filled with forebodings—fear of death, or of illness or that their case is hopeless and incurable—mental depression—despondency—timidity, with sense of fatigue—vanishing of thoughts while reading or writing—can not control thoughts—at times seems to be deprived of thought—sadness, anxiety and dread of labor—great inward uneasiness and anxiousness—repeated attacks of fearfulness during the day (with pain or without)—oppression and anxiety on awakening up in the morning (at night, syphilis) when the weather changes (sycosis). In psora, when these restless mental spells come on they are compelled to move about. In syphilis, it drives them out of bed, inducing symptoms of suicide. Psora is relieved by perspiration, syphilis aggravated by it. The mental anxiety of psora often makes its appearance about the new moon, or at the approach of the menses in women. Weeping often palliates these patients for a time. Dread of labor, of being alone, of the dark (dread of night, syphilis), sudden transition from cheerfulness to sadness, or to peevishness without any apparent cause. When we see these symptoms appearing frequently, we may take them as a sign of psora being disturbed, or the soon appearance of some outbreak of it, in some part of the organism. We have often observed this in severe forms of hysteria, the attacks would grow more frequent and more severe, previous to the development of tubercular disease. When they come frequently and severe, especially in young girls or young women under 25 years of age, you may be sure that there is a profound pseudopsoric disturbance, and that a prescription based upon the totality of the nervous symptoms will seldom do more than palliate the case. The least mental disturbance unbalances them, the nervous system becomes exhausted from their repeated attacks, when it is followed by tubercular manifestations, due to the lowering of the nervous forces in the organism. Melancholy, violent beating of the heart, anxiety and extreme nervousness often follow the awakening of psoric patients from sleep. Pulsations in different parts of the body is common in these cases, feeling of constriction about different parts, especially at certain nerve centers, or points of reflex, arterial excitation, flashes of heat, organisms of blood, excited images, fear, etc.

Hahnemann, in a foot note in chronic diseases, says: "This kind of mental or moral disease, which originates from *psora*, does not seem to be sufficiently attended to. A certain feeling of insanity induces those patients to kill themselves, although they have no anxiety, no anxious thought, and seem to enjoy their full understanding." *Nothing can save them*, except the cure of this *psora*. Psoric patients are easily frightened, often by the most trifling causes, their fear often begins with trembling and shaking of the body, followed by great weakness and muscular prostration and often with copious perspiration. They may have chills or chilly sensations, fainting spells, headaches, nausea, vomiting and a host of symptoms follow attacks of fear, even to convulsions, epilepsy and spasms. They become dizzy or faint in a crowd, or when they meet strangers, or when any unusual ordeal is about to take place, they have headaches, faint spells, nausea, vomiting, or they are suddenly taken with diarrhea. They are easily bewildered, inclined to be irritable, cross (sullen, morose, syphilis), or sensitive to many impressions, such as odor of flowers, smell of cooking foods, to atmospheric changes, bad news, joy, or they are very easily disturbed mentally. How easily they fly into a passion, and yet in a moment again they weep and are penitent. In their fits of anger, you will usually notice that they tremble in their rage, and when it is over they are greatly prostrated and often sick for a time. The true psoric patient is bright, active and quick in his movements. The latent syphilitic is dull, stupid, heavy and obstinate. The psoric patient is usually exalted, the syphilitic depressed, although when the psoric patient has the dumps, everybody knows it and can see it, while the syphilitic patient keeps it to himself, and the first thing you know he has committed suicide by jumping in the lake or river. The syphilitic patient does not worry his friends with his troubles much; he is a close-mouthed fellow, while the psoric patient is a constant annoyance to his or her friends; they are often in trouble, often found complaining, fault finding, unsatisfied, never well, and yet often quite able to locate their troubles. The psoric patient is a chronic complainer, a chronic grumbler, fault finder, never satisfied with his conditions in life; they are the abused ones, the neglected ones, and yet at the same time every one is doing all they can for them. They are anxious when ill, apprehensive, despondent, melancholy, sad, changeable in their moods (syphilis, fixed in their moods). Moodiness, where they are very changeable, is quite pathognomonic of psora.

Time goes too fast or too slow. The psoric patient is absent minded in a general way, but the sycotic patient is absent minded only in certain things; he forgets words, sentences and previous lines that he has just read—he wonders how the simplest word is spelled—he has momentary loss of thought, or he loses the thread of his discourse frequently—he is constantly stopping to find it, which causes him to repeat. Often this is due to his inability to find the right word. In the delirium or mania of psora, there is no end to his words; words are multiplied and he has no trouble in finding them; his thoughts run so fast and words are so multiplied that he does not know what to do with them. This is just the reverse of the sycotic patient, who can not find words and if he does he is not certain if they are right. If he is writing he is not certain whether he is using the right words or he is in doubt about his spelling; he drops words or letters or uses the wrong ones. When he is giving his case to the physician, he has difficulty in giving his symptoms, or he is afraid that he will not give them right, or that he will forget something. In speaking he is always afraid that he will forget something, or that he will use the wrong words. This is painful to him and causes him much annoyance and suffering. This is not so of psora; he may be so depressed that he can not speak, but when he is able to speak he is at no loss for words; in fact, they come to him in mental troubles faster than he can speak them. In reading or any mental effort, it is apt to produce pain in the head of a sycotic patient. Psoric patients, as has been said, are in severe or marked cases, sad, joyless, despairing, moody, downhearted, depressed, melancholy, and forboding evil. A recovery of their health seems an impossible thing; they do not look for it, or have any hopes of it. This is especially true in patients suffering from suppression of any kind and if often does not disappear untill the suppressed condition is re-established, when all will suddenly clear up.

Such is the power of suppression of one of the miasms over the mentality of the patient. See *Hahnemann's Chronic Diseases*, Vol. I, and from page 34 to 50, you will get some idea of the fearful ravages and profound action of a suppression upon the human organism. In psora we have mental delusions of all kinds, yet I doubt if they are so real under psora as they are under sycosis and syphilis. They are more apt to be temporary or flighty in psora, while in sycosis they are likely to be more fixed or permanent. Quite often you can reason a psoric patient out of his hallucinations or imaginations, but not so in the syphilitic or sycotic. There is a certain obstinacy of mind in a syphilitic, while in psora the mind is over-active and very acute. In the psoric diseases, the delirium and the action of these patients is often disgusting and they have more foolish fancies than they would have in true delirium.

In syphilis and sycosis, the reasoning powers are slow and they are constantly condemning self; while these symptoms may be present in psora, they are constant in a mixed miasm. The desire to kill or to destroy life is seldom a purely psoric mental symptom. The suicidal patients are, as a rule, the patients whose organisms are tainted more or less with syphilis or sycosis. Often we find the syphilitic patient morose and mistrustful; there is also a desire to escape or to get away from self. This often drives them to suicide. If you will study the well-proven anti-syphilitic remedies, you will find that this destructive and suicidal element runs throughout their action. In sycosis they are as a rule always cross and irritable and disposed to fits of anger, recollection of recent events is difficult, while things long past are well remembered; this is quite a constant mental symptom of sycosis. In the syphilitic patient, his thoughts and ideas vanish away from him and he has not the mental ability to bring them back; he reads over and over again a verse or a few lines, but he can't retain it; in a moment it is gone from him; there seems to be a sort of mental paralysis; he even forgets what he was about to utter. Sometimes we see this so marked in tubercular children all through their school days, and often we attempt to whip them into line with other children whose minds are clear and strong and who have no such mental depression or devitaliizing element in their organism. It is here we ought to say to ourselves, "Canst thou minister to a mind diseased?" and shall we not be very charitable with these children who have within their very life that which devitalizes and deteriorates their mental and physical powers. The syphilitic and sycotic patients are relieved of their mental stress and their mental disturbance, like psora, by some external expression of the disease, for instance a leucorrhœa or a gonorrhœal or catarrhal discharge of any form returned, relieves a sycotic patient at once. Of course this is in the secondary stage, for in the tertiary stage he may be relieved by an eruption of warts, or by fibrous formations or growths of any kind. How frequently I have seen the mental symptoms, even those of acute mania, subside in a very brief space of time by a reproduction of the discharge in a sycotic patient or in a syphilitic patient by the breaking forth of an ulcer, or some old sore that had been healed over by some local nostrum. I have seen irrepressible anguish and extreme suffering from pain, due to inflammatory conditions, relieved in a few hours by a gonorrhœal flow or by the appearance of a syphilitic eruption; this is often the case, also in brain stasis in syphilis. How frequently we have seen fearful suffering in women at the menstrual period, before the flow makes its appearance. How often we have seen a severe neuralgia clear up in a moment, in tubercular patients, with a hemorrhage from the nose. She is happier when she has a leucorrhœa and vice versa, as we remember under the proving of Murex, which is a purely anti-sycotic remedy, like Sepia. Her pains, her aches, her sufferings, both mental and physical, alternate often with a vaginal discharge which eliminates the sycotic element from the organism. The headaches, the weariness, the confusion of mind and disposition clear up by the renewal of some catarrhal discharge that has been suppressed or has been temporarily suspended. New feelings, new life and vigor comes with the moment of the establishment of the miasmatic elimination from the organism. We see a patient moaning with pain, or with fever, or in a delirium, and we give him a few drops of aconite or arsenicum and it ceases at once. Why? Because it has at once induced an elimination of that which was culminating within, which forced that condition upon that organism.

Our remedies only deal with miasms, not names of diseases. *The law of similia is only co-operative with that which disturbs life, not the organism as a part*, and we have learned that the miasms are the persistent disturbers of life. "The miasms are the maggots that are born within the brain," as Shakespeare says, and those maggots never die until overthrown by similia.

Psoric attacks of all kinds are relieved by some physiological eliminative process, such as diarrhea, copious urination, or perspiration. These are not apt to relieve a syphilitic or sycotic patient, although we may find temporary relief in pseudo-psoric cases, as is seen in offensive foot or axillary sweat of the tubercular patient, which when suppressed often induces lung trouble or some other severe disease. Sudden anxiety with strong palpitation of the heart, with people suffering from gastric or liver troubles, is quite a positive psoric symptom. The liver becomes inactive, often due to overeating, when the patient becomes much depressed, irritable, disinclined to work, with sudden loss of energy, no desire to do any mental or physical labor. This condition of things is often relieved by some form of cathartic which gives them immediate relief for a short time, but the same set of symptoms soon returns; the same treatment is repeated until it finally fails, then they are compelled to look elsewhere for help. Of course many symptoms, outside of the mental, accompany these cases, such as constipation, accumulation of gases in the alimentary canal, headaches, vertigoes, offensive taste, desire to lie down, moroseness, despondency, laziness, lassitude, aversion to all kinds of work, disinclination even to think, with general apathy. These symptoms are modified or changed in the different individuals, by virtue of the power of their constitutions, mode of life, diet, climate, race, sex, hereditary predisposition, education, tendencies of the mind and morals and occupation or vocation. The mental symptoms arising from moral insanity usually arise from a mixed miasm, and *sycosis* combined with *psora* figures largely in the criminality of our country. Men and women who commit suicide today (and you know how it has increased within the past ten years) are, generally speaking, sycotic, occasionally syphilitic. It is not uncommon for us to hear women say (especially women inexperienced in crime) "I will kill myself if I do not soon get rid of this loathsome disease," meaning the discharge, and they too frequently carry out their threats. Quite often from suppression of both syphilis or sycosis (subacute or chronic) a basilar meningitis is set up, which induces all forms of mental aberrations. The degenerate and all his kin is either sycotic or syphilitic, usually sycotic or deeply impregnated with a sycotic taint or a syco-psoric one. The epilepsy of psora or the true insanity of psora is usually of a tubercular nature, that is latent syphilis and psora. Malignant cases have of course, all the miasms present. Sycosis implanted upon a tubercular back ground, gives us, of course, all the miasms and if the tubercular taint has been latent ever since he was born, it is as a rule very apt to be aroused when the patient contracts the malignant miasm sycosis. The life force as a rule can not retain the three in an inactive state. That mysterious protective principle or power in the life force seems over-balanced by the addition of sycosis to the tubercular element; before its addition the protective principal in the life force seemed to correlate the tubercular element and hold it under bonds, but that bond is separated and broken by the presence of the true element of sin. It can not be harmonized in the acquired state, and even in the hereditary it will break forth. The pathological in any marked degree, seldom, if ever, comes from the psoric miasm; it is more of a functional disturber. It is when it is combined with syphilis or sycosis that we see the pathological begin to develop; that is especially true of internal lesions of the body, but we meet few human beings, today, who are purely psoric and free from any combination of other miasms. Of course psora has changed in its character

THE CHRONIC MIASMS.   175

and action since Hahnemann's time, but yet there is no telling what combinations were formed at his time, that produced those international epidemics that assumed the form of plagues, which swept over and over the old continents of this world. As we study the symptoms that Hahnemann has given us in Volume I of his "Chronic Diseases," we see the mixed miasm in the symptoms that he has tabulated under psora or that he calls purely psoric symptoms. Indeed it is difficult to separate them as symptoms. We can with a clear knowledge, however, of these miasms discern even the faintest latent tracings of latent syphilis or sycosis inter-blended with the psoric element. "Often we have to treat our psoric cases for some time," as Hahnemann has said, "before we can discern another miasm is present in the organism" and it comes to the surface or rather begins to manifest itself as the primary element, *psora*, begins to disappear; that is, two latent miasms seldom become active at the same time. If they do we are liable to have a malignancy on our hands. This work is like the work of an artist, it is a study of lights and shadows, or a study of symptomatology in all its shadings and in all its peculiar features, bearing upon the action that the different miasms produce upon the life force, either singly or in combination with each other. Knowing the primary, secondary and tertiary action of each we at once recognize their presence, in combination with others in any of the above named stages of action or of existence, for the signs are many and they are all in opposition to physiological life and law. Therefore the truth in the physiological law of life must reveal them to our senses, so we may feel them, see them touch them in their multiplied expressions, hear them often as they multiply and exaggerate the life action in the organism, yea, taste them, for every miasm produces its own peculiar taste in our mouths as we will see later on. Thus we have a panorama of dispositions, pains, sufferings of all kinds and all the multiplied and varied expressions that can be produced by their various actions.

SENSORIUM

Hahnemann speaks so frequently of the vertigoes of psora and they are indeed many and quite often very peculiar. He speaks of vertigo in walking, moving, looking up quickly or rising from a sitting or lying position. Whirling vertigo with nausea is very common in the so-called bilious subjects. Vertigo with momentary loss of consciousness, when things appear too large or too small; vertigo with eructations, with rush of blood to the head or face, with headaches, prosapalgia followed with temporary blindness; vertigo as if intoxicated; especially is this true in the morning dullness of intellect and confusion, with nausea and vomiting of mucous only; vertigo when stooping and with lightness of the head, as if swimming, sensations as if floating in the air; sensations as if the head were larger than the body, as if turning in a circle; vertigo with digestive disturbances of all kinds, with nausea, vomiting, disturbances of the portal system, and constipation; vertigo on reading or writing with confusion of mind or with specks or stars before the eyes, or sensation of a veil before the eyes; vertigo on closing the eyes, on falling asleep; vertigo with sensations of falling or as if in a boat; vertigo on riding in a boat, or at sea, with nausea and vomiting, or when riding in a street car or in a carriage. Psoric patients can not be disturbed much, they prefer to remain quiet when sick unless the mind is affected. The brain becomes anæmic easily, therefore they are subject to kinds of vertigoes. Vertigoes beginning in the base of the brain are more apt to be of a sycotic or syphilitic nature or may be of a tubercular origin. Vertigo with flashes of heat and with perspiration which often relieves, vertigo in a warm room or when the air is not good, vertigo when stooping, in walking, with roaring in the ears and confusion of the senses, heaviness of the head and weakness of the lower extremities and palpitation of the heart. Vertigo on turning over in bed, or closing the eyes.

Head.—Morning headaches, constantly returning, persistent, frontal usually. (Headaches at night, syphilis, worse at night or the approach of night, basilar) psora usually worse as the morning approaches. Syphilitic headaches get better in the morning and remain better all day until evening when they grow worse as the night advances, then grow better towards morning. Psoric headaches grow worse as the sun ascends and decrease as it descends. Psoric headaches are sharp, severe, paroxysmal; syphilitic, dull heavy or lanceolating, constant, persistent, usually basilar or linear, or one-sided. Psoric headaches are usually frontal, temporal or tempo-parietal, sometimes on the vortex, although quite often a vortex headache is a sycotic one.

Headaches occurring every Sunday or on rest days have often behind them a tubercular taint. They are worse riding in a carriage or are due to the least unusual ordeal as preparing for examinations; meeting with strangers and entertaining them. Headaches with deathly coldness of the hands and feet, with prostration, sadness and general despondency, have often a tubercular history. Headaches with bilious attacks, nausea, vomiting, coming once or twice a month, are usually of psoric origin. Headaches better by quiet, rest or sleep are apt to be psoric; headaches made worse by warmth, rest or while attempting to sleep are apt to be syphitic. Headaches with red face and rush of blood to the head, or at certain hours of the day, usually in the forenoon; headaches relieved by rest, quiet, sleep, eating, are pseudopsoric. A headache relieved by nose bleed has a tubercular taint behind it, in fact any disease that is relieved by nose bleed is tubercular. Headaches better by hot applications, by quiet, rest, sleep, are *psoric*. Prosapalgia or persistent headaches which are not easily relieved by treatment are usually of a tubercular origin, that is, the tubercular taint is present in that organism. A sycotic and a syphilitic headache is worse on lying down and worse at night. Generally speaking a syphilitic headache is basilar; a psoric, temporal or frontal, a sycotic frontal, or on the vertex; both the sycotic and syphilitic are worse at or after the midnight hour.

The headaches of sycosis in children are more common than we think today, they are worse at night, produce feverishness, restlessness, crying, fretting and worrying. The sycotic headache is always relieved by motion as in all sycotic diseases. Keep the children in motion in every sycotic disease and they are comparatively quiet; keep them quiet in psora. A tubercular or syhilitic headache will often last for days and is very severe, often unendurable, sometimes accompanied with sensations of bands about the head. Many of them are due to effusion. The patient often has a weak feeling about the head, can not hold it up, and sometimes we find them so severe as to produce unconsciousness, rolling or boring of the head into the pillow, ocular paralysis, moaning, with feverishness and restlessness or the patient is stupid, dull or listless, even semi-conscious. Other symptoms are rush of blood to the head or face, with roaring in the ears, with determination of blood to the chest, hot hands and feet, have to bathe them in cold water, as we find under Phosphorus or Opium. Occasionally the tubercular headaches are aggravated by heat which is not so true of psora. This shows the amelioration to be found in the syphilitic miasm by cold. In the syphilitic or tubercular headaches we see children striking, knocking or pounding the head with the hands or against some object. This is not true of psora in any sense, as psora is better by rest and quiet and sleep. Such a peculiar symptom as great hunger before headaches has its origin often in a tubercular taint and is not purely psoric. Headaches from repelled eruptions or suppression of any skin eruption, hunger before or during headache are apt to be pseodo-psoric.

OUTER HEAD

Hair.—Hair dry, lusterless, tangles easily, breaks and splits easily. (Hair moist, glues together, offensive odor from the head, tubercular). Hair becomes white in spots, aversion to uncovering the head, dry eruptions on the scalp; hair dry, dead-like, full of dry, scaly, bran-like dandruff which can be shaken out like a shower of bran; hair falls out generally, worse after acute fevers or acute diseases; hair falls out in bunches or in spots usually beginning on the vertex (syphilis, latent). Hair dry like tow (tubercular or latent syphilis;) hair dry, dead like the hemp from an old rope, tubercular or latent syphilis. Falling out of hair from eyelashes and eyebrows, syphilis, hair falls out in little circular spots in sycotic diseases of the scalp ; hair very oily and greasy, latent syphilis or tubercular ; hair falls out after abdominal and chest diseases or after parturition tubercular and psoric ; hair becomes grey too early, psora, especially if it is general over the whole head ; hair fetid, oily, sour smelling (syphilis ;) falling out of hair on sides of head and on vertex, latent syphilis ; hair falls out generally in psora, not so in syphilis. The beard is seldom affected by psora nor are the eyebrows and eyelashes ; stubby, dead, broken hair in the beard, sycosis ; hair falls out in beard due to skin eruptions, sycosis, syphilis. In latent syphilis and pseudo-psora are seen the crooked, curved or bent and broken hairs of the eyelashes even when no other marked symptom is present ; red eyelids, stubby, broken or imperfect eyelashes are found in syphilis or in the tubercular taint ; red eyelids, granular lids, often accompany this condition of the hairs. The eruptions in the hair of true psora are usually dry (moist, tubercular or latent syphilis). Severe itching of scalp with dryness, psora ; severe itching with moist, offensive, matted hair, pseudo-psora ; a fishy odor from the hair, sycosis; musty like old hay, tubercular; child smells sour, sycosis ; fetid, sour, oily, tubercular or latent syphilis ; hair mats together (plica polonica), tubercular or syphilitic ; head a mass of thick crusts of dried pus and excrement, tubercular or syphilitic.

SCALP

Psora; dry, scaly dandruff on scalp with much itching, dry, crusty eruptions (moist, thick crusts, syphilis); pustular eruptions, tubercular, thick, yellowish bland pus, tubercular; small popular eruptions on the scalp, psora; offensive discharges from behind and about ears, tubercular; cracks about ears, tubercular as seen under Hepar Sulphur, Petroleum, Tuberculinum, etc. Dry, eczematous eruptions about scalp, psora; moist, tubercular or syphilitic. Tubercular skin eruptions are aggravated by bathing, working in water, or washing; cold open air aggravates (better syphilis). Scalp is dry in psora; moist, perspiring copiously in syphilitic and tubercular children. Head normal in size and contour, in psora; large, bulging, often open sutures, bones soft, cartilaginous in syphilitic and tubercular children. Painful pimples on the scalp with much itching, which is relieved by scratching but is followed by burning and smarting; itching worse in the evening and by heat of bed, psora. The scalp eruptions of true psora are usually dry, when they are moist with copious pus formations they will usually be found to be tubercular, the scales and crusts of psora are usually dry, if moist the discharge is scanty and either of pure serum or bloody serum. A thick, heavy, yellow crust is quite apt to be of syphilitic or tubercular origin. Pimples in psora inflame, and are very sensitive, and often painful, but do not suppurate, or, if they do suppurate the discharge is scanty. Heat of the head may be either psoric or tubercular, usually tubercular being worse at night ; can not comb the hair until it is wet or moistened it is so dry, *psora ;* it will not remain in any position it is so dry, must comb it often. The aversion to having the head uncovered is a tubercular symptom, as a true psoric patient can not bear much heat about the head, while they like heat generally speaking. There is seldom any sweating about the head of a psoric patient, indeed they seldom perspire. The scalp always looks unclean like the skin of a psoric patient.

EYES AND VISION

The eyeball is seldom affected very profoundly by psora, usually syphilis is the miasm that makes serious inroads upon the structures of the eyes. If the vision is affected at all, it is found in the simpler forms of refraction, while the latent syphilitic or tubercular gives us such changes as are found in astigmatism and other marked refractory changes due to malformation or to hereditary changes in the ball itself. Changes in the lens are always syphilitic or tubercular, as are such changes as we find in the sclera, choroid, ciliary body and iris. It is syphilitic or tubercular processes that change organs and gives us perversions of form or shape and size. Psora does give many eye affections but never change in the structure of the eye itself. We also have aversion to light, even quite marked photophobia in psora, but nothing like that found in tubercular or syphilitic patients. Disturbances in the glandular structures or in the lachrymal apparatus are always syphilitic or tubercular.

Pustular diseases are apt to be tubercular as found in many cases of granular lids. Hyperemia of a chronic form may be of a psoric origin, but granular lids are quite often tubercular. Ulcerations and specific inflammations are sycotic, tubercular, or syphilitic, although corneal ulcerations in young people come often from a sycotic taint. Chronic corneal ulcers in children, where no trace of syphilis can be found, are usually of a sycotic origin and of course of a hereditary nature based upon a tubercular diathesis. (Sycosis never gives the true ulcer.) Ciliary blepheritis is, whether acute or chronic, either syphilitic or tubercular. Scaly, red lids, angry looking, crusty lids are never of a true psoric origin; they are either syphilitic or tubercular. All stys are tubercular or have, as we understand, a tubercular taint behind them, as they are a granular change whether they contain a sabacious matter or the cheesy formation.

Syphilitic or tubercular patients dread artificial light more than sunlight, although they may be aggravated by both. Thick copious pus formations or discharges, especially if of a greenish or yellowish-green color, are distinctly tubercular or sycotic. Ptosis is never psoric. Ciliary neuralgias are so apt to be either tubercular or syphilitic. Great dryness, itching and burning of the eyes are to be found frequently under the psoric miasm. The psoric eye has a great intolerance to daylight or sunlight when diseased.

Often in psora we have reflex eye troubles or nerve disturbances, of course all the diseases of the eye may depend largely on the psoric basis or psoric state as do other diseases, but what we mean is, that these diseases originally developed through and from the syphilitic and tubercular processes. We have many arthritic and rheumatic troubles with the eye, which do depend on sycosis, combined with the psoric miasm. The neuralgias and pains about the eye are often distinguished by their character and periodicity. The syphilitic pains are worse at night or after the sun sets and are aggravated by heat; this may be often true of the tubercular, although they are never, as a rule, relieved by cold or by cold applications; generally they are relieved by hot applications. This is not so of psoric pains; they are relieved by heat and are worse as the morning approaches and as the sun rises towards the meridian. Sycotic pains may come on at any time, but they are worse by barometric changes, or by moisture, rainy or stormy weather.

Conjunctival troubles are often of purely psoric nature, especially when there is an ardent desire to rub the eyes, much itching in the canthi, constant, not relieved by rubbing. A chronic dilatation of the pupil in children or women, is quite characteristic of pseudo-psora, or when a tubercular basis is present. When pseudo-psoric patients are affected with exanthematous fevers of any form, there is a strong tendency to inflammatory stasis of the eye, and serious eye troubles are apt to follow. In the visionary field in psora we have fiery, zigzag appearances around the objects, or dark spots, followed with streaks of light, unsteadiness of vision, or the vision is blurred; letters run together in reading. Usually the inflammatory troubles involving the eyes are accompanied with much itching and burning of the lids, with great desire to rub them. The pains and neuralgias are usually worse in the morning, or throughout the day, and are relieved by heat.

EARS—HEARING

The psoric difficulties in hearing are usually of a reflex origin or of a nervous character. All organic ear troubles are either tubercular or syphilitic. Suppurative processes and destruction of the ossicles of the ear are quite apt to be tubercular.

The ear is often a safety valve in tubercular children; it relieves them of many serious troubles liable to occur during dentition. Abscesses of the ear often relieve many quite severe meningeal difficulties in children. They show themselves so frequently in measles, scarlet fever and such diseases. Here the tubercular element comes readily to the surface in the form of a suppuration of the middle ear. The tubercular element is more frequently aroused from its latent condition by fever than by any other means. All of the blood vessels of these patients with a tubercular element in their organisms, are abnormal from the capillaries to the arteries themselves, their walls are all defective and usually unduly dilated. This we can readily see on examining the upper layer of the skin, where they are to be found lying beneath the surface of the thin skin, usually of a bluish or pinkish color. The circulatory system might be compared to poor plumbing that will not endure any unusual pressure, therefore, when it is disturbed we have intense febrile states that are prone to congestions of parts and the formation of pus cavities and abscesses. The peculiar carrion-like odor from these aural abscesses is so characteristic of the pseudo-psoric patients that we can not well be mistaken; often the discharges are cheesy or curdled. Such remedies as Hepar sulphur, Teucrium and Psorinum will represent the character of this pus found in tubercular abscesses of the middle ear. Seldom is the ear affected in a purely psoric condition. A tubercular or syphilitic taint is always to be looked for in these cases. Of course, psora is the medium that arouses into action all other latent or chronic miasms and becomes the basic principle of the acute as well as of the chronic condition. The auditory canal in psoric patients is always dry and scaly, dry bran like scales are constantly forming and falling off into the canal.

Quite often the serumen is greatly increased or diminished. Itching is a constant symptom in many cases. Markedly psoric patients are oversensitive to sounds or noises, as is seen under Coffee, Opium and such remedies. The eczematous eruptions about the ears and especially the humid eruptions, pustules, fissures and incrustations behind the ears are generally of a tubercular origin. The porches of the ear look dirty, dry and scaly in psora. In tubercular or latent syphilitic patients the ears look pale, white, often old, and in some cases translucent, almost, with the blood vessels enlarged, bluish in color or bright red, and their course traceable in the tissues. They are often unduly large and distended when the tubercular diathesis is very marked. All these symptoms are absent in a purely psoric patient, the ears are normal in size and shape, of dirty color, which washing does not make clean, that is apparently clean, but this fact is quite general over the epidermis of the entire body. The tubercular child is constantly having abscesses in the ear, due of course to the same tendency to congestion which is ever present in these patients. If they are free from ear troubles they invariably suffer from throat affections, especially the tonsils, hence are forever having tonsilitis.

We can not well mistake these tubercular ear troubles of children and young people. In the day time they appear well, free from pain, but at night their sufferings begin, often they awake out of sleep screaming with the earache. They may begin as early as the first year, even earlier, and continue more or less until past puberty. The least exposure to cold or slightest draft brings on an attack. Occasionally we have prolonged febrile attacks with great suffering which is suddenly relieved by the breaking of the abscess. Quite often their general health improves even when the ear is discharging copiously of this tubercular foul smelling pus.

NOSE AND SMELL

There are many symptoms pointing to psora and pseudo-psora in the nose. Psora greatly increases the sensitivity of smell. Patients are unusually affected by odors of any kind, which will even awake them out of sleep. They are troubled with odors of cooking, the smell of flowers, perfumes, paints, plants, etc., as they induce nausea, vomiting, headaches, loathing of food, fainting, sickness of stomach, vertigo, loss of appetite and many other annoying symptoms. Some times the smell may be diminished or lost but this comes more frequently in syphilis or sycosis, these have complete loss of smell and taste, also of hearing.

Hemorrhage from the nose is not a purely psoric symptom. When this occurs in young girls and boys, it will be found to depend on the tubercular and the cause is similar to that described in the febrile state of tubercular patients. We so often find in these patients rush of blood to the surface, to the face, head, neck or to the hands and feet, inducing great heat to the part. Papular eruptions and pimples about the nose, as is seen in simple forms of acne, not the acne indurata or the tubercular form, but the vulgaric form. A red nose with enlarged capillaries depends on a sycotic element or over-stimulation of the organism. Acne rosacea is so frequently found to be tubercular. The bones of the nose are never destroyed from any other miasm than syphilis. Snuffles in children are dependent on sycosis or syphilis. Syphilis produces ulceration, large thick crust, known as clinkers, often filling the whole nasal cavity; frequently they have to be removed, but soon form again. The snuffles in sycosis is unusually moist and there is no ulceration and no crusts, the discharge is mucus usually in sycosis, or if purulent, very scanty and has the odor often of fish brine or stale fish. The crusts of syphilis are dark, greenish, black or brown, thick and not always offensive. The catarrhal discharge in tubercular patients is thick, usually yellow, and of the odor of old cheese or sulphate of hydrogen and is constantly dropping down in the throat. The stoppage in sycosis is due to local congestion and thickening of the membrane or enlargement of the turbinated bodies due to congestion, the discharge is yellowish green, scant, except in fresh colds when it is a copious thin mucus. A tubercular child will have a hemorrhage from the nose from the slightest provocation—blowing the nose, a slight blow, or washing the face even will produce it in some people. The hemorrhages are profuse, bright red, difficult to arrest and are relieved by cold applications. Over-exercise, over-heating will often bring it on. These headaches, vertigoes and congestions to the head and brain are often relieved by nose bleed. In the worst forms of hay-fever, where there is much sneezing, and with much local trouble, we find it often depends on the tubercular taint with an acquired latent sycosis ingrafted. Of course psora is greatly magnified in all of these cases, but purely psoric cases are easily cured by the homœopathic remedy, while where the mixed miasm is present, it is extremely difficult to cure. The psoric colds, when they affect the nose, begin with sneezing, redness, heat, sensitiveness to touch when they have blown it for some time; the discharge is thin, watery, and acrid. In the tubercular subject it soon becomes thick, purulent, and sometimes bloody. In the sycotic cases the discharge is scanty, usually mucus; generally they can not breathe through the nose or blow any mucus from it, but the slightest amount of discharge relieves the congestion and stopped-up feeling. Painful boils, pimples and vesicles are common to psora, occurring in the septum; often they are extremely painful and sensitive and seldom break or discharge much pus. The septum of psoric patients looks dirty or sooty looking. In rhinitis it is often dry, hot, burning. In lupus of the nose the three miasms are usually present.

FACE

There may be no appearance of psora in the face and again the face may be a plain indicator of its presence in the organism, although it is usually in more advanced cases that we notice it in any marked degree. The face may be pale, sallow, earthy, sometimes the eyes have a sunken appearance, with deep blue rings around them, but this is also found in the tubercular diathesis. Circumscribed red spots on the cheeks is quite a positive tubercular symptom whether found in an infant, child or adult; usually these spots appear in the afternoons or evenings. We see them in such conditions in children as dentition, worms, febrile states, colds, etc., and in adults when tubercular troubles are just beginning to develop or when they are in full force. Flashes of heat to the face or head and chest have no doubt a tubercular element behind it disturbing the circulation, although the hot flashes at the climatric period is purely a psoric symptom, and is relieved by anti-psoric treatment. Red lips are found in a very psoric patient, or in extremely marked cases where the blood seems to be ready almost to ooze out of them, are tubercular. Often we find the face and lips blue and congested in patients with poor, slow, circulation. The lips often look parched and dry with a sooty coating. In syphilitic patients the face has a greyish, greasy appearance. Usually the skin on the face of a very psoric patient is dry, rough and pimply, often it has an unwashed or unclean appearance. Reddish, millet-seed sized papules that appear on the nose, cheeks and chin, ulcers in the corners of the mouth are apt to be tubercular; vesicles about the mouth, small, white, transparent and accompanied with much itching are psoric (hydro or cold sore).

Deep fissures in the lips are usually syphilitic but of course can be tubercular. Swelling and burning of the lips or burning, itching, is found under psora. We find edema swelling or puffiness of the face, lips, eyes and eyelids in tubercular people, especially is this found to be true in the morning or after sleep; erysipelas of the face will be found to have the psoric and sycotic element combined and we may have to begin the treatment with an anti-sycotic remedy such as Rhus-tox, although we may have to use a purely anti-psoric remedy as Sulphur to finish the cure, and vice versa; but as this is true of this disease so it is true of all diseases; of course all warty eruptions are sycotic, moles and papillomati may be either sycotic or syphilitic. In psoric fevers the face becomes very red, hot, and shiny, in tubercular patients it is more apt to be pale or have a circumscribed redness of the cheeks. Paleness of the face on rising in the morning or after sleep, and even after eating is found in tubercular patients, or that one cheek may be red and the other pale, one hot, and the other cold, is also common in these patients in either latent or active stages of the disease. In syphilis we often see that grey ashy appearance on the face of an infant. It looks old, puckered, weazened, dried up, wrinkled like an old man. The tubercular face is either round, skin fair, smooth and clear with that waxy smoothness of the complexion, eyes bright and sparkling, eyebrows and eyelashes soft, glossy, long and silken, thin lips, or we have the high cheek bones, thick lips, almost like an African; in some cases the skin of the face is rough, voice coarse, deep, often hollow, eyelids red, inflamed, scaly, crusty, lashes broken, stubby, irregularly curved and imperfect; in these cases the syphilitic or tubercular element predominates in a latent form of course. They perspire freely about the face, often we see large drops like pearls about the face, nose and lips, usually the skin of the face is pale, cool, perspiring, while in psora we have not such changes, physiologically speaking, and the skin of the face is dry, pimply, rough, complexion bad, dirty and of an unwashed appearance. In the tubercular patient, physiologically speaking, the face and head is often seen to be of the shape of a pyramid with the apex at the chin. The nose may be well shaped in this special form, the features sharp, the eyes unusually bright, often sparkling, the nostrils are small, the openings narrow, the least obstruction in the nose induces them to breathe through the mouth which causes an imperfect expansion and filling of the lungs. We many not see the flashes of heat or circulatory expressions we see in other expressions of the tubercular face, indeed the face looks fairly well even in the last stages of the disease, when other parts of the body become emaciated and show marked signs of the disease

CAVITY OF THE MOUTH, TEETH AND GUMS

Probably in no other part can we find as many symptoms of the syphilitic and tubercular diathesis as we do in the mouth and the organs of the mouth. Such diseases in children as thrush and stomatitis are of psoric origin, but when we see the true ulcer in the mouth or on any of its adjoining mucous surface, we must not attribute them to psora, for the true ulcer is of syphilitic or tubercular origin, as is also the swelling and indurations of the glands and such pathological changes as we see taking place in the teeth or dental arches are of a syphilitic or tubercular diathesis. When we come to hemorrhages of the mouth, excessive bleeding of the gums, we must attribute it to the tubercular diathesis unless syphilis is actually present. Often they will bleed at the slightest touch, again we see them receding from the teeth or they are soft and spongy and bleed at the slightest touch even when brushing them. The dental arch is imperfect, irregular, or the teeth are imperfect in form, club-shaped or come in an imperfect or irregular order, often decaying or becoming carious before they are entirely through the gums, or before they are perfectly developed. They appear often with much pain and suffering, accompanied with constitutional disturbances often of a marked degree, such as diarrhea, dysentery, spasms, convulsions, febrile states, abscesses of the middle ear, disturbances of digestion, meningeal congestions and meningeal inflammations. I now recall a case in a male child of 16 months who has had meningeal congestion with severe pain at the base of the brain at the eruption of each tooth. It would beat and pound its head against any object that was near it, or with its little fists; usually when these attacks came on it would scream for hours, with pain; they came on mostly at night. Diarrhea, nausea and vomiting of its food were quite constant symptoms; at the same time the gums were greatly swollen, hard and cartilaginous like, which of course prolonged the eruption of the teeth. Accompanying these symptoms was profuse perspiration about the head and face, dampening the pillow on which it had lain. The perspiration had a strong, musty odor. For these symptoms Stannum met. was given, which relieved many of the symptoms. This remedy was followed later on with Cal. carb. It is only of late years that we have recognized that these symptoms are of a tubercular origin. These white skinned, pale, flabby muscled children, as a rule, all have a tubercular family history. So, many of them die in these cycles of physiological stress or development. Their frailly constructed organisms are often overpowered by these unusual efforts that nature necessarily has to put forth in the development of these tubercular children. There is always something wrong with these children, if it is not one thing it is another. They can not endure either extreme heat or cold or any extremes of temperature; a few hot sultry days in July or August followed by cool nights throw them into diarrhea or dysentery or they have sudden arrest of digestion with marked gastric disturbances which often endangers their lives. We have no assurance of them at any time and should they survive the ages of infancy and childhood, they are prone to be partakers of every child's disease that comes along. Observe their large pyramidal shaped head, which gives the face a small appearance, the prominent forehead, the flabby, over fleshy baby, or in other words the phlegmatic babe with its copious sweating about the face, head and upper part of the body. Its enlarged cervical glands; the wilful, positive nature, the stubborn disposition, etc.

TASTE

The taste of a *psoric* patient is either sour, sweet or bitter and some times it is designated as bad taste, but the three forms above mentioned are to be found quite constant in *psora*. A putrid taste or a taste of pus or blood will be found in the tubercular patient, and in those suffering from a tubercular taint. Expectoration of pus that tastes very sweet is tubercular; some times the patients have a salty taste, or a rotten egg or sulphate of hydrogen taste. Any of the miasms may have a partial or complete loss of taste. A bitter taste with yellow coated tongue points strongly to psora. A putrid, musty or fishy taste will be usually found under the miasm sycosis. All metallic tastes make us think of syphilis or that the tubercular element is present in the organism. The saliva of a syphilitic patient is ropy, cottony, viscid, metallic or coppery tasting. After eating sweet things taste sour or the patient may have a sweet, sour or bitter taste in psora. Psora has much perverseness of taste, for instance bread tastes bitter, water has an abnormal taste, occasionally foods of all kinds are rejected because of their abnormal taste. Tasting of food recently eaten, or eructations, tasting of food or of grease, fats or oil, etc., is a common psoric symptom. Some psoric patients are extremely sensitive to taste. I can now recall a patient, a woman about sixty years of age, who could taste for days any application that was made to the skin, such as coal oil, turpentine, lard, liniments, and the different compounds which might be used as local applications in such diseases as rheumatism. The taste of blood is a peculiar latent tubercular symptom often to be found in women with a tubercular diathesis. It may or may not appear during the menstrual period, but is present frequently in the morning. The taste of a psoric patient is often bitter in the open air as we see under the remedy Psorinum. A burnt taste is only found under psora. A foul taste may be found under any miasmatic basis. Of course any of these tastes may be found in some degree in pseudo-psora, or where the psoric element predominates, nevertheless, the taste is of psoric origin. The miasms produce perversions in every expression of life, therefore our tastes, likes and dislikes are not exempt from them.

Naturally the taste in the mouth should be neutral. We should taste nothing but our food and drink and that should be normal, but it is the latent or active miasms that falsifies all things, even taste. Not infrequently we find a certain periodicity about it; it may be worse in the morning as seen in the foul, bad taste of nux vomica or the bitter taste of bryonia. Nat., mur. and phos. has a bloody taste. Washing out of the mouth does not even relieve in some cases; even pure water will taste bitter to some people, where the psoric or pseudo-psoric miasm is present. No remedy has a more bitter taste than Aloe, yet it cures an inky taste in the patient's mouth. Elaps cor. has a bloody taste before coughing; Mercury, a metallic taste; Hepar and Tuberculium, Pyrogen, a taste of pus when coughing. I mention these peculiarities of taste to show the endless variety of perversions we may find in this sphere alone from miasmatic action. It all comes, of course, through perverted nerve impulses; but they are basic miasmatic symptoms, because they are largely from a central nervous center, therefore they are very important in making up our case. I never neglect them in prescribing for my patients and always keep a repertory quite convenient that I have prepared for this purpose, that I may consult it when any of the special senses are perverted by miasmatic action. It is always a profound disturbance and demands more than a casual recognition in taking the case and making our prescription. I have frequently had patients (who were suffering from exhaustion due to hemorrhages or seminal losses) have a sour or bitter taste; this then we say is distinctly of psoric origin, just as the metallic and bloody taste is of tubercular or syphilitic origin. We can not afford therefore to overlook the miasmatic perversions of taste and they will grow in importance as you look into this miasmatic mystery.

HUNGER, DESIRES AND AVERSIONS

Morbid hunger or unnatural hunger is a very important and quite a constant symptom of *psora*. Hunger at unnatural times during the twenty-four hours; hunger an hour or two before eating or hunger in the night after sleeping; hunger immediately after eating; hunger is not satisfied when stomach is full; hunger with weak, gone sensations before eating; hunger with great prostration after eating; eating makes them sleepy; eating causes profuse perspiration, after eating, much distention and fullness, with flatulence and distention of gas; hunger that is not satisfied by eating, psora; although faint if hunger is not soon satisfied or extreme hunger with all gone, weak, empty feelings in the stomach is apt to appear more in the tubercular diathesis, although it is of psoric origin. They sometimes have constant hunger and eat beyond their capacity to digest, or they have no appetite in the morning, but hunger for other meals. Often the tubercular patient has a great desire for certain things, but when he receives them he does not want them, in fact they are repugnant to him. We see this symptom in the child more than in the adult; he will ask for things, then, when he receives them, will cast them from him with anger.

DESIRES AND AVERSIONS

The psoric patient has longings and desires for sweets, for acids and for sour things; the tubercular patient likes these things also, but it is the psoric taint that produces it. The tubercular patient likes hot or real cold things; they are extremists in the matter of heat and cold in many ways, one part of the day they are chilly and the next part they are too warm. Their longings are often for indigestible things, as chalk, lime, slate pencils, etc. It is a noticeable fact that if the system is not assimilating certain things, they will crave that thing. This is seen more particularly in young girls, in children, and in women in the pregnant state. They are great cravers for peculiar things; they crave salt, and will eat it alone from the dish; they use much salt in their food, more than the whole family put together.

The trouble with these patients is that they can not assimilate these things; they have lost the power of assimilation, and the more they become affected with the internal workings of the miasm, the less power they have to assimilate them, until it falls far below par. Again these tubercular patients, who have never taken stimulants, often have a longing for them, especially for beers, wines, ginger ales or hot aromatic things. In fevers the psoric patients have craving for butter milk, acid things, pickles, cabbage and indigestible things, things that they should not have. So it is the same in the pregnant state, the patients long for things often never eaten before, and will do almost anything to procure them. These desires usually depart after childbirth and then a loathing and dislike follows; they loose their desire and taste for these things and care no more for them. (Often these longings are conveyed to the child, and remains with it for many years of its life.) They have unnatural fancies for things that they would not have any desire for in the non-pregnant state. Sometimes the psoric patient will have desires for fats, greasy things, rich pastries and sweetmeats, which when eaten induce bilious attacks and all sorts of gastric disturbances. Indeed, those bilious states are often ushered in by these longings and desires; they are forewarnings of internal gastric warfare. Often the things that were very agreeable and palatable to them, become repugnant and they take a great dislike to them; for instance, the tobacco user;

he suddenly takes a dislike to his pipe, or his accustomed chew, and for a time it is impossible for him to use it or to even touch it. After this condition passes away, which is usually in a short time, he resumes his old habits again with renewed vigor and relish. We see in these things, disturbances of psora : all toxic drugs become sooner or later prime disturbers of psora or the chronic miasms in general, but particularly psora. In syphilis or sycosis we know how rigid are the rules laid down by the regular school of practitioners with reference to diet ; all stimulating or irritating foods are prohibited as are also narcotics of all kinds ; beers, wines, liquors of all kinds are strictly prohibited. Why ? Because of their positive action in restoring the eruption or the gonorrhœal discharge ; they know full well that they can not suppress it while the patient partakes of these things. As this is true in disease, it is also true in health ; the difference is only in the difference of the organism's sensitivity, the organism, being more sensitive and more easily aroused when diseased than in health. Often in health the patient may be able to use tea, coffee or spirituous liquors for many years without being especially disturbed, but when diseased or after some severe illness, they may never be able again to partake of those things, which were apparently harmless before, without suffering or disturbance from them. There is another thought that I wish to bring forward, and that is that the desires and the cravings for the unnatural things to eat, together with the desires and cravings for narcotics, such as tea, coffee, tobaccos, or any stimulant for that matter, have often their origin in psora or pseudo-psora, that is, the miasm so weakens the organism or so lowers its vitality that the great life centers are unable to supply the necessary nerve force ; hence, the call for those things which fill temporarily force these central impulses to increased activity, and for a while the demand is satisfied, until a reaction comes, as it always does in time. Then follows a lagging of these centers as they no longer can respond to the stimuli, which has to be increased ; but the time comes when it fails and a new stimulant has to be selected and so on until stimulants fail entirely. Thus a patient may begin with meat and follow with tea, coffee, then tobacco and finally end with intoxicating liquors; partaking of the greater, as the lesser fails to satisfy, fails to bring the nerve force up to the desired standard. This often is the beginning of a history of an intemperate life, by simply yielding to the demand of the organism which should have or might have been brought up to a perfect standard of health through the law of cure. Psoric people like sweets, syrups, sugars, candies, while the tubercular craves potatoes, meats of all kinds.

These cravings, desires, likes and dislikes of our patients are symptoms that stand high in therapeutic value in making a selection of our remedy, as they are basic miasmatic symptoms, next in importance to the perverted mental phenomena in disease. They all however belong to the phenonena of perverted life action, and I am glad to know that they can not be attached to pathology and do not come under any of its forms. Besides all these, there are cravings and longings for travel, change of place, vocation and manner of living; they want something and they know what that something is, which is characteristic of these despondent, weak, debilitated, psoric patients, who seem to never gain any strength and whose disease can not be located.

STOMACH SYMPTOMS OF PSORA AND PSEUDO-PSORA

An organ of so complex a function as the stomach has, of course, many symptoms that acknowledge the presence of psora in the organism. We will only attempt to give some of the more prominent ones, or those that may be considered characteristic, or to a great degree, pathognomonic of the psoric or tubercular patient. Usually the action of the miasms is quite marked in some other parts of the organism before its action is seen upon the stomach.

We must look deeper and farther than the gastric function for the phenomena of indigestion. Indigestion has behind it, as have all other disturbed functions, a distuned life force; and a gastric expression is as much a secondary expression as in erysipelas, eczema or any eruption on the skin; or in other words, a gastric dis_ turbance of any nature, whatever, is nothing more or less than the attempt of nature to, in some degree, eliminate the effects of miasmatic influence in the organism. Indigestion begins in the very cell itself, in its molecular movement, which is from its periphery to its center, from the vitalizing nucleus to its circumference, and as the vitalized point receives the non-vitalized or new food matter, it vitalizes it and projects it outward. Thus, this continuous process is kept up as long as life lasts. In diseased conditions, or in people who are over fed, these vitalizing centers are overworked, and the nutrient or food material is rushed too rapidly through these vitalizing centers and the result is an imperfectly vitalized tissue, which is soft, flabby, lacking the strength and vigor of a healthy structure ; and indigestion, gastric disturbances arise in all their disturbing forms and varieties. We sometimes see this condition arise where healing processes are taking place in wounds and ulcers, where the granulations are stimulated by local measures (or by local remedial agents, such as Calendula, Balsam of peru or any similar local stimuli). This over-action appears in the form of false granulations which break down suddenly, being unable to form a healthy and permanent tissue. Sometimes we see such nervous symptoms arising in psoric and pseudo-psoric patients, "as weak, all-gone feeling in the stomach," demanding food at unnatural periods. "Hunger at night" is so prominent a symptom in very psoric patients that it can always be relied upon ;

hunger soon after partaking of food is also peculiar to psora; hunger with an all-gone sensation in the pit of the stomach at 10 a. m. or between 10 and 11 a. m. will be found in pseudo-psoric patients, or when the tubercular taint is marked. This is very peculiar, but it is very frequently met with in general practice. But it is just such strange perversions that are to be found under the action of this deepest of all miasms, pseudo-psora. On the other hand we meet with just the opposite symptoms, in very psoric people, such as fullness, bloating, great distention due to the accumulation of gases or to flatulent conditions and food fermentation; rumblings, gurglings, and all such commotion due to the formation of gases, are found not only in the stomach but throughout the entire gastro-intestinal tract. Any other miasm of course can be present in the organism, but still these symptoms are of purely psoric origin. Sour or bitter eructations come up in the throat frequently; sometimes these risings from the stomach taste of food recently eaten, or they may be oily or greasy; not infrequently they are accompanied with heartburn, with nausea, faint feelings at the pit of the stomach, with a conflux of saliva to the mouth (waterbrash), acid eructations with burning in the œsophagus, with or without hunger, with hunger relieved by eating ever so little. This is sometimes followed with fullness in the stomach, chest or throat. Psoric patients have repugnance to boiled foods; they want everything fried, if possible, and highly seasoned; they like highly seasoned foods. Tubercular patients crave meat; they will eat it from infancy and nothing satisfies their hunger or cravings but meat. I am fully convinced in my own mind that meat is not a natural food; it is very unnatural; indeed, it is more of a stimulant than a food. Its prolonged use as a food induces similar conditions in the organisms to that found under the use of alcohol, that is, where it is used excessively. The capillaries become engorged and distended, the heart action weak, soft, the pulse easily compressed, the muscles of the heart soft, or the action of the organ becomes imperfect, the face flushes easily and the blood piles up in the lungs and brain when they exercise, attempt climbing heights, or run fast, such as running for a car of for a train. Human beings will live longer, endure more hardships, cold or heat when meat is not used in their diet at all. The porters in China and Japan have probably as great endurance as any people in the world, yet they subsist entirely on a vegetable diet, largely rice.

When these meat eaters come to me suffering with bad heart action or gastric difficulties, I at once cut out meat from their diet, and it is surprising how quickly the heart action improves, the food in the stomach ceases to ferment, the foul breath disappears, and the gaseous formations soon no longer exist. Meat, grease, and vegetables do not mix well in these psoric or tubercular patients. Before they are past puberty they are employing a physician for gastric difficulties. I speak now not only from experience in practice, but from a personal standpoint. I have eaten no meat for six years or flesh of any kind except at long intervals small quantities of fish. Previous to my taking up the vegetable diet, I had poor heart action ; a run of two blocks would almost take my life, caused from labored heart action. Now I can run a mile if necessary. The heart action began to improve at once, there is no more headache, no belching, no sour eructations, no gases, no unpleasant taste in the mouth, and above all there are no unnatural cravings or desires for highly seasoned food or fancy dishes. My diet consists wholly of vegetables, fruits, cereals and nuts. The mind is always clear, the appetite regular and normal in every way. Meat, then, we see, is a disease producer through its stimulating qualities and through its power to disturb or arouse latent psora, to say nothing of the great probability of the meat itself being diseased ; hence psoric patients should eat sparingly of it, if not avoid it entirely, when psora or sycosis is very marked.

Returning to the symptoms of psora in the stomach, we notice the constant gnawing at the pit of the stomach, cold, or hot sensations, sensations of weight, of fullness, of tightness, of goneness ; sensations of heavy weights, as of a stone or lump in the stomach, beatings and pulsations, throbbings, sensations of constriction, oppression after eating, shortness of breath, vertigoes, giddiness, anxiety, epigastric tenderness ; sweat breaks out after eating, weary, heavy, sleepy, drowsy after eating, falls asleep, can not keep awake after a meal ; eating causes pain, colic, nausea, vomiting, or is followed by diarrheas and gastro-intestinal disturbances of many forms and varieties.

Most of the aggravations of psora in the stomach are after eating, for instance after meals the patient suffers with headaches, flatulence or flatulent dyspepsia, weariness, sleepiness, nausea, vomiting, beating of the heart, coughing, pains in different parts of the body, especially in the region of the liver. In the hypochondria or epigastrium, they have pains often of a cutting or colicky nature ; very many of the stomach symptoms are temporarily relieved by eating, by hot drinks, by hot applications, by the belching of gas and by gentle motion. A sycotic patient, especially a child, is worse by eating any kind of food, whatever, and is relieved by lying on the stomach, or by pressure over the region of the stomach, and by violent motion, walking, rocking, shaking, etc. The stomach pains of sycosis are always crampy or colicky, paroxysmal, and relieved by motion and by hard pressure. A psoric patient is afraid of being touched when he has pain, even the slightest pressure cannot be endured. There are very many other symptoms of psoric origin referring to the stomach ; especially those with reference to the malignancies, which will be fully dealt with in Vol. II of this work. In conclusion of this subject, a few words might be said with reference to the diet of a psoric patient. They can digest meat even better than a sycotic patient. Meat in the sycotic, stimulates or assists in developing the uric acid and the gouty diathesis ; they, too, do better under a vegetable diet. If nitrogenous foods have to be given to a sycotic patient, they had better be in the form of nut foods, beans and mild cheese, etc. The tubercular patient thrives better on fats and fat foods than do those suffering from any other taint ; he also requires much salt in his food ; indeed the tubercular patients are the great salt eaters ; starches are not easily digested by them, and frequently their use has to be avoided almost entirely ; this is especially true in young infants. Tubercular patients crave meat, as has been mentioned, never getting enough of it ; many of them, however, reject fat meats, preferring to eat the lean portions. The psoric patient craves sugar or sweets of any kind, he can never get enough of them and he is forever filling his stomach full of sweetmeats ; this purely psoric symptom is very frequently found under Sulphur.

The reader will remember that his attention has alrady been called to this fact "that the cravings and longings of the patient, are basic miasmatic phenomena of great therapeutic value"

A syphilitic patient has an aversion to meats. In febrile states or in liver troubles, psoric patients often take a great aversion to sweets and crave acids of all kinds, fruit acids, lemonade, and buttermilk, otherwise they love sweets; they are just in their element when partaking of the sweets of the soda fountain. Sycotic and psoric patients are relieved by hot drinks and prefer their food hot or warm, while syphilitic and tubercular patients frequently desire cold things to eat or drink. Sometimes a tubercular patient will crave salt meats, salt fish, such as cod-fish, mackerel or salt herring, smoked ham or smoked meats. He likes these forms of flesh, largely for the salt they contain. Potatoes are another article of diet the tubercular patient craves. He will let you cut out any other article of diet but potatoes. The child 20 months old will gorge itself on this article of diet. A sycotic patient would prefer beer, rich gravies and fat meats but prefers to have it well seasoned with salt, pepper, etc. These patients herein described are, of course, typical cases, and any modification of these pictures can be found in mixed miasms.

CHEST, HEART AND LUNGS

As no part or portion of the organism is free from the presence of the miasms, when they are at all present, so the chest cavity with its contents is a fruitful soil for both these benign and malignant shadings of miasmatic action. The regular seat of the pseudo-psoric miasms is often found in the respiratory organs, developing into those malignant states known as phthisis-pulmanalis, tuberculosis, consumption, and other names which denote prolonged and fearful histories of sufferings and death. So many times we find these miasms lying in an incipient state of slumber, and many of us are totally ignorant of their presence in the organism until (as it seems to us), with scarcely any warning, they break forth like volcanoes from their slumbers. This should not be so. We should make ourselves acquainted with their latent expressions, and the symptoms of their presence, long before they have taken such a deep hold of this vital organ, the lungs. This we can do by becoming acquainted with just such phenomena as have already been presented; we must know something about this physiological difference which distinguishes the *psoric from the pseudo-psoric.* They are vastly unlike when we study them separately and yet we can not separate them fully, as they owe their existence to this combination, as expressed in the word *pseudo-psora.* These pseudo-psoric or tubercular symptoms, I say resemble both psora and syphilis, as a child may resemble both parents, and yet that distinction is often difficult to demonstrate, if we were called to do so. But as we have studied the head, face, ears, eyes and the different parts, and notice their distinguishing features, so can we study the chest, itself, as well as the chest organs. First of all, we must repeat to ourselves the rule "*that psora itself gives us no physiological changes of structure, that another miasm must be present in order to procure a physiological change in the structure or shape of a part or organ.*" With this in view and armed with the additional knowledge that syphilis is the only miasm that can, or does give us false physiological expressions or changes in the organism (any miasm may give us pathological changes, but not physiological changes), even to changes in the bony framework itself. Examine a tubercular bone or see the resemblance to syphilis, see the changes of structure and form, see the false formations and false expressions in that osseous structure; but we have shown this more fully under our heading of scrofulosis, versus syphilis, so we will hasten to give the psoric and pseudo-psoric symptoms and changes of the region coming under this heading. If we examine very psoric patients, we will see no changes in the lines, curves, and contour of the chest, they are natural; but let us see what we can find when we examine the tubercular chest; the curves and lines are imperfect, the chest is often narrow, lacking not only width laterally, but depth antero-posteriorly, the subclavicular spaces are hollow, or certain areas are sunken or depressed, quite often one lung is much larger than the other, or the action of one is accelerated and the other is lessened; one side is fuller than the other, showing a better development and a greater respiratory area, often the expansive power of the lung is greatly limited and the amount of residual air lessened. The breathing of these patients is not so full and resonant, although there may be no impediment or obstruction in the air cells or air passages. The shoulders of these patients are rounded, inclined forward, infringing on the chest area and the free lung action. They are as a rule all poor breathers, in fact they have no desire to take a full respiration; seldom do we find them breathing diaphragmatically, thus the lung never comes to its fullest expansion and the air cells are not all brought into use and simply become diseased from lack of that life giving principle they should receive from the oxygen. For lack of work or use, they atrophy or become useless; the least obstruction glues them together and destroys their office. Soon we find infiltrations with all the history of hepatic changes and finally complete destruction of such portions as are involved. These great air pumps, with their wonderful aerating machinery, should never be neglected, as they furnish to the commerce of the red blood corpuscles that invisible, vitalizing principle so necessary to life. So long as this free exchange of commodity goes on between the atmospheric air and the red blood corpuscles, we are safe, but as soon as it materially decreases the vitalizing principles also decreases as our invisible food supply diminishes.

Disease is largely a matter of imperfect oxidation, no matter what miasm is at the bottom of the trouble; any and all of them affect this process in some manner or other; the psoric, through neurotic processes, as in anemia; the tubercular as has been demonstrated, in faulty nutrition, and death of the commercial red corpuscles; the sycotic, in imperfect oxidation of the food products and their deposit in the tissues in the form of gouty concretions and lithic formations. These tubercular patients have not energy enough to take a full breath and besides they are afraid of cold air, especially if there is any exposure or chance of chilling the body. It is surprising how long they will endure a bed-room atmosphere, in which the lungs have partaken of the air over and over again. They should be forced, if possible, to live consistent with their miasmatic taint, and to promote health and strength. No wonder they improve when they take the open air treatment, as it is given in the Adirondacks and such exposed open air rest cures. Indeed these patients, suffering with the tubercular taint, need an abundance of fresh air ; they should always be in some ozone belt where oxygen is not at a premium. The devitalizing action of the blood in pseudo-psora demands constant purification of the life stream by coming in contact with large volumes of pure oxygen, or it soon becomes overwhelmed with detrite material that a lowered vitality is unable to take care of. Of course there are thousands of patients today who die of many diseases other than lung trouble, that are not classified under the tubercular disease, but which nevertheless are based upon this pseudo-psoric miasm. Often we notice a single symptom in these tubercular patients that may be persistent for years and on the least exposure to cold, they become hoarse ; it is not the simple huskiness of psora, it is a deeper thing, the voice is coarse, deep, with base-like chest tones, the throat is slightly sore at times, a rawness and a croak-like sound develops in the voice, there is a constant desire to hawk or clear the throat of a scanty, viscid mucus. The sore throat of Hepar and Phosphorus remind us of it. The coughs of psora are dry, teasy, spasmodic, and annoying, and are bronchial ; but the cough of the tubercular patient is deep and prolonged, giving us the lower chest tones ; it is worse in the morning and when the patient first lies down in the evening. The expectoration in psora is mucus usually, scanty and tasteless, while the tubercular expectoration is usually purulent or muco-purulent. In advanced cases it is greenish yellow, often offensive and usually sweetish to the taste or salty. The salt or sweetish taste can usually be depended upon. Sometimes it smells musty or offensive, or it is heavy and sinks in water ; again, it may be bloody or followed with hemorrhages. Quite often the cough of the tubercular patient is deep, ringing and hollow with no expectoration or none to speak of. The syphilitic is recognized by one or two distinct barks like that of a dog. The tubercular may assimilate it somewhat in those early dry coughs, before any breaking down of the lung tissue has taken place. We are all familiar with the rales and sounds peculiar to this disease, they are numerous and often peculiar to these tubercular changes. These coughs are often so dry and tight that they induce headaches, or the whole body is shaken by their explosive like paroxysms. Frequently these patients, who have suffered for some time with one of these chronic coughs, become surly, cross and ill-disposed, yet we know that they are the most hopeful of all patients as to the outcome. They seldom give up or think of death, in fact it is the last thing they think of and sometimes it is very difficult to convince them that they are incurable; indeed, they are apt to dispense with your services if you insist upon it. They are the last ones to give up the ship, always hopeful, always looking to the physician for help, always asking when they can be cured and how long it will take, even when dissolution has far advanced and life is at a low ebb. They are always planning for the future, building air castles, ever ready to accept any proffered help or promise of a cure; they are seldom sceptical of results and, therefore, often become a willing prey to the charlatan, the quack and the miraculous healer; thus they become a victim to every and any form of treatment that may be presented to them. We all have met this mental picture, although we may not all have fully recognized its meaning, or the persistency or the constancy of its presence.

We have not spoken of the glandular changes that take place in this disease, especially in the cervical region which is so positive a symptom of a tubercular diathesis, and which often precedes all other symptoms referring to lung changes; nor yet have we spoken of the oppressions about the chest, the weakness, the anxiety, the difficult respiration or the labored inspiration, the pain, the neuralgias and the suffering that only the afflicted ones can tell for themselves. It is a study in itself to see these tubercular patients struggle for the restoration of their health; they will do most anything, climb mountains, when they ought to be at rest, exercise when they should be quiet, take journeys by land and by sea, when they should be at home enjoying their last days in peace and quietness. They stop at nothing—drugs, diet, climate and treatments of all kinds, until everything has failed and often all their means exhausted, they even then have hope of a cure or of prolonged life. There are many other latent symptoms that have not been mentioned, symptoms that are often wrapped in mystery, symptoms of which we do not always comprehend their meaning or value ; some of these are that sense of great exhaustion, easily made tired, the least over exertion exhausts beyond that which is natural; they are always tired, never seem to get rested; "I was born tired," we hear them say ; tired at night, tired even after sleep ; as the day advances, they become better, or as the sun ascends in the heavens, their strength revives a little, as it descends they loose it again. How frequently I have examined the urine as well as making a careful physical examination of the whole organism, hoping in vain to find the cause of this loss of strength, and in the end decided that my patient's failing strength was due to a tubercular taint which was sapping, slowly but surely, the life. Again these patients suffer with neuralgias, prosopalgias, sciatica, insomnia, hysteria and all forms of nervous affections that are persistent and have a specific nature about their action, that is peculiar to a tubercular diathesis lying behind them, which lends them their dominantly persistent aspect. For years a persistent headache may be the only active symptom we find outside the many physiological expressions of the disease ; again I have seen a profound hysteria develop and remain with the patient for years, before a pulmonary lesion was discovered, and when the lung lesion made its appearance, the nervous affection departed and vice versa as the lung improved; often a severe form of dysmenorrhoea kept back or for a time stayed the development of the disease in the lung itself. Of course many of these intermediary expressions are often of a psoric nature, or the psoric element will dominate until it has fully aroused the tubercular element. Many a case of insanity has developed from a tubercular meningial inflammation, either from a diffuse tubercular infiltration or from tubercular growths on the pia mater. This is another way of saving the lung; the maniacal paroxysms often increase or decrease with these tubercular crops that come and go upon the membrane. We get meningial pain in children; it is frequently from this cause that they scream or cry out in the night as soon as they fall asleep.

But to return to the latent premonitory symptoms of lung trouble, we will continue our study of latent miasmatic symptoms. The aggravation of symptoms in the tubercular patients shows the parental nature of its old syphilitic basis. Tubercular patients are often worse in the night, which they dread, and they long for morning, as also does the syphilitic patient. Look out for disease that has a persistent nightly aggravation, as it means much sometimes, no matter what the pathology may be; it has a deeper meaning than the ordinary aggravation suggests.

Another thought that suggests itself here, is the non-resistance of the tissue in tubercular subjects, the slightest bruise suppurates ; the strong tendency is to pustulation or to the formation of pustules. The same may be said of the expectoration from the lungs ; its pus-like nature and its copiousness are features to be considered. The strong tendency to the enlargement of the lymphatic glands, the overworked lymphatic system, and indeed, latent hereditary syphilis bears the same relation to these pseudo-psoric subjects, that sycosis does to gout or to the gouty diathesis and lithic deposits. I make no distinction between the tubercular diathesis and the scrofulous, they are quite the same—the only difference is in the degree of the psoric and the tubercular combination, with probably the conditions of climate, race and other similar associations. In an article headed "The Scrofulous Versus the Syphilitic," I have endeavored to demonstrate that fact. The multiple expressions and modifications of the disease, often interferes with our seeing the two relationships.

Some members of a family will escape the chronic blepharitis or the ophthalmia of a latent tubercular condition and often the throat or bronchial catarrhs are the only active expressions of the disease. This is often due to the changes and defense of a strong, healthy parental influence, a fact which we must keep constantly before us in our study of these latent tubercular individuals, or we may be easily turned aside from a true conception of their true miasmatic state.

HEART

In our study of this organ, we find few tubercular diseases or manifestations. The psoric and the sycotic element strongly pervades in organic or even functional disturbances of the heart. Here is where the *syco-psoric* element predominates, especially in valvular and cardiac changes, which so frequently bring about a fatal issue in our own day. We have many psoric symptoms that manifest themselves in sensations, such as sensations of weakness, goneness, fullness, heaviness and soreness about the heart. A rush of blood to the chest, in the young or rapidly growing youth, is often a tubercular symptom, just as they have a rush of blood to the face or to any part of the body. Violent palpitation with beating of the whole body, is found in both the tubercular and psoric patients. In psora, they have violent hammering and beating about the heart, due to reflexes, such as gastric disturbances, flatulence and uterine irritation. Sycosis produces the same, from reflex rheumatic troubles, especially if local applications are employed to relieve the pain. Sensations as of a band about the body in the region about the heart, may be said to be due to psora. The mental and heart symptoms often alternate and vie with each other. It may be said that the majority of psoric heart symptoms can be attributed directly to psora, while in sycosis or syphilis, they are secondary or are due to secondary causes. A psoric patient suffering with cardiac troubles, has more or less anxiety, more or less fear in heart diseases, while the syphilitic or the sycotic have very little mental disturbances, none to speak of, even at critical periods of the disease. They may have heart trouble for years, which causes them no special inconvenience, save perhaps occasional dyspnoea, or some pain. These patients die suddenly with no warning; they are those whose lives snuff out like a candle. Very many of the *psoric* heart troubles are functional, and are accompanied with much anxiety, mental distress, with pain and neuralgia, often of a sharp, piercing, cutting nature. The heart troubles of tubercular are accompanied with fainting, temporary loss of vision, ringing in the ears, pallor and great weakness, worse sitting up and better lying down; the psoric patient is better by keeping quiet, lying down usually; the sycotic patient is better by motion, as walking, riding, gentle exercise. The tubercular patients, suffering with heart troubles, can not climb mountains at all, as the disturbed circulation affects the brain and they become, dizzy, faint, often fainting away when they reach a rarified atmosphere. The brain becomes anemic at a high altitude. The oppression and anxiety of psoric patients is worse in the morning, usually, and their pains are worse from motion, laughing, coughing, etc. The stitching pains almost kill the patient when he moves. Heart affections from fear, disappointment, loss of friends or overjoy are psoric; these patients think they have heart trouble and are going to die, but the sycotic and syphilitic patients as a rule deny that they have cardiac troubles, or they are usually unaware of it. We have psoric heart difficulties from eating or drinking, generally worse in the evening or soon after eating. Heart difficulties at night, palpitation on lying down, after eating or during digestion, which are relieved by eructations of gas, but worse on going to sleep and lying on the back ; heart pulsations shake the body, and are accompanied with great anxiety and sadness. In sycotic heart troubles, we are more apt to have less demonstration of action than in psora. We have fluttering, throbbing with oppression and difficult breathing at intervals. There is seldom much pain or suffering, unless in rheumatic difficulties, when we may find severe pains, but they are not so constant or persistent as those of psora. Under sycosis we may find much soreness and tenderness which is often worse by motion of the arms. Pain from shoulder to heart, or from heart to scapula, in rheumatic cardiac troubles, is quite frequently met with in sycosis. Often in sycosis the pulse is soft, slow, easily compressible. We notice it is full, bounding in psoric fevers ; and small, thread-like and quick in the tubercular. In fevers of sycotic patients, we do not find the tone or tension as seen in the psoric. Under the prolonged action of hereditary or acquired or tertiary sycosis, the valves become roughened, due to the acid condition of the system, the walls enlarged, the muscles flabby, soft and lacking power, therefore the pulse lacks that tension and that thrill is not present when we press upon the radial pulse. The sycotic patients are as a rule, fleshy and puffy; their obesity often lies at the bottom of their dyspnea and they are constantly gaining in flesh. In the heart troubles of the pseudo-psoric patient the reverse of this takes place and there is a constant and gradual falling away of flesh, rush of blood to the chest and face; frequently the sycotic face becomes blue, cyanotic indeed, there is apt to be a venous congestion or rather stagnation. The dyspnea of the psoric or the pseudo-psoric is often painful, which is seldom the case in the sycotic. The dropsies, or the anasarcas, of psora or pseudo-psora are always greater than the sycotic, they smother or drown the patient before death takes place; but not often so in the sycotic, their life is snuffed out when you are not looking for it and when you least expect it; they drop out of existence as quickly as an electric light is turned off, perhaps with one or two severe thrusts of pain, or without pain. We hear of just such cases every day in the higher walks of life among the wealthy. Of course this state of things is hastened or intensified by diet, especially when much meat is consumed, or in wine drinkers. Whiskey or beer does not affect the gouty diathesis as do wines, especially imported or spiced wines. Beer is less harmful than the other drinks mentioned, as it is more apt to prevent the deposition of salts of the blood, that deposit themselves in the tissues in the typical tertiary sycosis or gouty diathesis, although all are decidedly hurtful to the organism in the end. This will be more clearly seen in Volume II, as we take up the study more fully, studying each disease under this miasm (that is of sycotic origin). In psora, we must study the pulse, the circulation, the pains, the tension, the neuralgias, the palpitation and the thousand and one sensations. If the beat is not regular in psora, he soon finds it out, where in sycosis, he may never discern it until the case is far advanced and becomes truly organic, then we have the fear of psora, the restlessness, the anxiety, and the cardiac dyspnea, the pain and many other symptoms already dwelt upon so fully. There are many other symptoms to which we might give attention, but space prevents us from dealing with them farther, as we have a number of other subjects with which to deal.

ABDOMEN

In this region we have many symptoms that are quite similar to those recorded of the stomach, such as fullness, distension, flatulence, rumbling of gas, constant commotion and movement in the colon, that keeps the patient awake at night ; pain may, or may not, be one of the symptoms, but if so, the pains are often sharp, shooting or colicky. The true colic, or colic in its worst form, as found under Plumbum or Colocynthe, is very apt to have a sycotic element present. We see this in the colicky pains of Rheum and Chamomilla and in bowel troubles of children. Often the simplest kind of food produces colic or pain in the abdomen or throughout the intestinal tract. The abdomen feels full after eating; in psora, and the pains are often accompanied with a feeling of distension or fullness. These symptoms are more apt to be worse in the morning, and are often found in children. We may find empty, gone feelings in the abdomen, similar to those found in the stomach and soon after eating they appear. Again we find a stuffy, full feeling in the abdomen, preventing the patient from eating the normal amount of food; or we sometimes find sensations of constrictions, of bands or cords about the abdomen, pressure in the lower region of the liver, stitches on stooping or bending the body, audible rumblings in the bowels, sensation as if the abdomen were greatly distended or as if it were hanging down, heavy dragging down sensation, crawling, creeping before a chill, sensations as if diarrhea would set in, especially in the morning, rumbling and gurgling in the abdomen as soon as they eat or drink anything, cramps from eating certain kinds of food, or drink, such as the drinking of milk or cold water, etc., or the eating of potatoes, beans and many other foods that do not agree with these patients. Many of these patients have a tubercular diathesis, but of course, psora predominates throughout their lives, or at least it is the basic principle of their disturbances.

Hernia, while there is a strongly psoric element present, is seldom found outside of the tubercular organism. We most frequently find hernia in flabby, soft-muscled people. Hernia is due to this lack of tone of the muscular system throughout the whole abdominal region; it is not a true psoric development. The lymphatic envolvement is also pseudo-psoric, as is messentary complications. The shape of the tubercular abdomen is saucer-shaped or like that of a large plate turned bottom side up. The muscles are flabby and have an inclination toward muscular weakness. All the abdominal pains and sufferings of psora are relieved by heat, and many times by gentle pressure. Peritoneal inflammations and other difficulties are tubercular, even secondary envolvement (unless infection due to sycosis or other cause is present). The colic of sycosis is better by bending double, by motion or hard pressure; this it not so of psora; we often find the worst forms of constipation or inactivity of the bowels in psoric or pseudo-psoric patients. Sometime in disease states of the abdomen, the patient is very sensitive to motion. In psora we often have a beating or throbbing as of a pulse in the abdomen, while in tubercular patients, you can often feel the beating of the carotids through the abdominal walls. In tubercular children, we find ulceration of the umbilicus with a yellowish discharge, which smells offensive, carrion-like or similar to a Hepar-sulph. pus. We have this same thing in a sycotic child, with the tubercular element present, but the pus is yellowish, green, watery, thin, excoriating and offensive, often of a fishy or fish brine odor In menstrual difficulties, we may find reflex pains, spasmodic symptoms and bearing down sensations, especially in the tubercular patient. The skin in the tubercular person is pale, with an underlying bluish tint, showing the venous stagnation ; often the veins show quite distinctly beneath the integument. The psoric or pseudo-psoric patients are easily chilled about the abdomen, causing colic or diarrhea, dysentery and many severe bowel troubles to follow. Look out for the tubercular child during the first and second years of its life ; keep the abdomen and the solar plexus warm, as a chilling of the solar plexus means death to many of them. We were in the habit, in the past years, to attribute the so-called "summer complaint" to foods or to hot weather, but we were mistaken in this, as it was not the heat alone nor the diet in particular, but the much neglected protection of the solar plexus. The cold nights, or early mornings, are the cause of the majority of these cases ; the evenings and first part of the night being very warm, they uncover their little bodies to get relief, and sleeping soundly on until the earth becomes cooled and the atmosphere of the room chilled, and thus we have these midnight visitations, that lie at the bottom as a secondary cause of this great fatality in children, due to bowel troubles. A little flannel bandage, as a protection, would many a time have evaded all the trouble. All this tubercular element needs is a slight chillng of the body, or even a single part of the body, to arouse a tubercular inflammation or congestion (for that is what these dysenteries are in children), and set up a conflagration that can not be extinguished before it destroys the young and tender life.

THE BOWELS AND INTESTINAL TRACT

In this extensive region of unusual functional activity, we have a prolific field for miasmatic action ; for we find that where the function of a part is complex or multiple, the miasms often bring forth or manifest their most annoying symptoms ; this is especially true of the intestinal tract. Death in a very brief space of time has often resulted from some of the more malignant combinations of miasmatic action. Syphilitic children have died from bowel troubles from twenty-four to forty-eight hours ; tubercular, within a week. Often in hereditary syphilis we have seen the whole force of the disease center suddenly upon the intestinal tract and a watery discharge for twenty-four hours drain the system of its last vital drop, and death follow from exhaustion.

The diarrheas of psora are often induced by overeating ; the patient being always hungry, of course often eats beyond his capacity of digestion, thus the intestinal digestion is overcrowded, which produces one of nature's own catharsis. The movements are usually watery or consist of imperfectly digested food ; quite often they are accompanied with an offensive odor and with colicky pains or with a cutting colic. They occur usually in the morning, that being the general hour of their aggravation. We see this in the diarrheas of Podophyllum, Sulphur and Aloes. Tubercular patients may have this morning aggravation in bowel troubles, but it is nevertheless a psoric aggravation, and while psora patients are aggravated by cold, the tubercular persons are still more sensitive, and the effects of colds are more dangerous to life.

In the cholera infantum of syphilitic children, we meet with complete arrest of digestion, with purging and vomiting, with drowsiness and stupor, even to coma, or with spasms, convulsions and often death. A similar state of things is sometimes witnessed in the tubercular child; although the symptoms are seldom so suddenly fatal, yet the result is often very similar. In the psoric and the pseudo-psoric bowel difficulties, we often have gone, empty feelings in the abdominal region; sometimes it is a great weakness after stool, felt only in the region of the abdomen. In the tubercular patient, we have the general exhaustion or loss of strength, a feeling as if all his vitality is leaving him at each evacuation of the bowels. Usually the true syphilitic or tubercular patients are worse at night; they are driven out of bed by their diarrhea, sometimes this is accompanied with profuse, warm or cold perspiration, which is very exhausting and debilitating. In seven cases out of ten, the face is pale and earthy, eyes sunken, with dark rings around them, lips very red or bluish, loss of appetite, rapid emaciation, prostration and often accompanied with much thirst. As the disease advances the eyes become more sunken, the face more pale and the prostration increases until brain symptoms suddenly develop and death follows quickly. It is so characteristic of these tubercular children suffering from bowel troubles to develop a sudden brain stasis or brain metastasis of some form. Sometimes the tubercular manifestations in the brain alternate with a bowel difficulty, but we do not look for any such fatal issues in psora. No, psora is not so destructive to life ; no such developments arise as are found due to the mixed miasm, *pseudo-psora*.

Veratrum alba, Arsenicum, Camphor and Cuprum met are good types of such diarrheas or dysenteries, so characteristic are they of patients of a well marked tubercular diathesis. From a state of apparent health today, they are seized with a sudden attack of dysentery and within forty-eight to sixty hours they are dead ; look out for them in the month of August and the first part of September, when they are passing through that trying time of the year that tests whether they are tubercular of psoric. These cases will differentiate themselves readily, or at least with the varying of the thermometer, as the earth suddenly cools down at night after a sultry August day.

Podophyllun, too, is a remedy that fully represents a certain type of these cases, with their painless, copious, yellowish and very offensive stool, with its aggravations night and morning, as well as its aggravations from the use of milk. A tubercular child can't use cow's milk in any shape; the casein has to be modified before they can digest it at all. They thrive better on anything else than milk.

Every physician has had troubles of his own with

milk. How many times I have wished there was never such a thing as milk in existence, when these anti-milk children came into my hands. Give some of these delicate little tubercular patients a good dose of milk, and you can get a proving of anything you want out of it, from a dysentery to a convulsion or spasm, diarrhea, nausea, vomiting, colic and gastric pain of any order or degree, with febrile states, reflexes to the brain and anything to order you may ask for ; these children are no friend to milk ; indeed milk is their enemy.

We are at a loss sometimes to know just what to nourish them with ; often we are completely baffled, but for the ever present help we find in the administration of similia, we should often fail.

These tubercular children may have diarrhea every now and again from the day that they are born until they are two or three years old. The least error in diet or exposure to cold produces it, as they seem to have no resistive force whatever ; much of this is due to impaired glandular secretions in the whole alimentary tract, and often tubercular changes in the glands themselves, or to their imperfect action. Another marked feature of the tubercular babies (and what I mean by a tubercular baby in this sense is one who has any taint of the miasm present) is that when they begin the eruption of the first teeth the diarrhea often begins, or else if present, they grow worse and continue throughout the entire period of dentition, coming and going at the appearance of every eruption of a tooth. Sometimes these attacks are violent and prolonged and often endanger the young life. Co-operative with this state of things in these pseudo-psoric patients is that loss of power or inability of the system to assimilate bone-making material from the food. There is a close relationship between this non-assimilation of the lime or the calcarious agents for bone material, and the diarrheas of these children. The membranes covering the teeth are hard, firm and unyielding, requiring great pressure to soften them so that the teeth can push their way through. This great tension, if prolonged for any length of time, together with the deficiency of bone constructing material, induces often, it seems, reflexly this gastro or intestinal war, with all its suffering to the young life. In sycosis, we see none of this; sycosis usually gives us colic, until we are tired of hearing the patients cry of suffering ; occasionally it has diarrheas, but if so, they are of a spasmodic, colicky nature, and accompanied with a slimy mucus stool and with griping colic and rectal tenesmus. The stools of Rheum., Chamomilla, Mag, carb. are typical of this miasm. Psora also has a spasmodic offensive diarrhea, which usually relieves the patients of their sufferings, but they have no such exhaustion, no such persistency as we find under pseudo-psora or sycosis.

Croton. tig. gives us a stool that is found in these tubercular children, who are strongly tainted with sycosis. Sarsaparilla has, as a rule, all the miasms present, but sycosis is especially prominent. Sanguinaria, Phosphorus, Kali-carb., Tuberculinum and Stannum are quite typical of the tubercular discharges; the Mercuries, of course, representing the syphilitic, as fully as any.

These miasms are constantly expressing on the organism their own creative energy, which is of course antagonistic to life; sometimes we see it in lysis or by a crisis. In lysis as is seen in those slow and smoldering fires of some chronic malady, or by a crisis, overwhelming the already vitiated life force.

Sometimes in the tubercular child, the stools are ashy or grayish in color, showing lack of bile matter. Sycotic diarrheas have the most pain and the stools are forcibly ejected from the rectum. Croton tig., Chamomilla, Lauroccrasus and Colocynthis and that class of remedies represent this idea. The intestinal pains of sycosis as has been mentioned, are of an extremely colica nature, and they make the patient angry, as a rule. Sycotic bowel troubles, whether they be diarrheas or hemorrhoids, produce the same irritability. They are cross, irritable, with their pains.

I have often noticed that the stools are very changeable, usually greenish yellow mucus, seldom bloody (bloody stools, tubercular), greenish, watery, sour smelling, with cutting colic; even the child smells sour in marked cases of sycosis of a hereditary nature (child smells musty or mouldy, tubercular). In severe cases of bowel troubles of a low order in the tubercular, the child is fretful, peevish and whiny, and does not want to be touched or even looked at; prostration after stools, marked. This is not so in sycosis, and the little patients do not wish to be left alone, as when the tubercular element predominates, but are anxious to be constantly rocked, carried or moved about in some way; the colics are better by firm pressure or lying on the abdomen; they are aggravated by eating fruit, but the tubercular are aggravated by milk, potatoes, meat, by motion, or any disturbance by movement. In marked tubercular children we often notice before stools nausea with gagging; the child gags and tries to vomit, but often does not succeed. Although we have marked cases of nausea and vomiting of all of the contents of the stomach soon after eating and drinking.

Dulcamara has a typical sycotic stool, which is yellowish, green and watery, white or green mucus expelled with much force, is acid and corrosive, like all the stools of sycosis. It, too, is changeable and worse during a falling barometer; we have the same griping colic, the tenesmus, the impatience and the irritability. Psora has a diarrhea coming on from fright, grief, bad news or any undue ordeal; also when making preparation for any unusual event; it also has a diarrhea from taking cold or the slightest exposure (from getting wet, sycosis). The grass green stools of Ipecac, Mag. carb., Croton tig., Gratiola, Arg. nit., and such remedies, are apt to be of a sycotic nature. The true psoric stool may be any color, but it is usually modified in color, generally offensive and not very painful ; it is aggravated by cold, motion, eating and drinking cold things ; better by warm drinks and hot things to eat, rest, quite warm applications to the abdomen.

The constipation of psora is very marked ; it is stubborn, persistent and there is no action of the bowels whatever ; no desire to stool ; the stool is dry, scanty, hard, difficult of expulsion, sometimes we have alternations of constipation and diarrheas ; constipation with pains remote, such as headaches, pain in the liver or region of the liver ; constipation with basilar or temporal headaches ; constipation with drowsiness, sleepiness, stupor and heaviness, with no desire to work ; constipation with foul breath, foul coated tongue, nausea and loss of appetite ; constipation with no stool for days, although there is a frequent desire for stool ; stool hard, comes in round balls like the excrement of sheep ; stool looks dark and dry as if burnt ; where there is much slimy mucus, especially if it is constant, there is apt to be a tubercular taint; or where much blood passes after stool, will call our attention to the diathesis also. Hemorrhages from the rectum always call our attention to a tubercular element in the system, although we see bleeding hemorrhoids also in sycosis, but sycosis has great pruritis and usually has a scanty, thin, watery, discharge oozing from the rectum that has a fishy or fish-brine smell to it. Pin worms or intestinal worms are also of a psoric origin, but are found more plentiful in children with a tubercular taint ; sensations of crawling and creeping is quite characteristic of psora. Rectal diseases alternating with heart, chest or lung troubles, will be found to have a tubercular origin, especially is this true of asthma and respiratory difficulties; for instance, hemorrhoids, if operated upon or suppressed in any way, are followed by lung difficulties or asthma, and not infrequently by heart trouble. Strictures in the rectum, sinuses, fistules and fistulous pockets are all of a tubercular origin or of pseudo-psoric nature, but are greatly magnified by sycosis. Prolapsus of the rectum in young children will be found in tubercular also. Cancerous affections, malignant growths and such diseases have as a rule all the miasms present and especially the tubercular and the sycotic elements combined. Of course psora can never be left out of malignancies; no matter what other element may combine with it, it fathers them all. Indeed, it is first cause in all diseases or diseased states. The bowel difficulties of tubercular children are so frequently accompanied with febrile states, delirium, gastric disturbance, vomiting, purging, with exhaustive, copious stools. These tubercular children are easily and readily known by the numerous diseases they have to contend with in their childhood days. We know them by the severity of their diseases and the frequency in which we have to deal with all these acute and dangerous processes to the young life.

URINARY ORGANS

Throughout the whole urinary tract, we find latent symptoms of all the miasms. Of the true chronic miasms, psora and sycosis take an active part in the production of disease in these organs. The tubercular element, however, will be found to be not entirely absent by any means for it is the tubercular, plus the sycotic element, that gives us many of the so-called malignancies and severe diseases of these organs.

The tubercular patient complains of anxiety and much loss of strength after urination. Often in psoric children, we have retention of urine when the body becomes chilled; we see this also in old people; great distention of the bladder, with fullness, as if it was extremely full, is another symptom; sense of constriction, too, is often present. The urine in any psoric patient will pass off frequently involuntarily when sneezing, coughing or laughing. There is not much pain in passing urine in psora, generally a slight smarting, due often to acidity of the urine. After fevers in acute diseases, the deposit of psora is usually white or yellowish white, phosphates and similar deposits; occasionally it is pinkish or similar to iron rust. In the tubercular diathesis, especially in the nervous or neurotic patient, it is pale, colorless and copious with very little of solids present. Diabetic patients are, as a rule, strongly tubercular; you will find the tubercular physiology throughout them, with the diathesis strongly marked. If sycosis be present, these cases are of course more malignant in their nature and more fatal.

Fibrous changes in the kidneys also have the three miasms present; although the tubercular and sycotic are present in the majority of cases of Bright's disease. The urine of these tubercular-tainted patients is often offensive and easily decomposed, the odor is musty, like old hay, or it is foul smelling, even carrion-like. I have had them send it to me frequently for examination, thinking that they had some fearful and perhaps incurable kidney trouble. In tubercular children, it is involuntary at night (nocturnal enuresis) as soon as they fall asleep. It is also copious; they drench everything, it is so profuse. These cases are only cured by getting at the pseudo-psoric diathesis. This is why Calcaria carb, cures so many of them. Where they scream when urinating, as found under Lycopodium or Sarsaparilla, here we are apt to find a sycotic element present. The sycotic expressions are so numerous, that they can only be fully taken up in the second volume of this work. The majority of those painful spasmodic symptoms depend largely upon the sycotic element, which we find affecting the urethra and bladder. Hæmaturia will be found more frequently under the tubercular diathesis, but may be found under all miasms; nightly pollutions and all involuntary discharges of semen will be found to have the pseudo-psoric taint behind them. All such weaknesses and expressions are pseudo-psoric. They all are indeed profound expressions of the pseudo-psoric taint.

Idiopathic hydrocele can claim the same parentage; you may look for the same element in prostatic troubles, except where acquired sycosis is the exciting medium. In cases where we have a constant loss of the prostatic or seminal fluid, consumption sometimes develops. These are the patients who live in gloom, with depressed spirits, gloomy forebodings, poor digestion, loss of energy, want of memory and all that train of symptoms familiar to us. Often we see a livid or ashy complexion, appetite often voracious, as the system calls for more food than it can properly take care of, when finally gastric derangements follow until the organism fails to perform any function in a proper manner. Many of the urinary symptoms of psora are due to reflexes or other diseased states, or in other words, to secondary causes, and especially is this true in women. The majority of renal difficulties, as has been mentioned, have a pseudo-psoric basis, which can be demonstrated by a careful study of all the latent miasmatic symptoms of the whole organism.

THE SEXUAL SPHERE

In the males, many of these symptoms have already been mentioned, under our last subject, but many others may be mentioned. The action of psora upon the mental sphere, often centers the mind upon some part or organ of the body; this is especially true in certain nervous temperaments. Their organ of consciousness, which is the controller largely of fear, becomes greatly magnified and the mind centers itself upon some part or portion of the body; often it is upon the heart and they think they nave heart disease; again it may be upon the lungs or any organ, no matter where. This is frequently true in the sexual sphere and all sorts of syco-pathic sexual perversions develop in the psoric patients; probably they are even worse in the pseudo-psoric. The mind becomes fixed upon sexual subjects and they have no power of themselves to disengage the mind from this debasing influence, until many of them are dragged down to both physical and mental ruin, often to moral or even to true insanity, or to mania in its worst forms. Occasionally we see it take on some form of monomania, such as a desire to steal, burn or some other desire of a destructive nature. If sycosis is present, especially if it is acquired, it greatly magnifies these conditions. When we consider the loss of strength, the loss of energy, the lack of ability, or desire to make physical or mental efforts of any kind, save that of a mere existence, then we may have some conception of the degenerative power, that lies behind these latent hereditary productions, which are induced by the action of that hydra-headed monster psora and its co-operators, syphilis and sycosis.

In women we see probably no greater field for miasmatic action, than is found in the perverseness of the reproductive and sexual functions of that sex. In almost every woman we meet we find some form of dysmenorrhœa and so frequently in these sufferers we find that all their complaints are intensified at, or during the menstrual nisus. Disturbances, not only in the function of the uterus and its appendages, but not infrequently in almost every other organ of the body from the crown of the head to the soles of the feet, all of which are incurred by the presence of the tubercular element when it is present, and of course greatly magnified when the sycotic poison is tainting the stream of life. No function should be perverted in a normal, healthy organism ; no function should be painful at least, for pain is always a signal bell of disease, of perverted function. We should have no more than a simple consciousness of the presence of the function of any organ, and yet we find every degree of suffering, even to the anguish of death, in any organ of the body, as it attempts to perform its simplest function, when in a diseased state or condition.

Indeed the sycotic element has such a specific action upon the endometrium and uterine appendages that when we meet acute pain, acute or active inflammatory processes, we seldom make a mistake in attributing the cause to sycosis in some form. Syphilis seldom attacks the ovaries or uterus ; psora alone will not produce other than functional disturbances. Occasionally we find the tubercular pathology present, but it is so seldom that it is scarcely worth mentioning. We look upon diseases of the tubes now, as sycotic infections always. There are so many degrees or modifications of these sycotic inflammatory processes around and about the uterus and reproductive organs, that it is often difficult to say positively that they are or are not of sycotic origin. A few symptoms that are generally present, must be kept in mind, these are the spasmodic, colicky and often paroxysmal pains, the acrid discharges, the pruritis, the painful and often frequent urination, the fish-brine or stale fish odor of the catarrhal discharges together with the mental phenomena that are usually present. On examination we recognize the mottled appearance of the mucous membrane, so constant in this disease. There are many other symptoms that might be enumerated but as our subject is psora and pseudo-psora we must not depart too far from it other than is necessary in comparison.

The sexual and reproductive organs of women, are not the less free from the influence of miasmatic action; indeed they have become great centers of both physiological, psycological, pathological and therapeutic study for our profound consideration and most serious thought. Today the destructive action of the sycotic miasm upon these organs has become an alarming factor to our strongest therapeutists and our best pathologists. How often the surgeon has to be called in to remove a part or even the whole of the reproductive organs of women, who have gone beyond the power or help of the therapeutist, often because he is not familiar with the nature of the sycotic miasms action upon, not only the reproductive tract, but upon the whole organism of women. His therapeutic knowledge does not reach that far; the physician has for centuries been studying suppressive measures, which will dissipate the disease action of psora and pseudo-psora; when the new element (sycosis) appears, he thinks he can do as he has always done, suppress it, but later on, he finds that a suppression of its catarrhal manifestations gives it a new impetus, a renewed power and energy, and that new processes often develop of either a malignant, destructive or inflammatory nature, that baffles all his therapeutic efforts. Why? Because he is not dealing with the same slow insidious elements and processes he found present in psora and pseudo-psora; he, never having been schooled in the history, character, and action of miasmatics, can often distinguish them by name only.

The menstrual anomalies of tubercular patients, are in themselves often severe pictures of sufferings and of miasmatic action. The first to be thought of is an exhaustive and often a prolonged and copious flow to be found in these cases. The hemorrhages of bright red blood, are sometimes accompanied with vertigoes, fainting, and with pallor of the face, which is worse by rising from a recumbent position. Quite frequently they are too soon, appearing every two or three weeks; they may or may not be painful, but are always exhausting. She feels badly a week before they appear, suffering in many ways with headaches, backaches, gastric disturbances, neuralgias, etc. Occasionally the menses appear with diarrhea, with epistaxis, with febrile states, optical illusions, roaring in the ears, sensitiveness to noises, loss of appetite, abdominal pains, nausea and bitter vomiting. The psoric element is of course very marked in these cases, as well; usually flows of psora are bland, while in the sycotic they are acrid, excoriating, biting and burning the pudendum. After the menstrual flow the tubercular patient looks pale, with dark rings or circles about the eyes, or hollow eyed, with a worn and exhausted look upon the face. Hysterical symptoms frequently arise in these cases of any form or degree of severity and often they are the most difficult cases we have to treat.

Quite frequently the flow is pale, watery, and long lasting, as seen in Calcaria carb., Ferum, and such remedies. The extremities are usually cold and often the menstrual flow will induce general anemia in young women, whose ages range from seventeen to twenty-one. They become "chlorotic" as we say, due to the death of many of the red blood cells, which as we have already seen, was due to the specific action of this miasm *pseudo-psora*. Not infrequently the complexion becomes pale, assuming a yellow or ashy hue, accompanied with starchy or watery leucorrhœas, palpitation of the heart, faintness and loss of vitality generally; later on general weakness, flushing to the face, vertigo, ringing in the ears, hoarseness, dry, tickling, spasmodic cough, and finally a true tubercular condition develops. Many of these cases have mental symptoms accompanying those already given, such as great sadness, gloomy, anxious, full of fanciful notions, forbodings with much fear, extreme sensitiveness, nervous, irritable or inclined to weep. Occasionally they will pass through the whole menstrual period until its close, with very little annoyance or suffering, to be followed with prosopalgias of a prolonged and most distressing nature.

These are a few of the many symptoms that arise in these tubercular individuals, but volumes might be written in order to cover these cases fully. I have said nothing to speak of about the pains, neuralgias, spasmodic and reflex symptoms and sufferings of those patients, who suffer from retroversions, retroflexions and other malpositions of the uterus. Usually in marked cases of the diathesis, the uterus is retroverted or retroflexed and many of their sufferings date from some time soon after puberty, within a year or so at least. We have the same relaxed muscular system throughout; these patients becoming easily exhausted, easily tired, menses copious, too early and long lasting and accompanied with backache, headache, reflexes of all kinds and a long train of symptoms peculiar to this class of women. Their labors at childbirth are often difficult, severe, prolonged, exhausting, and many of them are unable to nourish their children at all. Displacement, prolapsus and all that train of symptoms are apt to follow with a history of subinvolution and general bad health.

This picture is not at all overdrawn; indeed we see it so frequently in our practice, that we often wish it were our good fortune not to meet these cases so frequently.

Hahnemann called these patients psoric, but they are more than psoric, they have combined with psora, an element that develops a train of symptoms that in which psora can only take a part. Most of these patients are of a motor or sanguine-motor temperament.

In psora, we may have almost any kind of a flow, but it never approaches the hemorrhagic form found in pseudo-psora. It is more apt to be scanty, indeed the patient will complain of its being of too short duration. It is generally offensive, often extremely so, yet it may have none of these characteristics, except that it is not as profuse as we found under the tubercular diathesis. We find not infrequently, an intermittent flow; it stops and starts. Indeed the dysmenorrhoea of psora, shows itself very early, at puberty and at the climatric period. The pains are usually sharp but never assume the colicky, spasmodic nature which we find in sycosis or when we find the sycotic taint accompanying the psoric or the pseudo-psoric combine. The menstrual pains of sycosis can well be understood from a study of some of our remedies, such as Colocynthis, Mag., carb., Phos., Crocus sativa, Sepia, Lac canium, Caulophyllum and others. There is another class that represents the rheumatic element in sycosis, which may be studied, such as Rhus tox, Bovista, Actea; rac Bry, Cham, Colch, Cyclamen, Dulcamara, Gelsemium, Phytolacca, Pulsatilla and others. Sulphur probably gives us a broader conception of the psoric diathesis, than any other remedy; yet it is such a deep acting remedy that it will cover even the pseudo-psoric constitution. The sycotic menstrual pains are spasmodic, extremely sharp, colicky, coming in paroxysms, the flow often only with the pains. It is offensive, clotted, stringy (psoric clots, small), clots large, dark, even black (flow bright red, the tubercular or light colored and watery.) The flow of sycosis is seldom bland, usually excoriating and acrid. patients with a tubercular taint we occasionally have cholera-like symptoms, such as nausea and vomiting, extreme purging from the bowels, with diarrhea or dysentery, fainting, cold sweat on the forehead, but the flow is seldom if ever clotted; it is usually fluid-like profuse, light red, watery and seldom offensive and not infrequently it has the odor of fresh blood.

The leucorrhœas of the tubercular are generally purulent but may be watery mucus. They are often debilitating and worse before the flow begins or immediately after. The leucorrhœas of psora are scanty, not exhausting, have nothing peculiar about their color, in fact they may be any color, but they have not the deep, thick, yellow or yellowish green of the tubercular individual.

The leucorrhœas of the sycotic patient are thin, look like dirty water, greenish yellow sometimes, scanty, acid, producing biting or itching and burning of the parts. The odor is that of stale fish or fish brine. Occasionally the leucorrhœas of the pseudo-psoric are lumpy, thick, albuminous or purulent, smelling musty. In sycosis they may be pungent or like that of a decayed fish; the patient is forever taking douches on account of the odor and the acridity of the discharge. Often the discharge produces little vesicles or excoriations on the pudendum, which are a source of great annoyance to the patient. In marked cases of the sycotic leucorrhœa often the mental symptoms are to be carefully considered as diagnostic in the differentiation of these different forms that come to our notice. We will have to study the other psoric symptoms of our patient, in order to get a clear picture of the menstrual phenomena. Many of the reflexes, such as headaches, heart difficulties, coughs and mental symptoms, are due to a deep psoric taint. Yet they are greatly magnified in a tubercular diathesis. Many of the ovarian or tubular symptoms that develop during the menses, are dependent more on sycosis than to any other miasm.

UPPER AND LOWER EXTREMITIES

Stiching, shooting or lancinating pains in the periostium or long bones of the upper or lower extremities, *syphilis*, shooting or tearing pains in the muscles or ioints, *sycosis*, pains in fingers or small joints; *sycosis*; neuralgic pains may be either psora or pseudo-psora; they are usually relieved by quiet, rest and warmth. The syphilitic pains are worse at night, or at the approach of night; they are also worse by change of weather, by cold and damp atmosphere. The sycotic pains are worse by rest and the patient is relieved by moving, by rubbing, stretching, and better in dry, fair weather; worse at the approach of a storm or a damp, humid atmosphere and a falling barometer or becoming cold; heat does not always relieve a sycotic patient; stiffness and soreness, especially lameness, is very characteristic of sycosis. They are worse stooping, bending or beginning to move. Psora often is worse by motion and better by rest and warmth Tubercular joint troubles have increased in osseous tissues, nodulor growths similar to syphilis. The bones are soft, rickety and curved, as seen frequently in bow-legged children. They lack the hard earthy matter necessary to make a firm bone. They are so soft and flexible, that many times in children they will not bear the weight of their body, therefore when children first begin to walk, the feet become deformed or the long bones become curved or bowed like a barrel stave. Nothing but the syphilitic element will make these changes as we find them in these pseudo-psoric children. The periosteal difficulties in pseudo-psora are due to periosteal inflammations or tertiary or tubercular changes in the bones themselves, while the pains in the joints or periosteum from sycosis, are due to gouty concretions, or chalky deposits in the tissues themselves, conveyed from the circulation. The tubercular and syphilitic bone pains are very similar, both as to their character and times of aggravation. In the arthritis of sycosis or rheumatism, we have an infiltration of inflammatory deposits, but it readily absorbs and is never formative as we find in syphilis and tubercular changes, which are permanent unless dissipated by treatment.

In the nails we have many inflammatory changes, due to syphilis and tuberculosis. We have in both, true onychia, though not of such a specific character in the tubercular process as in the tertiary syphilis; yet they are very similar in their nature. Paronychia is another common tubercular inflammation we may meet with in those pale skinned, anemic tubercular subjects. Pustules form often on the lower extremities or about the fingers or hands. The nails of those patients are brittle, break or split easily, often we have hang nails, which are so characteristic of a tubercular taint. It is an unfailing sign. In sycosis the nails are ribbed or ridged, but in syphilis or in pseudo-psora they are thin as paper, bend easily and are sometimes spoon shaped, that is, the natural convexity is reversed. Many of the tubercular nails are spotted or show white specks in them here and there. Sometimes the anterior edges are serrated or slightly scalloped. When we find this, we also find a thin spoon shaped and paper-like nail. Not infrequently, with no warning whatever, we have pustular inflammation about the nail. So often the nails drop off and grow again. The periosteal inflammation, commonly known as felon or periphalangeal cellulitis, is truly a pseudo-psoric inflammation as are other periosteal changes. We have many others, which will be dealt with under skin eruptions. The fingers of tubercular indivduals are long and do not taper gradually but are blunt or club shaped at their extremities. This long fingered individual with the lengths so irregularly arranged, is characteristic. Often the hand is thin, soft, flabby and easily compressed, usually very moist or often cold, damp, perspiring profusely.

The same thing may be said of the feet. This coldness of the hands and feet is very marked but the patient is not always conscious of it. In psora they are dry, hot, often with burning sensations in the palms and soles. Of course we meet with this often in the tubercular patient but it is nevertheless a psoric symptom. Occasionally this dryness and harshness is a source of great annoyance to the patients; we notice it as soon as we touch them; on the other hand, we can never fail to recognize the sign of the true tubercular taint, by taking hold of that long fingered, cold, damp and chilly hand, that almost chills you to the touch as marble would. The soft, flabby, non-resistent muscle, the clammy perspiration, the translucent nail, the flat imperfect curve, the uneven and ridged, pale matrix, the hang nail, the tendency to imperfect curves, especially in the nails of the feet, the ingrown nail, the tendency to ulcerations, and induration and abscesses where the system is very deeply impregnated with psora, the perspiration is sometimes very offensive, carrion like, rotting the hose often, which is a great source of annoyance to these patients. We see such types of pseudo-psora in the action of such remedies as Cal. cab., Baryta-carb., Baryta-iod., Iodine, Silica and that class of remedies, whose action is deep and long lasting partaking of both the tubercular and the psoric element. Notice their perspiratory secretions, their action upon the skin, glands and secretory apparatus, all of which are involved in pseudo-psora to any degree of physiological and pathological changes, due to the powerful action of these two miasms. Probably no other parts of the body reveal to us more typical demonstrations of their action, than that found upon the extremities, or parts remote from centres of circulation, which are apt to manifest their latent symptoms more clearly. Cramps in the lower extremities, in the calves of the legs, in the feet, toes, ankles and in steps are usually of a psoric nature, although found more frequently in the pseudo-psoric. In psora we have burning in the soles of the feet, numbness of the extremities with tingling sensations, feeling as if the parts were going to sleep, worse lying down or after sleep, or if any pressure is brought to bear upon the part, as lying lightly on the arm or crossing the limbs, etc., prickling or tingling in the fingers or extremities, due to poor circulation, coldness of single parts, as knees, hands, feet, ears and nose, etc. Often there is a constant chilliness in psoric patients, when suffering from any disease or slight ailment; we find them hovering over the stove or over the radiator. They can not leave it without suffering from cold. Again in the pseudo-psoric, the warm air of the room is extremely annoying to them; the pseudo-psoric can not endure much cold yet they can not endure much heat.

Chilblains are based upon all the miasms. We have the pseudo-psoric taint with a sycotic element as a basis; this is why they prove such a dreadful disease producing agent, when suppressed by local measures. Any expression of disease may follow their suppression, even to malignant or spasmodic disease. I have traced chorea and many other severe nervous disorders to a suppression of chilblains; more will be said of it and cases given to demonstrate this fact in Volume II of this work. Corns are found in the pseudo-psoric; these and like classifications of hypertrophies are found in the tubercular taint. Boils are usually psoric but they may depend on both the psoric and pseudo-psoric influences; the small, sensitive, painful and non-suppurating kind are truly psoric, but where we have much suppuration, we will find the tubercular element present. They are a good omen often, especially so after giving an anti-psoric remedy, although Sulphur will produce them if repeated often and they be mistaken for an idiopathic condition; paralytic disease, edematous swellings, anasarca and such diseases are either sycotic, syphilitic or pseudo-psoric; there may be any degree of a psoric element present, but what we wish to make clear, is that psora alone does not produce these diseases; there must be more than psora present to develop such deep destructive diseases. Talipes and such deformities in children are also pseudo-psoric or syphilitic. We might mention many other conditions in children due to this pseudo-psoric element, and yet not exhaust this subject. We find general muscular weakness or loss of power in the ankle joints among these children; they stumble and fall easily; they are clumsy and awkward and lack co-ordination or complete muscular control of themselves, thus they are forever falling; indeed they will stumble over a straw; they drop things easily out of their hands; they have no surety in themselves whatever; they tire easily in walking, and especially in climbing a height. The psoric patient can walk well, but it kills him to stand still; this is such a positive symptom of psora that it can always be depended upon. The tubercular patient is short-winded; a short mountain climb gets him all out of breath or the climbing of fifteen or twenty steps of stairs tires the patient out. They can always descend better than ascend. White swelling of the joints or idiopathic synovitis, even the rheumatic forms have this tubercular element very marked. Of course the rheumatic form has a mixed miasm or the sycotic taint, combined with the pseudo-psoric. We also find the pseudo-psoric element in what is known as drop wrist, or in all idiopathic weakness or loss of power in the tendons about the joints. In children and young people, we find the ligaments about the joints are easily sprained, the ankles turn very easily from the slightest misstep, the wrists show the same weakness in these soft and weak muscled individuals playing the piano or operating a type writer, causes swelling, soreness or pain in the wrist joints, and sometimes bursæ form suddenly from these causes; or they become lame easily or there is sudden loss of strength.

This muscular insufficiency is seen all throughout childhood and early youth ; these are the individuals that have no strength to develop themselves through physical culture or gymnastic exercises. Indeed they lack energy as well as strength, and although they may be induced to try these exercises, they soon give them up for lack of vigor and strength to continue them. Many of these patients look robust and well nourished, but when they are brought to the test they have no endurance. Their exhaustion is restored only by much rest and especially long sleeps. Many of these young people are forced to labor far beyond their strength, but because of their apparently well nourished and robust appearance, they do not get the sympathy they deserve. The basic principle of strength, is in the basic elements that the red blood cells have built up from having all the true protoplasmic elements present, that go to make up a healthy blood cell; but in pseudo-psora many of these elements are in excess and others deficient, thus limes and silicates are deficient in these patients, while we usually find the muscular and adipose tissues greatly in excess.

SKIN

We have already stated that all skin eruptions are either secondary or tertiary expressions of miasmatic action. The skin is the mirror or the reflector of the internal stress, the internal dynamis, the internal workings of this human machine. It has in the skin, its reflectors, its kaleidoscope, its kinetoscopic views of its internal movements, and its multiple shadings of disease, its lights and its shadows that go to make up a picture, thrown upon that human canvas, the skin, showing much of perverted life action in the organism.

Pathologically speaking, we look upon the outer man for signs, for markings or pencilings that tell of the kind of life within the organism itself. Sometimes these pencilings are like shadowgraphs, showing only faint tracings of the presence of a latent miasm, and again they may be well defined and well developed even to physiological changes of form, color and proportions.

When we look upon these lesions of the skin as local states or changes in itself, we simply ignore that co-operative principle that rules throughout the organism as a whole, and we attribute that power to a part and not to that which governs the whole. Therefore our therapeutic efforts are themselves misdirected and instead of directing the perverted life forces aright, we misguide them, bringing about nothing but *Babylon* or confusion.

It was upon the skin that Hahnemann first saw the true psoric vesicle; it was there he first became familiar with psora as it came forth or receded under the potent influence of the applied law (similia). It was there that the mysterious veil was rent or lifted and he was permitted to look into the psoric mystery and see the true etiology of disease. It was in his study of disease that he saw the *hemorrhage*, the *menorrhagia*, the *persistent local pain*, the *abnormal growth*, the *vertigo*, the *nervous attack*, the *spasm*, the *convulsion*, the *mania*, the *moral insanity* and a thousand other things that might be cited, disappear forever, as a local expression of an eruptive disease presented itself upon the surface of the skin; and as he watched these multiple presentations that appear often so mysteriously from within, so we today look for relief and for cure through the same natural processes or metamorphosis of similia.

The skin of a psoric patient is dry, rough, dirty or unhealthy looking, and not only that but it has an unwashed appearance, and the more you bathe it the rougher it becomes, as it can not endure water. In pseudo-psora, this is magnified in such diseases as eczema fissum and itching of the skin. Pruritis of the skin is always a psoric symptom.

There is very little suppuration in psoric skin diseases; they are apt to be dry, with scanty suppuration, seropurulent and occasionally bloody. Quite often the eruptions are papular in form, accompanied with intense itching. Sometimes the eruptions are papulo-vesicular in form, accompanied with intense itching. If pustular or vesicular, they are nowhere as marked in their suppurative process, as we find in the pseudo-psoric. The syphilitic eruptions are found about the joints, flexures of the body or arranged in circular groupings, rings or segments of circles. The color is significant, copper colored or raw-ham color, brownish or very red at their base. Psoric eruptions are as a rule the color of the skin, unless an inflammatory process is present. There is no itching in the syphilitic and very little soreness, itching is wholly a psoric symptom, the vesicle is also a psoric lesion when found in non-syphilitic cases. The scales and crusts of syphilis are always thick and heavy, while those of psora are thin, light, fine and small and usually quite general over the affected part; for instance, if the scalp is affected in psora, the scaly condition is quite universal, while in other conditions, like syphilis or sycosis, it is patchy or in circumscribed spots. Of course, such diseases as psoriasis have to be differentiated. Often the skin loses all moisture and becomes exceedingly dry and free from oil or from the sebaceous secretions; we recognize it by the touch in psora. If it is very oily or greasy, we will find the sycotic element present or the pseudo-psoric. Skin affections with glandular envolvement will necessarily have the syphilitic or the tubercular element to conform with the glandular envolvement. When we look into such skin diseases as Ichthyosis (fish skin), we will find all the chronic miasms present, and where we find them all present, we usually find an incurable skin disease, especially if hereditary.

In Ichthyosis we see the dryness of psora and the squamæ of syphilis, and often the moles and warty eruptions are present, showing the sycotic element. In the varicose veins we find the tubercular taint predominates and it is in these patients we see the varicose ulcer, the last skin lesion to make its appearance in a case of ancient or hereditary syphilis, that has already become and now is, largely pseudo-psora. In ecchymosis, or in fact, any form of purpora, we can easily recognize a pseudo-psoric basis. Even in continued fevers like typhoid, we see this in the petechial hemorrhage into the skin. The wondrous variations that we find in eczema are in themselves a miasmatic study and often a great problem to decipher as to their miasmatic origin, from the papular eruption of psora to the pustule of the pseudo-psoric. In eczema exfoliatia, we see all the chronic miasms reflected therein and more particularly the sycotic element. We often see them all present in such diseases as erysipelas, carcinoma, epithelioma, lupus; lupus always has the three miasms and the features of each are easily recognizable to the experienced student of miasmatics. In acute exanthematous diseases, we can readily detect the tubercular patient from psoric by the severity of the attack, the appearance of the eruption and the tendency to secondary complications. This is clearly seen in measles, scarlet fever and such diseases. Not infrequently we have cases where the vitality of the patient is so low that we are unable to assist nature in bringing forth the eruption. This lowered vitality is always dependent on a tubercular dyscrasia. Herpes are found in the tubercular and some forms, such as circinnatus and herpes zoster have a sycotic basis, which we have to deal with largely in our treatment of these cases. In most cases of litchen, I have seen this sycotic principle combined with a tubercular taint. Many forms of urticaria can be traced to patients who have a tubercular dyscrasia. Psoriasis has a syco-psoric foundation and this fact has been recognized by a number of pathologists ; of course they call it a lithic state, which means the same thing ; variola and that class of diseases comes under the same catalogue. In diseases of excretion and secretion, such as Hyperidrosis and Bromidrosis, we see them only in the pseudo-psoric. Anidrosis is of course psoric, but will be found also in the pseudo-psoric. In urticaria we see the psoric element cropping out in the pruritis, yet it is in the individual with a tubercular taint and especially in women and children, that we see the more marked manifestations of urticaria. In abscesses and ulcers of the skin, this element is always uppermost and of course is active in their production. Freckles upon the skin are also quite significant to these fine, smooth, clear and transparent skinned patients, with an underlying pseudo-psoric taint. Psora has no such a smooth, clear skin as we find in these freckled patients ; indeed, psora has just the reverse ; a dirty, dingy, muggy skin, showing more or less papules and other eruptions. Goose flesh, commonly so called (cutis-ancerino) is another pseudo-psoric state, induced in these easily chilled patients, who are disturbed by the slightest chilling of the surface of the body, causing the superficial circulation to recede. Indeed, their cutamous circulation is very easily disturbed, inducing colds and catarrhal conditions of the head and throat. Of course psora may be at the bottom of much of this, but what I wish to emphasize is, that this condition of the skin is found in the pseudo-psoric individual; Nat. mur. Hep., Silica and such remedies are a good illustration of this pseudo-psoric manifestation. Injuries to the skin, especially slight injuries, heal readily in the ordinary psoric patient, with little or no pus formation, but it is in the pseudo-psoric individual that we see the abscess arise, the ulcerative process, the copious formation and elimination of this pus element, far beyond that necessary in the ordianary healing process. The same thing can be seen in our surgical operations; if we study the miasmatic basis of our patient, we will readily see why we have stitch abscesses in one case of abdominal operation and not in another; by no means are the antiseptic precautions always at fault or the suture material to blame. These cases come where the closest attention has been given to these facts and where nothing has been left undone to make the work a success. If the sycotic element is present as it is in the majority of abdominal operations, the possibility of stitch abscesses or pus products is greatly increased. A few experiences of this kind, together with a careful study of the miasmatic basis of our patients, will reveal this truth fully to our minds. Condylomata anywhere in the skin have sycosis or are of a syco-syphilitic nature.

In gangrene or gangrenous spots upon the skin of an idiopathic nature, we will of course always find a syphilitic or tubercular taint in the organism unless it is due to medicinal causes. In the dry gangrene, of which I have seen a great number of cases, a syphilitic infection was always present. Of course this may not always be the case, but it has been my experience to find this true in every case I have examined. Insect stings from a bug or bee, etc., and like causes, affect these patients with a tubercular taint very decidedly, even more than they affect those suffering from a simple psoric condition. It is surprising, the reflexes that develop in these cases; this is also true in patients suffering from punctured wounds of the skin; they do not recover from these slight injuries and are so liable to tetanus, spasms, or some severe reflex condition that endangers life.

Impetigo is another skin eruption of an inflammatory origin and will be found, as a rule, in pseudo-psoric individuals. I have made a careful study of this disease and find it largely in these patients. Its unknown contagious principle, however, is likely to be found, from the fact that these psoric patients take every disease that comes along (as we often remark), whatever may be the basic element in its origin.

New growths are in themselves a life study; when I speak of new growths, I mean all of a benign or malignant origin; all are due to miasmatic origin and to miasmatic influence upon the life force. When we speak of new growths, we mean of course, false growths, abnormal growths, or falsifications in parts and organs of the body.

A perfectly healthy organism can and does nothing else than to fulfil and carry out its normal function in the organism. It is only when that function is disturbed that pathology is given its birth. Pathology is but a wrong way or a wrong movement in the life action, hence new growths are the results of false movements or false action, prolonged, of course. Now, while their primary or predisposing cause may lie in psora, we do not find false growths or abnormal growths in those patients that have no other miasmatic basis but psora. A close investigation will reveal other miasms to be present and to be co-operative with psora, and these are either the tubercular or pseudopsoric element, often the sycotic combined.

In lupus, we see all the miasms, both in the erythematous and the vulgaric forms.

In epithelioma, the pseudo-psoric is the prominent miasm or the tubercular ; it is seen in the tuberculosis of lupus, also. The sycotic poisoning always lends new vigor to any malignancy. These are the incurable cases that have all the chronic miasms co-operative in abnormal growths. How often we have noticed that people suffering from tumors, whether of a benign or malignant nature, have a thin, pale skin, or if the body is well nourished, there is a certain clearness about it that is characteristic of a tubercular taint ; in the skin there is also a certain transparency, the blood vessels, especially the veins and capillaries, reflecting through the tissues as they lie beneath. It is in the tubercular or the syphilitic that we see much scarring and an increase of cicatricial tissue; quite often the cicatrix is atrophic, or it seems to lie below the level of the surface of the skin, as if it was not completely filled in. It is in the tubercular constitution that such scarring and deformity after ulcres, burns and scalds are found and the ulcers preceding the scar are usually deep, destructive and have a copious exudation of pus.

In leprosy, we have another destructive process of tubercular origin, even to vicious and unprecedented deformity. It is in the lymphatic temperament, a temperament in which the tubercular element thrives very luxuriantly, and especially is this true when the lymphatic temperament is beginning to fully show itself (fortieth year) that we see our malignancies come to the surface. It is in the lymphatic that we find such a rich soil for that sexual disease, gonorrhea and syphilis; it is in the lymphatic that the glandular system is so frequently involved and in which rapid and destructive processes take place. It is in the tubercular we have so much difficulty to eradicate from it syphilis (acquired) or gonorrhœa. It is in these systems that we have the prolonged tertiary processes and the tertiary lesions, that are persistent and stubborn. The gonorrhœa runs into a gleety discharge and strictures, pockets and metastasis forms, or we have metastasis to the ovaries, broad ligaments, tubes, uterus, rectum and all such complications with which we so frequently meet. It is the tubercular diathesis that complicates all our skin diseases and make them so difficult to remove. In the fibrous growths, we have all the miasms present, the displacement of other tissues for the dense, white and fibrous formations which we find in fibroma, which is due to one of the deepest and most profound miasmatic changes conceivable. Not long ago I saw a case of skin disease in a young woman of about 30 years of age which consisted of fibrous growths all over the body from the size of a large pea to that of a cherry; on close examination of the case I found all the miasms present; although all were of hereditary form, there was the dilated capillaries of the tubercular or the pseudopsoric; the dry, dirty skin of psora; the verruca of sycosis; the moles with their hairy tufts of syphilis; the red pinhead sized sycotic mole, besides she had the family history of tuberculosis on her mother's side. It would require years of treatment to make any impression on such cases, in fact, many if not all of them are incurable. In *Nevus* or congenital markings of the skin, we see all these miasmatic elements present; these warty, pigmented growths, these wine-colored patches, all have an underlying stratum of sycosis, as well as of *pseudopsora*. We then see them all also in elephantiasis, in the vegetable parasitical pest as seen in tinea. We see the animal parasite in the psoric and pseudo-psoric; probably no skin diseases show such a special form of sycotic expression as we find in Tinea barbæ, Tinea tonsuraus, Tinea vesicular and similar diseases of the face, scalp and other parts of the body; when they are suppressed, they develop further sycotic difficulties of a sycotic nature.

Many forms of pruritis have all the miasms present and in severe cases we always recognize psora and sycosis, especially those developing about the sexual organs, or anus, and nose. I have seen some of these cases, especially those of anus and the rectum, so severe as to almost drive the patient to distraction; when the sycotic element was counteracted by a suitable remedy, the patient got immediate relief. Medorrhinum has often done this for me and there are many other remedies to be thought of, such as *Abrotanum, Aeusculus, Nat. mur., Rhus Tox, Rhus. Ven., Sabadilla, Sepia, Agaricus, Cannabis Sat., Dolichos, Gambogia*, and others. (See Pruritis, page 206 to 213, DISEASES AND THERAPEUTICS OF THE SKIN.).

Eruptions suppressed by local means have produced, according to Hahnemann, the following diseases and conditions that were observed in his own practice: Dyspnea, two died of suffocation, five had difficult breathing and general anasarca, where itch was suppressed; one had infiltration of the pericardium; one had pneumonia and died in about a week; many have died of chest diseases, says Hahnemann, where *scabies acarus* was suppressed; Tinea, suppressed, has produced asthma, convulsions and death in a number of cases. All throughout Hahnemann's experiences, the suppression of pseudopsoric eruptions produced hemorrhages, spasms, convulsions, coma and death. It has also produced reflexes of all kinds, nervous disorders, asthma, paralysis, stomach and intestinal disorders, catarrhal conditions, chronic coughs and such disorders. Where the tubercular taint is present we have had dyspnea, infiltration of the lungs, pneumonia, chronic lung affections, tuberculosis and especially chest diseases.

Where sycotic skin diseases were suppressed, we have had malignant growths, especially where the psoric taint was marked or the tubercular element was clearly present, cancer, lupus, vulgaris, and lupus erythematosis, cardiac difficulties, carditis, pericarditis, dropsy of the pericardium, valvular lesions of all kinds, epilepsy, apoplexy and lesions in all parts of the body. How careful we should be not to suppress any local manifestations of one of these chronic miasms, knowing not what the outcome may be; for possibly by so doing, we may have started the organism in its downward course to death, instead of directing it in the right direction, whereby it might receive the blessing of its healer, the true physician, and not his curse. Then let our work show for itself, let it demonstrate that it is of law, by its vivifying refreshing, recreating, uplifting, encouraging and healing process in the suffering one ; let the patient speak for the true process of healing by the cures we make ; yes, let the new power and new vigor given to the lagging life forces, *answer; God is in this work and it is His way, for His way is the way of law.*

"It is impossible," says Hahnemann, "that a rational

physician, after these examples shining clear as the sun, should still continue to assail the body as hitherto done." Then let us draw together, after having read this work, and if we can not fully imitate the Master Hahnemann, let us at least make an effort to know this law of cure, which like Portia's blessing, "blesseth him that gives and him that takes," for it becomes us better than a crown.

"Humanity is an army on the march," says Savage. "Many of them are sick." If the unscientific methods of today continue, the whole army will soon be fit subjects for the hospital or the camp.

When we take into consideration the false cures and the suppressive measures used in the eager attempt to satisfy, or to show results that approach in some degree the semblance of a cure, together with the lust for gold that has so lamentably taken hold of the physician of today, who should, above all men, be free from the power of its fetters and bands, little wonder that we desire a reform.

When humanity falls, we should lift them up, irrespective of nationality, caste, class, color, or race, for all are humanity and all are sick from the same cause, and have the same weaknesses, the same sufferings and deserve the same pity and the same help, for the same God ruleth over all, and if we are his true physicians, then these are all our children and we are subject to their cry for help.

If we would know the truth as taught by Hahnemann, we must get away from the influence of those teachers who have no faith, no experience and no knowledge of this law of cure. We must put ourselves under the influence of, and in personal contact with, men of large faith and of broad knowledge of this law, and who are enthusiastic in advancing the truth, who live out this truth in their practice and who will not yield to the temptation to resort to those uncertain methods, experiments and makeshifts of tradition or of modern medicine.

With such a foundation, we are ready to build our superstructure and do justice and honor to the cause of Homœopathy.

If our children (students) call for bread, shall we feed them stones? No, we can not satisfy their hunger with false doctrines, and should we attempt it the reflection is forever cast upon the false teacher and his false doctrines.

Friends of Homœopathy, wake up! The time has come for your light to shine. There are a few leaders who are working with all their might for the truth they represent. We can not all be leaders, but we can at least be supporters of those who are, lending a helping hand. False prophets are on every hand and we must "keep watch and ward," for as one has said, "eternal vigilance is the price of liberty."

There is no Golden Age coming to us; we must make it ourselves; the prophetic inspiration must be in you that have the light within you. Then let us keep our lamps burning at their full brightness, speaking the truth, living the truth and sealing it by our workmanship through the law, letting the voice of the healed one echo an answer down through the ages, so that the coming generations may know that we were lights in this world of darkness, and that we were known by our light.

We must have a greater and a larger faith, for true knowledge is only born of faith; sin, error, and confusion come in when faith goes out, and man recedes back to his own reasonings, "which are vain and imaginative."

The Greeks were the wisest people of their age, and even today their knowledge is our classics, yet we see that "the world by wisdom knew not God" (1 Cor. 1 : 21). When Paul the Apostle visited Athens, that great center of learning, he saw a sculptured image to an unknown God (which God was the true God) yet, through their wisdom they had lost sight of Him, therefore knew Him not. So the wisdom of this world comes in a cloud to overshadow the light, and we lose sight of God's laws and His principles, thus, in our blindness, we create false principles and false methods to take the place of truth. This is just what has taken place with the teaching of Hahnemann. Men would displace them, even his *mighty Organon of principle*, for their vain, unscientific reasonings and imaginings, until the teachings of these false prophets bring us as slaves to Babylon, until our Israel of power and truth would vanish from the earth. Then it is that our death processes multiply and pathology becomes more complex, disease more difficult to cure, and we become vassals to makeshifts ; the splints and the bandages of tradition are returned to us and we are disrobed of our former power to heal the sick, because we have lost sight of the basic principles of our law. When law disappears, doubt comes upon the throne and with doubt comes darkness and the vanishing of light.

A true Homœopathic education, however, knows no doubt ; faith takes the place of doubt, for nothing is brought into that education that savors of doubt ; nothing is brought into it but what strengthens our faith and builds up and makes strong. As we advance in its knowledge, every doubt disappears, every false teaching that we may have hitherto believed, is expunged. A new revelation comes to us. As we become followers of law, we become followers of light until we are lifted up beyond the clouds and misty exhalations of the world's knowledge, and as we enter the doorway of truth we see the falsity of all that which is not in harmony with Hahnemann's *Organon* of medicine, and with his precepts and principles. What I mean by world knowledge is the knowledge which we call empiricism, which has only man's experience behind it ; a thing not to be accepted alone in medicine. Mechanics is built on true principles, and has power, and is in agreement with true science and the mechanical laws. "It is the testimony of the few," says Dr. P. P. Wells, "who make and observe experiments which constitute the additions to the sum of human knowledge, as possessed by the many." This should not be so, but, nevertheless, it is true, yet how zealous are these men who do investigate for themselves; they become all of one mind and one accord, by virtue of all having the truth, for truth makes them as of one mind and as one man. Nothing but truth unifies, and when we take hold of truth, we place ourselves in the pathway of divine circuit, whereby we are able to analyze law, which is the wisdom of our Creator. Now, knowing law, we become as an Archimedes of power, drawing from the central source of power by our obedience to the demands of law; but being without law, we are simply powerless, a mere nothing, a vessel beached upon the sands, void of power. In fact, our ability in any sphere of life, is in proportion as we comply with, or as we draw upon law.

To be governed by these principles of Homœopathy is to be governed by truth; to be governed by truth is to be governed by law and to be governed by law is to be governed by Omnipotence.

Every student of Homœopathy is a student of nature, studying the phenomena of natural laws, and scientists in the laboratories of the force world, comparing the laws of biogenesis with the laws of similia, so that "every new development makes us stronger in the faith." Law is a something to be hated by an unlawful man; but, to the one who loves law, it speaks in whispers, yet loud enough to be heard by that humble listener, and in a language that is not foreign to him, yea, though often it is only in a symbol or a cipher.

As we apply law to disease, we become acquainted with these mysterious movements of disease; thus we know them as perverted law movements and changes, through perversions in the life force; and so, as we appeal to law, we can scientifically apply it to these perverted movements and changes in what is known as disease, for we call into effect all the forces governed by that law. The truth is this, he feels that he is ever "standing in the omnipresence of law and it has taken possession of him." It is guiding and directing him into these strange and mysterious by-ways of perverted life action, which he, through his limited reasonings otherwise can not follow, indeed he would become lost in this labyrinth of perversions and changes, due often to heredity alone. Law, you see, then, lifts that veil and enables us to see into that which seemed impenetrable and closed forever from our vision; thus we are led on from truth to truth, from mystery to even greater mystery, until life becomes clearly manifest in law. Our cures of disease are not to be found in Aconite, Arsenic, Apis and Aloes alone, but in their application to disease through the law of similia. Similia is not a disease nor a remedy nor a pathy, but a law. These miasmatic forces are in this way made plain as we study them from this standpoint, and we are prepared to give a reason for these many manifestations of disease, for we become viewers of nature through the telescopes of law. By diving down into the very spirit of things, we are enabled to awaken a spirit of research in others, so that they take a part with us, and these things that have ever been a mystery to us, heretofore, become intelligible, yea, we get a genetic view of things, untrammeled by prejudice, and truth becomes an exact correspondence in its subjective and objective relations. In this way we can open up doors of truth that have been barred during all time. Hahnemann did this as he brought forth his mystery of the miasms and the law of similia. The world often frowns upon this truth, but it shines all the brighter for it, and like the diamond, throws out its light from every angle. The influence of similia steals over us gently through this wonderful law and the law is fulfilled in itself. It expunges the miasmatic taint and through its creative power, it creates health, bringing forth all the attributes of health and strength. Indeed "Homœopathy partakes of that great pulse of nature that beats against the barriers of materialism." It is the pulse of love, and with each throb comes a new genesis, a new life.

From the true scientist nature cannot keep hidden her secrets, indeed her secrets and her mysteries are only hidden from him who tramples upon her laws and carest not to know her as she should be known. But to him who is honest and who earnestly endeavours to understand the truths of Homœopathy, all these truths are made manifest. No language is too old for him to read, it speaks to him in tongues of fire and he is allowed to escape from the "hear-says" of uncertainty in his study of life and disease ; so we are brought face to face with the true *Shekinah* in man and the secret of the diseased *ego* is made manifest.

HOW TO STUDY THIS WORK

In order to get a perfect understanding of this work careful study should be made of the history and action of psora and pseudo-psora, which is to be found in the first half of this work, included under pages 9 and 164. There should also be a careful analysis of each expression of the miasms given therein; this is necessary in order to be able to discern their presence in the organism. We are now prepared to take up the study of the miasms under the different headings as found under the Rubrics, pages 164 to 267. This study will be found to be an interesting one if taken from a clinical standpoint, the truth is we can only have these facts impressed on our minds by a clinical comparison and experience. As our patients come before us we should procure from them as clear and perfect a clincal history as is possible, going back into the family history of the father, mother, sisters, brothers and not forgetting the clinical history of uncles and aunts, which is sometimes of more importance than that of the father or mother, when we come to consider heredity. Sycosis and syphilis is of course never to be forgotten, whether it be in the acquired form or indirectly through heredity. We are to look for psora in the mental phenomena, in desires, aversions and habits of life; in their fears, longings, cravings, etc. We see it in the skin as we look upon it or touch it. The tubercular element can be seen in the circulatory system, in the arterial and venus expressions. In the physiology of the body in general, in the shape of the head, face, ears, nose, mouth, lips, teeth and in a thousand ways, as we come to study the different rubrics. All these things will have to be considered when we come to study a mixed miasm, therefore a comprehensive knowledge is necessary in order to discern their presence in latent forms in the organism. Each miasm has its own peculiar history, its physiological expressions, its mental phenomena, its aggravations of time and circumstances, its secondary and tertiary manifestations upon mucous surfaces or upon the skin. The repertory at the back of the book will also assist you very much in this work. If sycosis is present you will not be able possibly to get a perfect picture in all cases until you are in possession of the second volume* of this work, which will follow this in a short time, and will deal wholly with the sycotic miasm and its therapeutics.

THE AUTHOR.

*See part II, Chronic Miasms—Sycosis Vol. II.

REPERTORY

	PAGES.
Absolute in disease, seen in miasmatic action	42
Antipathic schools	10,11,39
Bacillus, declared to be *causus-morbi*	79
Bacillus, an appendage to the schools of Pathology	79
Bacteria, latent	77
Bacteria medium of conveying disease	77
Bacteria, knowledge of does not lessen mortality	79
Battle between dynamics of drug and disease	27
Bond of subversive force with the life force	42,43
Cachexias	26,37,148
Cell deified	10
Cell—the unit of life	10
Conflict of life force with miasms	93,94
Confined—we are to the study of phenomena in disease	95,96,97
Diathesis	149
Diathesis tubercular	23,57
Disease—a vibratory change	16
Disease—how shall we deal with it	114,118
Disease—Specific and malignant	23
Disease treated from a miasmatic standpoint	136,137
Disease when treated by local measures	132,133
Dr. Hughs' teachings	52,53,54
Dual—action of life force	91,101
Dynamics behind every expression of life	61
Dynamics—put a dynamic force in their physiology	104
Errors we are liable to make	34,35,36
Fibrous growths	267
Gonorrhœa	121,122,129

PAGES.

Hahnemann..16, 17, 18, 19, 21, 29, 31, 32, 34, 36, 51, 64, 65, 66, 67, 91, 101, 103, 109, 137, 209, 268, 269
Hahnemann discovered the miasmatic cause of disease.... 27
Homœopathy, a complete science 51,52
Homœopathy, distinction between false and true 52,53
Homœopathy remedy covers all phenomena in disease 77
Homœopathic education 273
Humanity—an army on the march 270
Humanity—when it falls 270
Idiosyncrasy enters into our hopes, fears, longings, cravings, moods and manners of life 149,150
Idiosyncrasy—its relationship to barometric changes.... 151
Idiosyncrasy—its relationship to desires, foods stimulants..153
Idiosyncrasy—its relationship to electrothermal changes.. 151
Idiosyncrasy—its relationship to miasms 152,158
Idiosyncrasy—its relationship to music 153
Idiosyncrasy—its relationship to predisposition 153,154
Inhibition, peripheral 25
Inhibitary point 25,26
Inhibitary point of disease set up by suppression of the miasm 25,26,27
Inhibitary center 97,98
Introduction 9,10,11
Knowledge of disease found in a study of the miasm.... 115
Koch, Dr., teachings 162
Law—a revelation 47,106,272,274
Law—a witness against itself 47
Law—all things are under it...................... 47,48
Law—all movements governed by.................. 48
Law governing life 80
Law—its application 275
Law of similias 63,64
Law of similias co-operative with that which disturbs life 172
Law—physiological 48,49,50

	PAGES.
Law—rules all invisible things	106
Law—uniformity of	95
Life—life force a dynamas	61,97
Life—inner life process	137
Life—magnified by continues by normal nerve impulses	84
Life—nature the complement of	108
Life—only understood by a study of its laws	106
Life—perverted life brought under law	107,108
Life—perverted life brought under law by anti-miasmatic treatment	105,106
Life—principles govern all truth	116
Life—workings of its invisible potens	84,85,86
Mental symptoms, basic	50
Miasmatic action	90
Miasms—acute could not exist, but for the chronic	75
Miasms—business is to kill	27,28
Miasms—causes illustrating	120-123
Miasms—co-workers with sin and death	28
Miasms—how aroused	29,30
Miasms—opposing forces in life force	108,109
Miasms—not to be treated locally	103,104
Miasms—suppression in the different forms	109-139
Miasms—the result of suppression	113,114
Miasms—the presence of in the organism	118-121
Miasms—the sin process	80-84
Miasms—the work of	28,29
Miasms—their action in the organism	44,45
Miasms—their action on mental sphere	44-50
Miasms—why should we know them	11-14
Organon	10,11,34,94,112,142
Pathological—prescription based on it	104,105
Pathological—does not fully represent disease	59,60
Pathological—fully understood by a knowledge of the miasms	70-73
Pathological in general	40,53,60,61

                                                              PAGES.
Pathological—finished work of perverted life action....58,59
Pathological—why should it constantly change.......... 58
Pathology—built by the perverted life force........86,87
Pathology—can it do more for us today............... 72
Pathology—its office 88
Pathology—its lesions not first cause in disease.......... 89
Pathology—its polymorphic presentations............ 69
Pathology—mixed miasms give up complex pathology..57,58
Pathology—mystery of disease hidden in the miasms..135,136
Pathology—not nourished by pathology.............. 64
Pathology—nothing but false eliminative points in disease88,89
Pathology—only understood by a knowledge of the miasms
                                                         70-73
Pathology—produced by disturbed function 84
Pathology—pathognomonic, symptoms of 59
Pathology—seen through the potential..............93,94
Pathology—Virchow's cellular 82,83
Potential 85,86,87,88,90,95,96
Predisposition—its relations to artificial disease........ 156
Predisposition—its relation to contagious diseases...... 156
Predisposition—its relation to disease in general..43,95,154
                                            155,157,158,265
Predisposition—its relation to the miasms.............. 157
Predisposition—its relation to temperament.......... 154
Psora—abdomen 226,229
Psora—aggravation of time 127
Psora—an arrest of elimination..................... 132
Psora—attacks relieved by some eliminative processes.... 172
Psora—bond with other miasms 23
Psora—bowels 230-238
Psora—brain stasis following suppression.............. 123
Psora—change of character 174,175
Psora—chest 202,221
Psora—chronic miasm 141,142
Psora—desires 201-204

	PAGES.
Psora—epilepsy of	174
Psora—eruptions	144
Psora—extremities	250-257
Psora—Heart	222-226
Psora—importance of	29,30
Psora—in general	35,36,40,41
Psora—local developments	30,31
Psora—records of	143,144,149,159
Psora—sensations	209
Psora—sexual sphere	241-250
Psora—skin	257-269
Psora—stomach symptoms	203-212
Psora—universal action of	26,27
Psora—urinary organs	239-241
Suppression—a single symptom	137-140
Suppression—an arrest of elimination	132
Suppression—cases illustrating	120-123
Suppression—dependent upon miasms present in the organism	118-121
Suppression—increases physiological stress	101-102
Suppression—internal disease formed	132
Suppression—malarial by quinine	125,126
Suppression—mental phenomena	123
Suppression—nothing can be suppressed but miasms	145
Suppression—resistance to life force	114,115
Suppression—reverses physiological action	137
Suppression—repeated involves new centers	98-100
Suppression—ring-worm	129
Suppression—the power of	169
Suppression—signs of	118-120
Suppression—syphilis	87,88
Suppression—ways of	109,110,111,113,114
Skin diseases	257-264
Skin diseases—color of in syphilis	260
Skin diseases—ecchymosus	261

	PAGES.
Skin diseases—gangrenous spots on	263
Skin diseases—herpes	261
Skin diseases—herpes zoster	261
Skin diseases—Ichthyosis	260
Skin diseases—Impetigo	264
Skin diseases—lumpus	161
Skin diseases—new growths	164
Skin diseases—pathology of	258
Skin diseases—psora	251,259,261

Sycosis ....41, 46, 69, 70, 75, 113, 118, 120, 121, 123, 128, 130, 131, 140, 146, 164, 169, 173, 174, 178, 179, 181, 188, 222, 223, 224, 265, 267, 276.

Syphilis and psora the parent of the tubercular diathesis..78

Syphilis in general ..46, 80, 160, 161, 162, 163, 164, 165, 167, 169, 170, 174, 177, 178, 179, 180, 181, 182, 184, 185, 186, 187, 190, 192, 193, 195, 198, 200, 203, 211, 214, 222, 230, 231, 243, 250, 251, 252, 255, 259, 264.

Syphilis—its dynamic origin	87-89
Sin—transgression of the law	133
Sin—wages of	133
Sin—process	140
Stasis of disease may produce abnormal growths	97,98
Teachings in the different schools	51,52
Temperament	30,154,155,156
Tubercular—process	80,81,135

Tubercular—suggestions of 28, 68, 69, 83, 99, 114, 121, 135, 160, 162, 163, 182, 183, 184, 185, 186, 187, 189, 190, 191, 193, 194, 196, 197, 198, 201, 202, 208, 209, 212, 217, 219, 220, 221, 226, 227, 231, 236, 237, 238, 240, 241, 242, 244, 245, 246, 247, 248, 249.

X-Ray	21,111

THE CHRONIC MIASMS

SYCOSIS

BY

J. HENRY ALLEN, M. D.

AUTHOR OF
"DISEASES AND THERAPEUTICS OF THE SKIN"

PROFESSOR OF
DISEASES OF THE SKIN AND MIASMATICS
HERING MEDICAL COLLEGE
CHICAGO, ILL.

VOLUME II

B. JAIN PUBLISHERS (P) LTD.
NEW DELHI-110055

DEDICATION

TO
THAT DEVOTED BAND OF PHYSICIANS,
NATIVES OF INDIA AND GRADUATES OF HERING COLLEGE,
WHO ARE SPREADING THE BENEFICENT TRUTHS OF HOMEOPATHY
AMONG THE THERAPEUTICALLY BENIGHTED MILLIONS OF THEIR
NATIVE COUNTRY, THIS WORK ON MIASMATIC DISEASES IS
DEDICATED, WITH HIS BEST WISHES FOR
THEIR SUCCESS, BY

THE AUTHOR.

PREFACE

In presenting this second volume of the CHRONIC MIASMS, (SYCOSIS) to the profession, we trust it will receive the same welcome as did Vol. 1, PSORA AND PSEUDO-PSORA.

In the production of Volume 1, we had the teachings of Hahnemann to aid us and the writings of his many followers to sustain us with their volumes of research and their many established truths, but in the construction of this work, we had but scant data to draw from. Hahnemann has given us but a page or two on the subject SYCOSIS. The literature is meager even in the Regular School of Medicine. That which has been brought forth, deals largely, if not wholly with the primary or gonorrhœal stage. Many no doubt have realized to some extent, its depth of action and the degree to which this terrible miasm has effected the human race. They have read between the lines in the great book of experience and have seen the profundity of its action, its persistent nature and its progressive movements and inroads upon the life force, yet have not brought their knowledge to the light of publicity. They have rather kept it under the proverbial bushel. I trust that my readers, after having read this work, will add to the literature of this subject, a knowledge of which, is of such vital importance to the human race and to the medical profession throughout the world, for what is of interest to the human race, should be of vital interest to the profession and vice versa.

The theory of the CHRONIC MIASMS, as being the sum total of the causes of chronic diseases, meets with two strong opposing forces, first from the pathological, material or chemical therapeutist who views life from its material side, and who is looking for finite or material causes in all that disturbs the living organism; secondly, from the therapeutists of symptomatology (the symptom doctor), they have their minds focused upon Section 18 of the Organon, therefore they maintain that the totality of the symptoms in a given case, should govern the prescriber in making a selection in every case, independent of any chronic miasm that might lie behind the grouping.

While we maintain these principles of the law of totality as the only guide in making such a selection, we also insist that the remedy that meets the true requirements of the law governing our therapeutics, should cover the symptoms of the active miasm, and especially is this true in cases of mixed or pseudo miasms. The author has dealt with this subject quite exhaustively and trusts that he has made himself clear to his readers on this important phase of the work.

The sycotic symptoms presented in the different stages of the disease, have been carefully observed and many times verified, so that we feel quite confident they will endure the test of further investigation. And we know that time and further acquaintance with the nature of sycotic diseases, will greatly add to their numbers and value.

In writing the therapeutics of this work, we have endeavored to give the indications of each remedy in as brief and concise a manner as possible, not to burden the prescriber with too many symptoms. The therapeutic index in the back of this work, will greatly assist in making a comparison of the different remedies and in some degrees take the place of a repertory.

THE AUTHOR.

INDEX

	PAGES
Sycosis	9-81
Complications of Sycosis in the first stage	31-34
Secondary Sycosis	38-49
Suppression induced by operative measures	49-54
Suppression by medicated douches and the use of crude drugs	53-58
Coughs of Sycosis	59-60
Tertiary Stage	61-64
Tertiary lesions	64-81
Chronic Miasms	81-119
Treatment	119-132
Gonorrhœa	132-162
Ways of infection	138-141
Source of the disease	141-142
Symptoms and Mode of Attack	142-152
Gonorrhœa of Females	152-155
Chronic Gonorrhœa and Gleet	155-162
Bacteria, their origin	162-165
Therapeutics of Gonorrhœa	165-202
Materia Medica of the Urinary Tract and Sexual Sphere	202-254
Dysmenorrhœa	254-263
Therapeutics of Dysmenorrhœa	263-358
Leucorrhœa	358-365
Therapeutics of Leucorrhœa	365-417

THE CHRONIC MIASMS

SYCOSIS

If that which is set forth in Vol. I of this work is of vital interest to every physician who is desirous of looking into the mystery of disease and of knowing its true etiology, this volume ought to be of still greater interest, as it uncovers the true etiology of the diseases that are so prevalent today, permitting us to get at the fundamental principles of the very basis of the diseases we meet in daily practice. For every earnest and thoughtful physician must have seen before being long in practice, that there is something about the diseases he encounters, that makes them difficult to eradicate; something that, lying as a basis, makes disease stubborn, persistent and positive in its nature and difficult to cure. These cases and these principles we wish to deal with in this little work ; and in dealing with this dreadful miasmatic scourge that is wrecking and destroying the race as no other disease is (excepting that of tuberculosis), we will not speak of it from its historic standpoint, nor from any sociological point of view, but simply from a miasmatic basis, treating with many of the factors pertaining to its action upon the human organism. Other writers have written fully and clearly upon the subject of gonorrhœa, therefore, it will not be necessary for me to even describe to you a typical case of gonorrhœa, save as it relates to the subject of Sycosis. We will deal with it simply in the relation it bears to other miasms and to disease in general, both acute and chronic.

We must treat it then, not only from an etiological, pathological, pathogenetic and nosanic point of view, but must also study it carefully from its therapeutic side, looking closely into the dangers of the unscientific methods of treatment of this dreadful disease, and the grave danger that lies in suppressing it in any stage of its action.

It was Dr. Charles J. Hemple who said that "Disease is the totality of the effects by which we recognize or perceive the action of a peculiar order of subversive forces upon an organism which has been specially adapted, or prepared for their reception." Out of these subversive forces comes, either directly or indirectly, all that which is known as disease. Hahnemann has recognized three special forms which he has designated as Psora, Syphilis and Sycosis. This triune of the subversive forces also called the chronic miasmata, are the vicarious embodiment of the internal disease, each having its own peculiar type or character by which its sole purpose and effort is to conform the organism to its nature. Each of these forces becomes a creative force, and at no time is the life force able to free itself from the bond of any of them (either alone or in combination with the others), without some other assistance. Just how these subversive forces, Psora, Syphilis, or Sycosis, combine in the organism, or rather with the life force, can probably never be explained or accounted for.

It is true, however, that their introduction into the organism (which has undergone a process of adaptation capable of receiving them) is followed by an endless history of subversive changes and diseased phenomena peculiar to each type. This is shown in Psora, and still more clearly in Syphilis, whose history we are fully able to prophesy with all its multiplied and polymorphic lesions, from its initial physical expression in the organism to its tertiary destructive processes in the bony framework of the body itself. As this is true of Psora, and Syphilis, so it is also true of Sycosis. It has its primary, secondary and tertiary stages, and a world of phenomena peculiar to itself, accompanying each stage or setting of the disease. But a small number of our medical men today have any conception of the great depth and the degree of action of this specific miasm upon the organism, or the frequency with which it is met in practice. It is the *prima causa* of much of the suffering and of innumerable ailments to be met with every day in general or special practice.

Very few Homeopathic physicians today contest the fact that Hahnemann's psoric theory is true, and all those who have carefully and honestly given the subject study will bear me out in this statement. Few are the physicians who have not frequently recognized the sudden and mysterious appearance of disease in the human organism, coming as it seemed from nowhere, and developing out of no apparent cause, coming as it were out of the unknown, out of the invisible, remaining either permanently or temporarily a functional disturbance, or developing into innumerable or varied pathological states, often causing untold suffering, and many times endangering the life of the sufferer. Yet how few have come to any positive solution of the subject in their own mind. Hahnemann has solved the mysterious problem for us, and today if we will but listen to his words of wisdom, we will learn whence cometh that sudden pain, the rheumatism, the eczema, the ulcer, the papular eruption or any of the multiplied expressions of disease.

They surely develop from the disturbances of the life force, due wholly to the action or continued action of these chronic miasms of Hahnemann. Thus arises the papular eruption, the inflammatory processes, the stasis in internal organs, the cough, the spasm, the convulsion, even all the multiplied phenomena of mind and body, tabulated and known as *disease*. All this falsifying of life and its processes, this anatomical and physiological deflection from that which is true, can be reasonably and positively shown to be caused by, and to arise directly or indirectly, from the three chronic miasms—Psora, Syphilis, or Sycosis, either singly or combined with each other in various degrees of combination. The oldest of these subversive forces, we all agree, I believe, to be Psora ; it therefore becomes the basic miasm, the first cause of all disease in the human organism. But

THE CHRONIC MIASMS. 13

there are other chronic miasms than Psora to be studied, and the miasm of Syphilis is one of those whose far reaching dynamis, whose slow but sure destructive action, is well known to every healer of the sick; and how closely pathologists have studied the complex and almost endless phenomena that are presented throughout the course or stages of its prolonged history. Its slow progress, its persistent nature, whether it be of its pains, its ulcers, or its gummatous growths, or in whatever presentation it may come, we cannot but have noticed the positiveness of its bond with the life force.

Sycosis is not a new name for gonorrhoea, neither is it gonorrhoea in any sense of the word. The well-known specific urethritis, presents only in its initial stage, similar phenomena to that of Sycosis, and the history of the two diseases differs widely in their constitutional developments and progress. Gonorrhoea simplex is not a basic miasm, while Sycosis comprises one of the chronic miasms of Hahnemann, and next to Psora it is the most persistent of the great triune of the subversive forces, Syphilis, Sycosis and Psora. Sycosis, implanted on a rich pseudo-psoric soil, develops into one of the most formidable enemies of the race, whose destructive power and depth of action upon the organism cannot be expressed by any combination of words. What the pathologists of today call gonorrheal infection, is what we term Sycosis. But it is not an infection from a supposed gonorrheal catarrh, for gonorrhoea simplex does not affect the organism as does gonorrhœal Sycosis.

The early history of gonorrhoea simplex is a history of painful and spasmodic symptoms, and of decided vesical irritation, of chordee, and marked specific urethritis, while the history of a typical case of Sycosis in its initiatory stage is lacking in many of the above symptoms, and should the symptoms be present, they are so modified that a casual observer can readily distinguish between the two. As a rule in Sycosis very little pain is present—sometimes but not always there is a decided soreness and some tenderness is felt along the anterior surface of the first third of the organ. The patient experiences more or less burning at the meatus, but it never assumes that degree of severity experienced in the spasmodic or simple form of the disease. The catarrhal discharge in the sycotic form is scanty, and as a rule mucopurulent at a very early date. The color varies in the different cases, but it is generally a dirty colored pus, yellowish green, or a mixture of brown, yellow and green. Quite often it is offensive, and in many cases has a stale-fish, musty, or fish-brine odor, and it maintains this peculiar offensiveness more or less throughout the various stages of the disease.

Its incubative period is from five to ten days, and these patients early show more or less mental anxiety, with a desire to frequently examine the organ. These are the first symptoms to present themselves, and they frequently follow the disease throughout in its various phases, usually developing into an over-anxiousness as their condition. This very noticeable and undue desire to give special attention in their case is decidedly, if not emphatically, impressed upon the attending physician, and it frequently embarrasses him and hinders a cure. The patient's anxiety sometime forces the physician to resort to means unprofessional and against his better judgment in his haste to dry up or suppress the discharge, which the patient thinks is the embodiment of the disease.

In truth it is but the eliminative process, for when the discharge is suppressed, a secondary stage of the disease develops, characterized by stasis to internal organs, more manifest in the pelvic inflammation of women —a field so fruitful of late, to the work of the modern surgeon. Should the disease not be cured by constitutional treatment, it will by no means end with the secondary stage, but usually within a period of from one to three years, it passes into a tertiary form (or true Sycosis), which if not cured, may last the entire life of the patient. Quite frequently, however, the disease runs into some malignancy, such as scirrhus of the different organs of the body, or cystic degeneration, fibrous growths, stasis in internal organs, chronic rheumatism, and gouty conditions. This last may be shown by gouty concretions of the joints, gout of the heart, stomach, or any of the internal organs. Mania, insanity, and many other mental aberrations can be traced to a suppression of this miasm. In fact, our jails and our prisons are filled with these poor unfortunates, far outnumbering the victims of Syphilis. Sycosis is more potent than Syphilis as a cause of mental diseases, of moral insanity, and of those degenerative processes which form a basis for much of the criminality of our own country as well as that of Europe.

Sycosis may be said to be the most venereal of all venereal diseases, as it is seldom contracted (outside of gonorrhœal ophthalmia) in any other way than through sexual congress. It is a disease of lust in the broadest sense of the word, hence the appearance of the mental phenomena in its early history. That monarch of the mind, the Will, is overthrown. *He thinks, he wills, he acts, and out of that false triune develops the lust disease.* A precept of the decalogue is broken, and man falls by virtue of the breaking of that genetic principle which is an epitome of the character of his Creator, after whose image he was formed. He at once becomes a victim to the false and disintegrative power of broken law and the true physiological process at that moment ceases, and a false one is set up within that organism. Yea, all its processes, whether moral, spiritual, mental, or physical, are interfered with, and in some measure they at once take on a retrograde metamorphosis; the miasm (Sycosis) becomes a force co-existent with the life force; therefore, the *life forces* are from that moment propelled forward in the direction of its influence and power which is always unfavorable to the good of the organism. What was at first a mental process, an unholy thought, implants the seeds of death within the physical organism and its presence with the life force is first manifest in the members that violated that divine precept. At first the disturbing element is **functional** as it is in all disease, to become later on an **organic disease**, and the *fons et origo mali* of many of the diseases of today.

So generally is this miasm, Sycosis, distributed among adult males that it is estimated that fully eighty percent are affected by it. Of course this estimate includes the latent as well as the active forms. No wonder that so many of our women are sufferers from pelvic affections, rheumatism or chronic gout. This large proportion is without counting heredity, for the disease is congenital, as is Syphilis and Psora. This will be understood more fully as we proceed in the study of the subject.

The majority of married women suffer in some way from Sycosis, either from the suppressed or imperfectly cured forms. Children born of such parents invariably show some form or manifestation of the disease and not infrequently ophthalmia neonatorum. If they escape this dread disease, they suffer with colic almost from the moment of their birth; not the ordinary flatulent colic, but one of a severe and specific nature, continuing often from one to three months after birth. The sufferings that these children have to undergo is simply indescribable; they writhe and twist and squirm with pain, drawing up their limbs and screaming often for hours at a time. The pain usually comes in paroxysms, or it is of a spasmodic nature, sometimes relieved by pressure or by the child lying upon the stomach or by being carried about in the arms of the nurse; again shaking or rocking gently seems to modify their sufferings. Heat gives temporary relief, but all foods greatly aggravate, even the mother's milk; although food when first taken seems to give relief for the time being. Gas is frequently expelled from the stomach or bowels with great force, and is often quite pathognomonic of sycotic colic. Many times I have relieved these little sufferers with a few powders of Lycopodium or Argentum nitricum. Both these remedies seem to be frequently called for in these cases.

Again if they should be fortunate enough to escape the colic, other manifestations of the disease are met with, such as indigestion, catarrh of the bowels, vomiting of food without apparent nausea; diarrhoea, the stools being sour smelling, acid and excoriating the infant about the perineum. Quite often these children escape the gonorrhœal ophthalmia and have in its place, snuffles, which makes its appearance a few days after birth. The mother or nurse will tell you that the child has taken a cold in the head, so closely does the disease resemble the ordinary coryza, yet on examination of the nasal passages, we will find a specific form or rhinitis, known as the snuffles. The nose is dry and has a stuffed up feeling; quite frequently the child will scream with anger in its attempt to breathe with its mouth closed; this is more noticeable when the child nurses. The disease may last a few days, or it may continue for some time, but is usually displaced by something else of a more severe nature, especially if local measures are applied to relieve it.

The history of the parents will reveal Sycosis that has been suppressed or imperfectly cured. The diarrhoeas of these children are usually of a greenish, sour, slimy, mucous nature. The stools of Chamomilla, Rheum, and Mag. carb. are very characteristic of Sycosis. Often the child itself will smell sour and no amount of bathing seems to sweeten it. I have sometimes noticed that a case of snuffles coming on soon after birth, would be followed by a case of purulent ophthalmia. The length of time between the suppression of Sycosis and marriage, seems to make little difference, for children born to these parents, always show forth the disease at an early age. The time to cure them is in infancy, or during childhood, as they then quickly respond to Homeopathic treatment.

I have noticed in a number of cases that children born of very sycotic parents, complicated with gout, were affected with gouty conditions in the urethra, ears, nose and even in the rectum and vagina. These children take cold at the slightest exposure and frequently suffer from an acute coryza; the discharge from the nose becomes copious, watery and often excoriating. You are able to make a diagnosis of Sycosis in these children, you need not look for speedy cures or rapid results from your remedies; you must in some way make the parents understand that you have a deep constitutional disease to deal with.

You are fighting for time, and you need plenty of it.

If the snuffles should suddenly leave and a good brisk case of colic develop, it will help you out, for you then can inform this impatient parent that the baby will suffer more or less from this for at least ninety days. If, however, you should be fortunate enough to select the right remedy you will put the colic out of business much sooner. You can easily do this, if you will study a little over your materia medica, and give a high enough potency. Give nothing lower than the 30th, and the 1m, 10m, 45 or 50m, and even cm. may be needed. It will take the highest you have to cure them sometimes, as it is a deep-seated disease. Remember that *potency means power*. You have no power curative, outside of potency, with which to cure disease. Whether you believe it or not, it is the truth nevertheless, and it will stand the test of every man who applies it through the law of cure which no Homeopath disputes. When you have found the right remedy (which will require a close study of the provings, until you get the true picture of it in your mind), give it and then wait on its action, only going higher up in the potency when the lower potencies cease to act, and so on until you have exhausted the action of the highest in your possession. You will get ten times more prompt action in this deep chronic diseases from the cm. potency than you will from the lower ones. In acute diseases remedies will work many of them, anywhere from the tincture upwards. Yet I have many a time stopped completely, on modified severe pain like that of neuralgia, rheumatism or pleurisy in from three to six minutes, with the hundred thousandth potency. I am not alone in making this statement ; hundreds of men who use these high potencies can testify to this fact. You limit your own power when you limit the power of potency ; you believe God is infinite in all things, do you not? Well then prove Him, and see for yourselves if this is not true. Let us remember that life in the beginning was but a breathing. Is it not so yet? It is not the body you are trying to cure, it is the distuned life, or that which cares for, sustains and animates the body. Disease puts it out of working order. Is snuffles the disease? Yes, to an allopathic physician, to a materialist, but not you, dear reader. We say Sycosis was the real disease, and the snuffles but the expression of its presence in the young life. But do not think for a moment that snuffles is confined to the infant alone, we find it all through the life of the sycotic individual. We see it in every cold he takes, in his many catarrhal conditions, and in some forms of hay fever. When Sycosis is present, the nose may be clear one hour, and the next he cannot get a particle of air through his nasal passages. We see it also in his Lagrippe, coryzas and winter colds. You will soon become familiar with sycotic snuffles by a careful study of the disease.

Gouty concretions, so frequently found in gouty adults, are also found at birth in the mouth, nose, ears, rectum, and urethra, and in the outlets of the body, in these babes of sycotic parentage. I call to mind, a case in a new born male child where it was unable to urinate until the gouty concretions were removed from the urethra. In fact a probe had to be used in order to remove the concretion, which consisted of the usual crystalline formation found in common gout.

As has already been mentioned, the disease is not ushered in by such painful spasmodic symptoms, as we find in the simple catarrhal form of gonorrhœa, but the main difference is that it shows no tendency to a spontaneous cure. The acute stage gradually subsides in from six to eight weeks, and the disease settles down to a scanty catarrhal discharge of a characteristic yellowish-green color, generally purulent, and more or less offensive. If not interfered with by local treatment, the patient suffers from no special pain, simply a slight soreness along the urethra, and the mental disturbances before mentioned, produced by the fact that he has a specific venereal disease that must be stopped at once, and at all hazard.

Quite often the discharge dwindles down to a single drop of a creamy consistency and greenish-yellow color. Now it is this apparently insignificant drop, which to the patient seems of so little consequence, that he thinks it ought to be disposed of at once. Little does he know of the nature of the specific virus contained in that small drop of purulent matter. Each corpuscle contains a virus as specific, as malignant and as far reaching in its profundity of action, as the little seropurulent drop from the true chancre. Behind it is that dynamis of death. Like the bloody spot on Lady Macbeth's hands, all the multitudinous seas could not wash it out, when conveyed to an unaffected organism. It is the "damned drop." It damns the body at its birth, and it condemns the organism forever after, until it is fully eradicated from it by and through that God given principle, "*the law of Similia.*" No other system of medicine yet known can remove the effects of that specific poison, from the organism, but the Homeopathic, with its well selected remedy. An attempt to cure by any other method has been fully shown to be impossible, we think, to the satisfaction of all Schools of Medicine.

The male is capable of infecting the female at any remote period in the history of the case, even years after the disappearance of the discharge, and their offspring will show symptoms of infection at birth, and all through their natural life, unless anti-sycotic constitutional treatment is given the mother before and during gestation. The latent infection in the wife now becomes an active disease manifest by the symptoms of pain, inflammatory changes, and more or less suffering in the multiplied forms in which Sycosis may now present itself. The history of that case is the history of suffering and ill health, well-known to every physician. We speak of the woman as having the part of the endometrium affected, such as the cervix or any special part, specifying the local condition, as if the disease could advance by extension.

Such may be true of an ordinary inflammatory process, but in Sycosis every drop of blood, every fiber in that organism is affected. We might say the same thing of diphtheria, or some tubercular inflammatory process. The process may be localized, but the whole organism, even the very life itself, is diseased. No part or portion is favoured. The whole Biotic life is a oneness, although its pathology may have its habitat, as the pathology of every disease has. Usually diphtheria selects the mucous membrane of the pharynx or the throat. What you see there is not the disease but the eliminative process. It comes out at that point; *it is but the waste gate, through which the disease of the polluted city escapes*. The potential is the disease, and the potential (the life force) is that which is disturbed. It is a similar process which creates a tumor, a gonorrhœa leucorrhœal, or catarrhal discharge. If a death-dealing element is put into the organism, the organism must deal with it as such; or if a life-giving principle, such as food, is put into the organism, the result is that of more life, more power, more energy.

Noeggerath and many other close observers have recognized this fact. One of the latest authors in his work on venereal and sexual diseases, says:

"The more carefully we study the pelvic diseases of women, the narrower their etiological field becomes, and the more frequently are they found to depend on gonorrhoea. Thus, when freed from pathologic and anatomic errors, pelvic inflammations are dependent, in the majority of cases, if not all, upon tubal disease, the tubal

THE CHRONIC MIASMS.   25

disease is unquestionably due to gonorrhoea and its congeners or derivatives."

How true this is found to be by those who have given the subject study and attention. These inflammations do not act like other inflammations, which are due to Psora or Syphilis. There is always a definite feature about them, a persistence and positiveness conspicuously noticeable. The pains and the aches of Sycosis have seemingly a mysterious origin. These patients often suffer from month to month, or from year to year, with very little relief in spite of the efforts of their physician. In fact, he does not seem to understand the case, nor can the patients give satisfactory reasons for their disease. Their parents were not found to be rheumatic or gouty, there is no such family history or record. It all seems a mystery, an enigma, and not until the physician goes fully into the history of the case, can he trace the effect to the cause. The patient usually gives you a good family history.

She has never had any serious illness in her life, except the usual children's diseases. In fact, she was well until after marriage. In a year or two a child was born, and since that time she has been suffering with pelvic pain, neuralgia, rheumatism, chronic back-ache, chronic bladder troubles, uterine or ovarian troubles, headaches, menstrual irregularities, and such symptoms. The truth is that she has never seen a well day since the birth of her child. The whole case is a history of pain and suffering, or general bad health, all due to that primary infection (and that, too, from a husband who was considered free from that disease) who for years perhaps showed no signs or symptoms of its presence in his organism. This is where we all err in looking for symptoms of the primary or secondary stage, for it has now passed into the tertiary stage.

These symptoms are foreign to the majority of medical men, who have not given the subject of Sycosis a careful study. The phenomena are now unfamiliar to them, especially when it has been suppressed by local measures, and the symptoms by no means represent gonorrhœal infection as seen in its first and second stages. This is the parting of the ways to many physicians who lose sight of the original disease. The new phenomena, growing out of the suppression, is an enigma to them as it has but little in common with the original malady. The attending physician will tell the patient, as soon as the discharge is completely suppressed, that he is a fit subject to marry, as he is cured. But this is not true, and he should delay marriage, indeed he should never marry until the discharge has been reproduced or re-established, and cured in a proper and scientific manner. Only then should he marry a healthy wife, for only then will she continue so and bring forth healthy children.

It is only the busy general practitioner who realizes the frequency with which women break down in a year or eighteen months after marriage with uterine or pelvic troubles. A close observer need not always go to the annoyance of getting the husband's early history, for the symptoms of disease and suffering found in the wife are sufficient.

I can best illustrate this by a typical case. Mrs. F., age 24, German by birth, well developed physically, bright intellectually, and of sunny disposition, married three years, no children, was pregnant eighteen months after marriage, but aborted the third month. Her treatment was curettment, after which she was confined to her bed for three months. She has been unable to look after her household duties ever since. On making an examination of the pelvic contents, the uterus is found to be very much hypertrophied, and extremely sensitive to touch. She complains of shooting pains in the ovaries and through the uterus, bearing down and continual aching through the pelvic region ; she has fainting spells during the menses, and much trouble with her heart, although on examination it seems normal; she suffers with a scanty musty smelling leucorrhœa and pruritis vulvæ. I decided at once from the previous and present history of her case, that she was infected with Sycosis, and told her that her husband would also require treatment, in order to make a perfect cure.

In a few days he came to the office and gave the following symptoms : Pain in the stomach after eating, of a dull, heavy character, accompanying the pain was a fear of death, or a fear that he was going to die. I said to him, "you have had clap within the last five years." His answer was, "How did you know, did my wife tell you ?" I said, "Your wife knows nothing about the case, whatever." Later on, he admitted he had had gonorrhoea five years previous to his marriage, and that he had not seen a well day since. He also stated that the treatment was medicated injections and some powerful internal remedy. I then informed him why his wife was ill and why he was ill himself. Further that the discharge would have to be brought back as it was in the first place, and cured in the right way. He demurred at first, but finally consented to have me treat him. His treatment was Nux vomica cm the first week for the gastric symptoms, but as it did not cover his mental symptoms, therefore, he did not receive any benefit from the remedy. Medorrhinum in the cm potency was then given, which caused the discharge to return and a complete cure followed.

A history of good health in the wife before marriage, and then a sudden decline (in non-tubercular patients) is a pretty positive sign of sycotic infection, especially where pelvic symptoms are present. When Sycosis is suppressed in a pseudo-psoric or tuberculous patient, the miasmatic union becomes one very difficult to separate. Indeed, this subversive force (Sycosis) has such a positive bond with the life force that the latter is unable to disengage itself. The life force, therefore, must become subservient to it. It is a law of all forces that they act or push out in the direction of least resistance, so Sycosis in the organism is modified by the kind of suppression and the constitutional pre-disposition of the patient whether tubercular, syphilitic, psoric, or whatever degree of perversion met with. So we see that the secondary phenomena arising from an imperfectly treated case may be almost anything we can imagine.

An organism so disturbed must set up an inhibitory point or a center of resistance somewhere, and the life of the patient then is dependent upon the nature of that inhibition, modified somewhat by the character of the poison and the constitution of the patient. Many cases that I have noticed have acute articular rheumatism, others suffer with the chronic and sub-acute forms, or they may later on in the tertiary stage of Sycosis take on a gouty nature, and the concretions in the joints or tissues increase their sufferings. Again, many of these sycotically affected patients, either in the secondary or tertiary stages, have attacks of appendicitis, a disease, I think, largely dependent on the sycotic poison. If the patient happens to have already implanted upon that organism the tubercular taint, the disease assumes a malignant type.

A case comes to my mind of a young man who eight months previous to his death was strong and healthy. No finer physique or better specimen of health could be imagined, but he had a faint history of tuberculosis in the family. He was suddenly taken ill with appendicitis The organ was removed, and within sixty days there was noticed a marked infiltration of the right lung accompanied with fever and cough ; a little later on malignant symptoms of phthisis developed, and death occurred within eight months. The history of this case was a history of suppressed Sycosis. I simply cite this instance, as being a typical one of many that I have observed in the past ten years. The pus, the local inflammatory process is similar to sycotic inflammations in other organs, and especially pelvic inflammations of women. The dirty, brownish or yellowish-green color, the odor so characteristic, the spasmodic pains assuming that of a colicky nature, and the characteristic adhesions besides the specific and septic character of the process in general all show that Sycosis is present. Whole families of tubercular patients are swept out of existence by our epidemics of LaGrippe and other acute expressions of Sycosis. When the disease is met with in tubercular patients who are already suffering from perhaps an acquired Sycosis, we have a case upon our hands that is certain to form a metastasis of the disease, to the lungs, bronchi, meninges of the brain, or some other organ. Many of us have overlooked the fact that almost every case of LaGrippe requires an anti-sycotic remedy such as Rhus tox or Gelsemium in the first stage of its invasion. The fever, coryza, and the acute rheumatic invasion are truly the phenomena of a sycotic element, of a contagious nature which the life force is vigorously endeavoring to throw off. Of course, if the psoric element is most prominent in the patient, a true anti-psoric may have to be selected, or a pseudo-psoric as the case may require. When we stop to consider carefully the specific nature and character of LaGrippe from its start to its finish, we will see that it has that specific and positive action which allies it to Sycosis ; it has the fever, pain, cough, catarrhal invasion of the nose, bronchi, lungs, eyes or other mucous membrane as does Sycosis.

COMPLICATIONS OF SYCOSIS IN THE FIRST STAGE

Complications in the primary stage are few and seldom dangerous ; cystitis of a mild form is often present ; severe forms develop only in cases where local treatment is employed ; these may go on even to abscesses about the neck of the bladder or in the urethra. Frequently I have met such cases where silver nitrate or mercury had been used in the injection fluid. Some of these abscesses were followed by hemorrhages. I have never seen gonorrhoeal orchitis except in cases that had been tampered with by the use of some local medicament. Even in the ordinary uncomplicated case, where a tubercular diathesis is present in the patient, gonorrhoea is slow and difficult to eradicate from the organism. But when the disease is suppressed in the above specified soil, you have a case on your hands of which you cannot prophesy the outcome, for unless the process is soon arrested there is no telling what complications may arise, or to what degree the tubercular element may be stirred up.

If the discharge is not re-established a cure can never be made and the organism may die from morbid processes and changes dependent upon the stasis due to suppression. Sometimes the disease, after its suppression, will develop secondary or tertiary symptoms at once ; again it may take years to manifest itself in any marked degree upon the life force. A cachexia does not always develop in those cases where the disease is suppressed, and this is where some of us are deceived. We do not always recognize the immediate effects of the suppression in all cases, but it will come later on in some form, often foreign to that which you are looking for, or that you would expect. It may be in the nature of the pain as neuralgia, rheumatism, ovaritis, again the digestive tract may be disturbed, or the brain, and mental changes and aberrations present themselves. Indeed, there is no telling where it may break out or what the nature or character of the new disease process, or change may be. By suppressing the disease we have wrapped up in the organism a death process, it is a deadly virus disseminated—the bite of the deadly asp, brewing its deadly potion in the innermost chambers of the Tabernacle of life. Therefore, Death's processes must come forth and will sooner or later open the doors and show you the mortuary changes within.

The first great change which Sycosis produces when suppressed, is to attack the blood and to produce anæmic states and conditions. It is not always noticeable, even when it is present in considerable degree. However, catarrhal conditions come after a while, and rheumatism, and gout, even Bright's disease may develop. Diabetes and kindred diseases have often their parentage in a suppression of the disease in this primary stage. Inflammations follow in organs and in soft tissues ; fibrous changes in any organ are to be met with, until the whole organism is overcome by this death-dealing process due to the suppression. But to return to our subject of primary complications, we notice buboes are sometimes present, as is the case in Syphilis. They may be of a suppurative or non-suppurative variety, yet they seldom come unless suppressive measures are employed. They are usually due to stasis of the disease in its primary stage or in the beginning of the secondary stage. Prostatitis is not uncommon, hemorrhoids come later in the disease, of which more will be said. Prostatitis is a very common lesion, and it may continue throughout all the stages of the disease. It is, indeed, as you know, one of the most stubborn and difficult conditions to combat. Of course it is not always due to Sycosis, but that element is frequently the origin of its apearance.

As has been seen acute articular rheumatism is apt to develop after a supression. You, no doubt, have noticed how prevalent rheumatism has become in the past ten years. Did it ever occur to you that ninety-four per cent of these cases were due to a sycotic infection or taint? It will pay you to look into this matter and to search diligently for a primary cause. We used to look for it in men more than in women. It appears in women now about as frequently as in men. Why should this be so? The reason for this, is that the rheumatism of twenty years ago was not often found to be of sycotic origin. Now eighty per cent of males are affected, and they, of course, affect their wives, so the rheumatic element is found to be very nearly, if not equally distributed between the two sexes. I can remember the time when rheumatic fever was a common disease. We seldom see it now, that is the true old psoric or pseudo-psoric rheumatic fever, where the temperature would rise each day to 103, 104, and even higher, where the joints become greatly swollen, and sensitive, and the patient developed symptoms similar to typhoid fever. We usually meet with such cases in youth, in young women, or in growing girls, with a tubercular element well marked.

The arthritis we meet today seldom has such a temperature, nor does it develop a typhoid character. In its place we have the true sycotic or gonorrhœal arthritis which usually presents itself in a sub-acute form with a temperature of 101 or 102, with one joint involved, and the swelling never of such a character as mentioned in the old-fashioned arthritis. The pain is usually sub-acute, although at time it does become severe, but there is not the high temperature, the sensitiveness, the swelling, the prostration as found in the old-fashioned rheumatic fever. Strange to say, the sycotic arthritis usually follows a suppression of some kind, and is relieved by the re-establishing of the original discharge, either from the urethra, or by the return of an old suppressed leucorrhœa. Much more might be said concerning the subject of suppression, but we will deal with it more fully later on in this work.

We will now take up *Secondary Sycosis* and on looking closely into its phenomena, we will see that the secondary and tertiary stages bear about the same relation to the first stage as those stages do in Syphilis. When Syphilis is treated homeopathically, we find but few secondary lesions and the tertiary stage is conspicuously absent. The tertiary symptoms do not develop and the same thing may be said of Sycosis when treated homeopathically; there are no secondary and tertiary developments. Therefore, all secondary and tertiary symptoms are the result of poor treatment. How necessary it is for us to become, not only familiar with the disease in its primary stage, but all through its developments. No honest physician will do work that is detrimental to his patients if he is aware of it. Indeed, it is largely for lack of knowledge, that men err. "My people perish for lack of knowledge," says the Divine Book; so is it true with the physician of today. There are many of us, who at times are like Pandora's Box, when all that was left in it was hope. Hope is a very good thing to be in possession of, but a knowledge of the truth is power for present use and for present action.

Contagion is said to be the transmission of the poisonous principle. So in the transmission of the sycotic virus, the result will depend largely upon the stage in which it is transmitted. The symptoms that follow, and the diseases that make their appearance, will correspond in some degree to the stage and age of the primary infection. That is, if the virus is transmitted during the primary stage, the symptoms develop in the newly infected one will be primary symptoms, or those found in gonorrhœa of the first stage. If the disease is transmitted in the second stage, there will be no primary symptoms to speak of. For instance, if the female is affected in the second stage, we may have no symptoms to begin with, save a scanty vaginal catarrh with perhaps a slight pruritis of the vulvæ. This discharge is so acrid that it induces the pruritis, which if suppressed by local treatment, will present sooner or later new and often distressing symptoms, such as inflammation of any of the pelvic organs, or some form of rheumatism.

Often a single organ like the ovary or a tube may become affected, and the whole force of the disease for a time be concentrated upon this point or centre. There is no telling what the outcome of the disease may be, or the endless line of chronic affections that may follow secondary infection. The patient, on the other hand, may show signs of infection only by the anæmic state of the blood. Anæmia is prone to develop in all stages of the disease, but especially in the second and third. This anæmic state of the blood is a profound state—it involves every cell and fiber of the entire organism. It increases the same as in Syphilis, slowly and insidiously, until the whole organism is engulfed in its profound intoxication. The face looks at times ashy, grayish, drawn, puffed, and even doughy in severe cases. This anæmic condition becomes the basis of deep destructive diseases such as cancer of the breasts and uterus, epithelioma, diabetes, Bright's disease, acute phthisis, pneumonia, cholera infantum if in children, and numerous other diseases of which more will be said. In cases of typhoid, scarlet, and other severe fevers, we see by their deep and profound action, their slow and tedious recovery, that some deep acting poison, already in the system, is being disturbed from its slumbers by the new miasmatic, "the fever," that gives to it a malignancy and a positiveness not found in other cases of the same fevers. How necessary it is for us to know what miasm lies behind these fevers, for no cure can be made until the right anti-miasmatic remedy is found.

The remedy covering the febrile totality of symptoms does no good, it does not even palliate or give relief. We must look into the mysteries of the miasm, and find out whether it is Psora, Syphilis, or Sycosis. A man came to me not long ago suffering from a severe pain in the muscles of the back, about in a line with the tips of the clavicles ; it was very severe, accompanied with great restlessness, and < at night. Rhus, in the different forms, was given, that is Rhus tox, and Rhus radicans ; Mercury and Arsenicum were also given with no relief. He was a clinic patient, and we lacked the necessary time to look carefully into his case. I invited him one day to my office where I examined him carefully, and found he had had Syphilis, which as he said "had not been cured." His body was covered with scars, many tiny spots of syphilitic squama were to be found on the skin on different parts of the body. Syphilinum cm was given, which cured his pain in a few days. His general health improved, and the skin lesions disappeared. I state this simple case, to show how necessary it is to become acquainted with the nature and action of the chronic miasms.

We have learned from a study of this chapter that, in Sycosis, the diseases or symptoms that follow infection are dependent on the stage, age, or time of the infection. How necessary it is then, to know all about Sycosis in its different manifestations and stages of actions, just as we are acquainted with the different stages in Syphilis and its polymorphic lesions. To know these things, is to be able to follow Sycosis in all its multiplied manifestations and in all its deceptive workings with the life force.

THE SECONDARY STAGE

The secondary stage of Sycosis has no definite period of commencement; it may occur as early as ninety days after infection; and again it may not appear as a secondary disease, sooner than one or two years. The constitution of the patient, his or her habits, and the treatment will modify this feature very much. We now recall the case of a young woman of eighteen, who had illicit intercourse with a man who was suffering from a latent form of the disease. Only occasionally would he notice a slight discharge from the urethra, never more than a single drop, and seldom was it purulent. She suffered in no way from the infection, except a slight burning and occasionally an itching about the vulva. Medicated douches were prescribed for these symptoms, when within a short time she began to suffer with a pain in the right foot, growing in intensity from day to day, until a severe case of sub-acute rheumatism had developed, which confined her to her bed for three months. She had about given up in despair of being cured, when I was called. Suspecting infection from the history, specific nature and persistence of the symptoms, I questioned her closely, when she gave me the above mentioned history.

Medorrhinum was prescribed upon this history, and from present symptoms ; it soon developed the old symptoms of itching and burning, together with a scanty, dirty, watery colored discharge from the vagina. This was followed by Bryonia which cured the case. She has been perfectly well since. She since married and has one child, that up to this time shows no symptom of the disease. In this case there was no history of rheumatism in the family, nor of taking cold or in any way becoming chilled, besides she never before had employed a physician, nor to her recollection taken any medicine. The specific and intense character of the disease, the persistence of the symptoms, together with her previous good health and that of her family history, called my attention to the possibility of the case being due to infection. This case is a typical one, where the secondary stage of Sycosis presents itself in a sub-acute gouty form of rheumatism.

Almost every disease in the secondary stage of Sycosis, is of an inflammatory nature of some form or other.

These inflammatory changes may be either acute, subacute, or chronic; of any degree of severity, from the mild, wandering rheumatic pains of the muscles to that of a severe, specific, acute arthritis. The most frequently met with sycotic inflammations are to be found in the pelvic diseases of women, better known today as the surgical diseases of woman, or pelvic inflammations. Some of these might be mentioned, such as inflammation of the ovary, or ovaritis in its various forms. As the different structures of that organ are involved, hydro-salpingitis, cysto-salpingitis, and pyo-salpingitis, and abscesses of the tubes are not at all uncommon. Cystic degeneration of the ovaries, cervix, and uterus, are some of the more severe changes due to these inflammatory conditions.

We may also have peritonitis, cellulitis, pericystitis, cystitis, metritis, perimetritis, or inflammation of the endometrium. Appendicitis, as has been mentioned, has frequently a secondary Sycosis as its primal cause. Indeed there is a remarkable coincidence between the increase in appendicitis within the past ten years, and the spread of Sycosis; the increase is truly alarming to say the least; with it there is an increase of malignant diseases of all kinds, as well as that of the tubercular.

On close examination of the tissues involved in these local inflammations, we find the mucous membranes have a mottled or spotted appearance, or in other words they appear patchy or blotchy, one part of the tissues being of a dark reddish color and another part of the natural color. These dark venously congested spots are often covered with a thin purulent secretion, having an offensive odor; occasionally they are sensitive to touch. Again, they may be of a dark bluish tinge, showing the peculiar bluish congestions common in sycotic inflammations. The discharges are common to the sycotic inflammations in other parts—dirty-colored, and offensive. The odor alone is frequently diagnostic of the disease. The patients frequently notice it themselves, and no amount of douching and washing will remove it. Often it is pungent, musty, or of a dead fish odor. Even the perspiration in these patients has an extremely rank and unpleasant odor. Locally it is more noticeable about the axila, thighs, and external genitals; they are forever washing and scrubbing the body.

They are subject to erythemas and chafing of the skin, which pours out the peculiarly offensive sycotic discharge. Especially is this true in fleshy patients. The affected surface is bluish red, and the pus dirty, brownish-yellow, or yellowish-green. Frequently it excoriates the unaffected parts as it passes over them. This symptom is quite a constant one in young babies and is present soon after birth. The urine and feces excoriate, as has been already mentioned; a result due to their acidity. Often the whole perineum is found inflamed, hot, very sore and painful, due to the urine, and the child will scream after urinating. These children always require great care to prevent excoriating of the parts mentioned, and frequent bathing and dusting with the emollient baby powders.

Thus on examining any mucous surface where these sycotic catarrhal conditions exist, we are to look for this mottled condition of the tissues, also for the oozing from these dark venous congested spots. It will at once be seen that the mucous membranes have lost their normal pinkish hue so characteristic to those tissues. There are many other secondary pelvic processes that we might refer to that assume a more malignant character, when the system is tainted with Sycosis, such as pelvic and peritoneal adhesions, pelvic and peritoneal abscesses, and mucous cysts attached anywhere to the external uterine walls. These vary in size from that of an egg to that of a distended bladder. The contents are a yellowish or straw colored water. They have pendulous attachments : every abdomenal surgeon is familiar with them, for they are of such a common occurrence as to be met with frequently.

I recall one case in which a young woman of twenty-five was infected from her husband immediately after marriage ; she suffered with a scanty vaginal discharge, which was accompanied with vulvar itching. No special attention was paid to it, however. This was about the fourth month after marriage. Soon after noticing these symptoms, she became pregnant, and then suffered with uterine pains, and a profuse vaginal discharge of such a nature as to show fully a specific form of Sycosis. At the end of the fourth month of her pregnancy, her pelvic

THE CHRONIC MIASMS. 43

pains increased, and the gravid uterus was discovered to be three times the normal size, for that period of pregnancy. She came to Chicago to consult a surgeon ; he advised an exploratory incision, which was performed a few days later. As was suspected she was found to be pregnant, the uterus was fully four times the natural size, of a dark bluish-black color, with nodular growths all over the external walls. Many of these nodules were two or three inches in diameter. Again, others were as small as hickory nuts, and when opened up were found to be of a fibrous nature.

Attached to the pelvic walls of the uterus were fully a dozen cysts, from the size of a small egg to that of a full extended bladder ; they had thin translucent walls, and were filled with a light straw-colored serum. A number of them were so large and distended with the fluid that their contents had to be removed before they could be severed from their pedicle-like attachment. Very few fully realize that these cysts are secondary processes, due to sycotic infection or secondary Sycosis. Yet this truth is coming now, more fully to the light, and to the minds of the profession, and while such symptoms have to many, a mysterious origin, and they are unable to cope with them therapeutically, yet such marked and clear-cut developments, as may be seen in such a history as has been given above cannot be overlooked. Some physicians today, of all schools, are brave enough to come out boldly and say these conditions are due to gonorrhœal infection.

The history of the above case did not end with the removal of the uterus and its appendages, as was prognosed by the surgeon who so skillfully and successfully performed the operation ; for in those days (which was about twenty years ago) the operation was a wonder to all who witnessed it, especially as she finally recovered from it and again took up her household duties. Being a friend of the family. it was my good fortune to follow the history of this case, more or less closely through all those years, which was as follows : One month after the operation, she was removed from the hospital to the home of a friend, where she convalesced slowly. At the end of six weeks she broke out all over the neck, arms, and trunk, with an eruption of warts, small, slender, sessile, pointed, thickly grouped together, from the size of a pin head to that of a grain of wheat, of the filliform variety (verruca filiformis). I called her attention to them, and suggested she should have a homeopathic remedy for them, as there was a marked relationship, I thought, between the eruptions and her pelvic trouble ; but she had already spent much money, and replied she did not feel like spending more at that time.

For three or four years I did not meet her or hear from her, and so lost sight of the case. Then I heard she was suffering from rheumatism and stomach trouble, and had found no permanent relief from the many forms of treatment which she had employed. She was then residing on the shores of Lake Superior, and on account of the cold and dampness, was compelled to move farther south to a less inclement climate, as the cold and dampness of the northern lake region greatly aggravated all her symptoms. It was then I again met her in Chicago. I now found that she had developed a chronic stomach trouble and a well marked case of diabetes mellitus, which is speedily sapping her life force. The history of this case is a typical one ; one in which the infection was of a very specific nature, probably made so by being ingrafted upon a very psoric constitution, with a history of a tubercular taint in the family on her mother's side ; but as she was born with all the characteristics of her father and her father's people, she was probably greatly fortified against any tubercular out-break.

This case is worthy of our further study. In the first place, she did not have homeopathic treatment, and the discharges were suppressed by local medicated douches, and an inflammatory stasis of the whole pelvic circulation was the result. A secondary suppression of a more serious nature, was produced by the operation, which of course at that advanced stage of the disease (that is the secondary or inflammatory invasion), could not well be avoided. Nevertheless, an operation is often the worst form of suppression as the life force sets up an inhibitory point in the organism, when it is diseased ; this point may be either functional or structural, and if treated according to the law of Similia, is removed in a natural way by virtue of the removal of the miasmatic basis, or that which compelled the life force to set up the inhibitory point in the first place. But by operative measures, this inhibitory point is mechanically removed, and the life force suffering still from the same perversion due to the same taint, is compelled, by virtue of this same law of action and reaction on which all life and all motion is dependent, to set up another inhibitory point or center, which is only fulfilling the law of self-preservation. Therefore, that inhibitory point must be, according to the law of progression of the forces, located in a great center of that organism, at least in some great center or organ.

Our case can be no exception to this rule. So we find the nervous system greatly involved together with the stomach. She has lost the power to digest her food, which previous to the operation, was never disturbed in any way, and now she has developed a marked case of diabetes mellitus, which will soon destroy her life. Such is the history of thousands of young and promising women, although, perhaps, not so many advance along the lines given in the history of this one, but along lines which although dissimilar, are equally as severe and destructive to life.

Another case might be cited, to show the destructive and malignant action of Sycosis, when implanted upon an organism with a tubercular history. Mrs. B., age 32, dark hair and eyes, of the brunette type, contracted Sycosis from her husband soon after marriage. Two years later a child was born, after which she was sterile. Soon after the birth of the child, the disease became active, and she suffered with metritis, accompanied by the usual vaginal discharge of Sycosis which was treated with medicated lotions. Retroflection and adhesion of the uterus to the rectal wall followed ; four years later she was sent to me from the state of Indiana, where she lived, for examination and counsel as to whether an operation was advisable or not. On examining her, I found the pelvic cavity filled with a shapeless cancerous mass, the growth projecting from the vagina about an inch ; the uterus, rectum, ovarian tubes, and broad ligament, were all involved in this chaotic mass, as if they had been fused together. She was then suffering beyond description, with the usual pains and hemorrhage of the disease in an advanced stage, of which she soon died ; the disease was too far advanced to offer anything promising in the way of an operation. Sycotic abscesses are so common, that every physician can testify to the frequency with which they are met, in married women.

The great danger lies in any local interference with the discharges of these sycotic patients. As a rule no stasis will take place, unless this is interfered with, and there are so many ways by which it can be suppressed— by medicated douches, or the local application of crude drugs, such as Hydrastis, Boracic acid, Nitrate of silver, Zinc sulphate, or other suppressive medicaments. Even hot or cold douches may force the acute inflammatory processes up through the cervical canal into the uterine cavity and finally into the tubes, until the septic process involves all the endometrium. In men, we do not have this great mucus surface in the pelvis to become involved, as we have in the female, therefore a suppression induced in the male in the primary stage, does not necessarily produce such disastrous effects, or such prolonged or intense suffering. Neither are there such complications and such destruction of tissues, or such a demand for surgical interference. We do have, however, rectal complications, the pus pockets, the hemorrhoid, and many other difficulties of that organ.

In the male we have many cases of orchitis, and epidydimitis and of cystic troubles, besides an infinite number of cases of sycotic arthritis, and sub-acute forms of gout, rheumatism and gouty states of the system. The full stress of the disease, seems to fall upon the male organism along these lines; still, it may produce even more profound impressions or more dangerous complications, such as mania, true insanity, heart lesions, stomach difficulties, gastro-intestinal diseases, pneumonia and other inflammatory processes. How frequently we meet these cases suffering from a suppression of the disease in our clinics! they are of common ocurrence; and sad to relate, many of them are the work of so called Homeopaths, who are ignorant of the true methods of cure, and who therefore resort to old school methods. This combination of unskilful Homeopathy often induces a more profound suppression, and more dangerous complications than the treatment of the regular or old school. Oh! that the gospel teachings of Hahnemann might take a deeper hold upon those men who pose as followers of him, that they might not be forever learning, "yet never come to the knowledge of the *truth*."

SUPPRESSION INDUCED BY OPERATIVE METHODS

Modern surgery is another great source of suppression of this disease, and the consequent prevalence of secondary and tertiary lesions. Indeed, the increase of Sycosis during the past twenty years has enriched the specialist and the surgeon of abdominal, pelvic, aural and throat diseases. A great proportion of this class of surgically or mechanically treated diseases, now so common, is dependent upon Sycosis; causing those specialists to derive a large income from the suffering public, without really knowing what they are treating. Why should this be so? The majority of these men would not deal in this way with Syphilis—no; they are extremely careful, and cautious how they approach or operate upon syphilitic lesions, no matter how serious their character or the seeming necessity of operation. Why? Because they have learned the lesson well, their past experiences and the past records of such procedures, have proven to them, over and over again, that the results are disastrous; that the disease returns or retaliates against them, in some other part of the organism; besides, they have found out that the so-called anti-syphilitic or constitutional treatment is safer and far more satisfactory in the end.

Then why should not the same thing be true of Sycosis? Is it any less virulent? Any less specific in its destructive action upon the human organism? We think not. It is in some ways more destructive, more positive, more speedy in bringing to a conclusion, its death processes. Syphilis will often take years to accomplish what Sycosis will begin and bring to a fatal conclusion in a few months, even in a few weeks. The great reason is, that men fail to see the true relationship between the act of suppression, and the new diseases, and new processes that are forthcoming. This is because they are not familiar with the workings of the sycotic miasm; they seem to know scarcely anything about the secondary or tertiary steps, or the symptomatology that develops from a suppression in the primary or secondary stages. This is true of all schools of medicine who have not studied miasmatics. Pneumonia may suddenly develop and take away the life of the patient, yet it appears to be no different to them from the ordinary form of that disease.

Peritonitis makes its appearance in women, after the suppression of a leucorrhoea, or after an operation upon some of the pelvic organs that were effected with Sycosis, and the special relation between the secondary inflammatory process, and the suppression of a specific venereal leucorrhoea is not seen; neither could they see why one case of peritonitis is speedily cured and another runs on to pus pockets, extensive adhesions, and perhaps perforation. We must become acquainted with a sycotic lesion, with sycotic pus, sycotic inflammations in general before we can recognize the true processes as they develop from one condition to another, in so positive and so destructive a manner.

We must know the true character of the sycotic poison, and all its processes, especially when it is suppressed and the effects of the virus dammed up in the system, with all the eliminative processes barred and sealed up. The closing up of a sinus, that is freely discharging purulent matter, such as a fistule or burrowing abscess, will often develop into some severe stasis of the original disease. I have seen Sycosis which had been latent for years stirred up by the repair of a lacerated cervix, lessening the drainage of the uterus. I have seen ovaries or tubes often become involved after a curettment. The uterus becomes enlarged and a chronic hypertrophy follows curetting or the use of sounds or other instruments, being forced into the uterus; abortions, child-births, and their after effects, will frequently stir up an old latent sycotic difficulty that is very hard to eradicate.

These cases ought to be carefully treated before childbirth, in order to remove, if possible, that specific character of the disease that is so liable to become active at these critical periods in the patient's life. Operations on the rectum, removal of hemorrhoids, the suppression of hemorrhoids by salves and medicated suppositories, rectal injections are all modes of suppression and should not be employed, as many cases of hemorrhoids, proctitis, and other diseased conditions in the rectum, are due to a gonorrhoeal stasis. More especially is this true of itching piles, so frequently met with in men and which are sometimes so severe as to almost drive the patient frantic. A slight oozing from the rectum of a fishy odor is not uncommon in hemorrhoids due to Sycosis. Rectal pockets and blind pouches are often present, although there is not that tendency to burrowing or formation of fistules so commonly found in tubercular or syphilitic patients.

Warts and warty growths are common, although what is known as condylomata never come from Psora or Sycosis alone. A careful investigation of these cases will reveal both miasms Syphilis and Sycosis to be present in the formation of condylomata, verruca accuminata, pointed papillary growths, coxcomb, and warts; this is not true of the common wart (verruca vulgaris) which is frequently met with about the rectum and sexual organs. The removal of any of these sycotic expressions of a verrucous nature (more especially those above mentioned), by local measures, potash, strong acids, by actual cautery, or electrolysis, is a fruitful source of suppression of the disease out of which arise many of our worst forms of malignancies. These warty growths on close study will show that specific nature, that persistence of character, that stubborness so characteristic of the sycotic element. Their nature is also shown by the response to the action of anti-sycotic remedies.

The majority of my readers have no doubt seen the bad effects from suppression of this venereal miasm Sycosis, but it is my intention to give a number of clinics, in which I shall endeavor to show, and demonstrate the bad effects of suppression. We will also try to show you the positiveness and persistency of the disease when suppressed, as well as its malignancy and diversity of action; We will show how secret and non-assuming it is, in its beginning, in its inroads upon the internal organs and parts remote and unassociated with the disease in its primary stage. Here is a patient who has had the gonorrhoeal discharge suppressed in the first or second stage, who tells you he has never been well a day since he was cured, as he calls it. Another has had stomach trouble or some form of indigestion, yet another suffers from gouty conditions, swelling of the joints; at every change of weather, he is lame or suffers with stiffness of his muscles; some have heart troubles, valvular diseases, or rheumatic difficulties about the heart, or in the cardiac region; again we have kidney affections, pain in the back and about the loins, or they have ailments that the patients say are indescribable; something is not right, either in the physical sphere or perhaps it may be found in the mental. *There is somehow, somewhere, a something wrong. It is the old story of Hahnemann's distuned and disturbed life force.* This abnormal sensation experienced by the patient is but the preparation before the onset, a gathering together of the forces before the storm breaks out in its fury and in its miasmatic strength. As yet we have no pathology, but pathology will come later on. The character and manner of its coming will be similar to the clinical cases we will now present to you.

Case 1. George H., age 37, sandy complexion, and of a pleasant disposition, contracted Sycosis eight weeks ago. The disease was suppressed within a week or ten days, and was followed by an outbreak of intense nervousness. He says he is so nervous and irritable that there is no living with him. His other symptoms are stiffness and lameness in the muscles of the back, dull headache, loss of appetite, sleeplessness, constant restlessness on lying down. The meatus is red and swollen, urine scalds him much, he is afraid something fearful is the matter with him. Medorrhinum was given in the 1m potency. Four days later a slight discharge from the urethra appeared, the nervousness was much better, sleeping better, not so irritable ; continued the remedy. This patient will continue to improve until a complete cure is made. Mental symptoms first to improve, discharge returned before physical symptoms became any better.

Case 2. William B., age 40, dark hair and eyes, weight 140, of an even temperament, slow in his movements ; gonorrhoea three months ago, suppressed with injections ; since then temporal headaches every morning. He feels $<$ in the morning and better as the day advances ; constipation, dry scanty stools, better by heat, ankles and feet greatly swollen and painful. Diagnosis—gouty rheumatism. Nux vomica 50m, two doses. Second visit one week later. Improvement ; constipation better ; not so chilly ; feels better in every way except the rheumatism ; continued the remedy. Third visit next day ; rheumatism worse ; feet and ankles very painful ; thinks he had better go to some mineral baths ; parts not so painful when he kept quiet, but very sensitive to touch and to pressure when standing upon them. Medorrhinum c. m. cured him in two months.

Case 3. Mrs. W., age 35, looks pale and bloodless, suffered for two or three months with a severe pruritis of the vulva, some pain and bearing down on urination ; treatment—douches of cold water ; a little later on, swelling and much pain in left ankle joint. Treatment for next ten days hydrotherapy, locally, hot packs and fomentations ; took internally antikamnia in order to get sleep. At the end of twelve days, I was called. The symptoms were, dull pain in the ankle joint, joint greatly swollen, could keep the foot still in one place for only a few minutes, she was constantly changing it on a pillow ; *color dark*, *puffed up*, and *sensitive*. She had no other pain, no appetite ; had eaten nothing for many days with the exception of oranges ; weeps with the pain, weeps at the least annoyance or whenever her case is mentioned. Pulsitilla 1m is given. In 48 hours there was relief from all pain ; improvement continued for one week, then a relapse. Symptoms—great sensitiveness of the part to touch ; color of tissues over joint very *dark*, almost *black*. Joint had been greatly reduced in size but now was much swollen and painful again. She was extremely nervous, sleepless, worse after sleep, had bad dreams ; dreamt of dead people and of falling into deep dark water ; had great fear when alone at night ; sees *faint outline* of *images of people* and *things ap-*

proaching her, and cannot go to sleep because of them. Lachesis cured the case in two months, the pruritis or vaginal discharge did not return, hence the slowness of the cure.

Case 4. Albert R., age 35, contracted gonorrhoea in the fall of '94, which was suppressed by injections of some specific, sold by druggist for that purpose. Soon after he began to suffer with a severe form of indigestion, which increased from month to month, and finally developed into cancer or scirrhus of the pyloric end of the stomach, from which he died. No other symptoms of Sycosis ever appeared after the suppression of the discharge.

Case 5. Arthur B., age 24, blond, expressman, contracted Sycosis eight weeks ago, treated with injections of mercuric chloride 1 to 1,000; fifth day after the use of the drug, began to have severe pains about the neck of the bladder, followed with fever and restless nights. His symptoms were always < at night; a day or so later, an abscess broke and discharged bloody pus for some time, until cured by the homeopathic remedy.

Case 6. Jacob F., age 29, dark complexion, with a nervous temperament, and tubercular diathesis; has had the disease for some time. Has taken oil of Cedron and numerous medicated injections, but with no apparent lessening of the discharge; was advised to use some French preparation with which to irrigate the canal, this was followed in one week with abscess of the neck of the bladder, which took many weeks to cure.

Case 7. Wm. B., age 20, dark complexion, nervous bilious temperament, suppressed the discharge in the first week of the disease which caused orchitis and later on inflammatory rheumatism, confining him to his bed for three months.

Case 8. J. P. H., who was a travelling salesman, had the disease suppressed during the second week. Orchitis appeared in a few days, complicated with bubo of the right side and followed with a severe and stubborn form of cystitis. Neither of these cases was relieved until the discharge was re-established.

Case 9. Mary M., age 20, contracted the disease three months ago. The usual treatment with medicated douches was tried and caused a suppression of the vaginal discharge, which in turn brought on an abscess of the tubes. Fully one hundred cases similar to this could be cited that have occurred in my clinical work. These cases are of common occurrence in the practice of almost every physician. One of two things usually occurs in a woman when the disease is suppressed in the first stage. Either the disease is reflected to some of the pelvic organs, or a gouty or rheumatic condition develops in some part of the body. Should these conditions not arise, you will find a metastasis farther on in the tertiary stage. It may appear as a severe form of gout, not infrequently delayed until the climactric period, when it is first seen in the joints of the hands, usually the index finger being first attacked. Again, we find deeper and more destructive forms in the disease appearing later on in life, such as diabetis mellitus, or Bright's disease, complicated with heart or stomach troubles.

Another case might be cited, in which the disease Sycosis would not be suspected by the ordinary observer, and which shows to some degree the diversity of its forms and manifestations. Mrs. Chas. E., age 54, sandy complexion, quiet disposition, tall and spare of flesh, contracted the disease from her husband in the secondary, or gleety stage. It is at this stage of the disease, that so many physicians tell their patients that there is no longer any danger of contracting the disease. But this is not true, for gleet is the secondary stage of Gonorrhoea, or a sub-acute state of the primary disease, that may develop in the newly effected patient, either primary or secondary symptoms.

Occasionally they present to some degree symptoms of both stages. This was true in Mrs. E's case. Since infection (which was about fifteen years ago) she has suffered with the following symptoms, more or less modified of course, none of which she had before infection. She takes cold easily, beginning with sneezing, followed by a copious watery coryza. In two or three days the disease settles on the bronchial tubes, a cough follows of a raspy, teasing nature, the whole chest becomes raw or sore, often with much weight or distress over the region of the middle sternum. These symptoms continue for an indefinite period, unless relieved by a remedy. Small papilla dot the posterior wall of the throat, which seems to keep up an irritation and cough. She has to live in some southern climate during the winter and in the summer she migrates back to Chicago again, only to return south again in the early autumn. When the cough is better there is a frequent desire to urinate with much soreness and burning, often only a desire with some burning. When this is relieved, she will suffer with hemorrhoids and acidity of the stomach. No acid of any kind can be tolerated by the stomach, neither concentrated sweets.

The cough of Sycosis has very little expectoration, usually of clear mucus; occasionally it is ropy, and may also be of a cottony nature. A great deal of coughing is often required to raise it, hence the prolonged, teasing cough. This case is a typical one; one that we often meet and are unable to help with any degree of satisfaction. These are the cases that anti-psoric or pseudo-psoric remedies fail to cure, but only palliate. We do not understand why they are so unresponsive to our remedies, but this is the way Sycosis secretes itself behind an impenetrable wall. In the treatment of this form of Sycosis (which is tertiary) one remedy will seldom cure the case. We have to take them back over the way they came, no matter how circuitous the path.

The treatment I give this case will better illustrate what I mean. Lycopodium was given, which relieved all the gastro-intestinal symptoms and the cough improved somewhat. After the fourth week under this remedy the bladder symptoms grew much worse, and the hemorrhoids also became very annoying. Later on Thuja was given, and the case is improving under that remedy slowly. The cough and urinary symptoms are persistent but the general health improves. These cases go from pillar to post, from specialist to specialist, one part, or organ is treated for a while until its symptoms are palliated, then others grow worse. It is necessary to tell these cases what you propose to do, your plan of attack upon the disease, so that you may secure their confidence and hearty co-operation, or you will fail in your purpose and they will pass on to others, as they have in the past. Both of the remedies given in the case just related were anti-sycotics; the first acting decidedly upon the whole gastro-intestinal tract and digestive field, the second upon the mental sphere and the urinary tract. Both remedies were slow but progressive in their action, corresponding to the chronic state of the disease; both are capable of producing profound functional and pathological changes. If these do not cure the case, it is not at all likely that further anti-sycotic remedies will be called for, but some anti-psoric may be necessary to complete the cure.

We will deal more fully with this subject or suppression, as we take up the study of the third or tertiary stage of the disease. It is a subject of vital importance to every healer of the sick. This is a matter of justice and judgment. No physician should be ignorant concerning this matter of suppression of disease. We should know how to proceed towards a cure, and understand the difference between a suppression and a cure. Fully fifty percent of the so called cures of Sycosis are suppressions, the sequelae of which are new developments and new processes of disease. Venereal diseases are not at all to be dreaded if they are treated properly. They are only peculiar expressions of a disturbed life force, and should be treated by the law of similia. A secondary and tertiary stage in Sycosis or Syphilis, are the results of no treatment, or poor treatment. All pathology is due to the suppression or loss of control of the disease in the initial stage. The same thing may be said of scarlet fever, typhoid, or any severe acute disease.

TERTIARY STAGE

There are many things to be considered as influencing the vital force in bringing about the tertiary stage of Sycosis. First and most important is the suppression of the disease either in the primary or secondary stage. If the disease is suppressed in the primary stage, it may without showing secondary symptoms at all, go on to the tertiary stage, although in most cases, especially in the tubercular constitution and in women, the secondary stage develops in a few months after the primary suppression. Usually tertiary lesions, due to primary suppression, do not make their appearance sooner than from one to two years. In cases where the vitality of the patient is good, and where there is a strong reactive force in the organism, it may be delayed for many years. Sometimes we see it appearing as a malignancy, after forty years of age or at the climactric period of women. Of course functional disturbances are as a rule found to be present in the majority of cases soon after suppression. These functional disturbances may be almost anything, headaches, neuralgia, rheumatic pains, gastric troubles, mental difficulties, menstrual irregularities, aggravations from cold, climatic changes and barometric risings and fallings.

Returning again to our subject we find the things influencing the appearance of the tertiary stage, are early suppressions, the drying up of the discharge by any means either from local irrigation or the introduction of strong drugs into the system such as Copaiba, Cubebs, Gelsemium, Ergot, Potassium bromide, the fluid extract of corn-silk, sandal-wood oil, Balsam of Peru; the Saw-palmetto, and many others. The most profound suppressions, however, are produced by the use of irrigation with such drugs as potassium permanganate, nitrate of silver, hydrastis, zinc sulphate, besides compounds of ingredients too numerous to mention. Operations in the secondary or inflammatory stage of the disease, such as curettments; the removal of a diseased organ, the uterus, ovarian tubes, or any of the pelvic organs, are methods of hasting the third stage of the disease; also the suppression of secondary inflammations such as cervicitis, leucorrhoeas, orchitis, acute rheumatism or catarrhal difficulties of a secondary character, wherever found.

The fourth means of tertiary invasion, and probably the most fruitful cause, is the suppression of gleet by medicated douches, medicated pencils, the local treatment of strictures, by dilitation, incision, or other operative measures. The patient suffering with gleet is a sick man in every sense of the word. He is always complaining, never well; his complaints are numerous and his symptomatology as variable as the winds of March. His system is thoroughly poisoned with the gonorrhoeal taint, that has so long been dammed up in the organism. Indeed gleet is sub-acute gonorrhœa. You may call it gleet or any other name you will, but it is as much gonorrhoea as it was in the beginning. It may be subdivided into the different forms and given scientific names, but it is nothing more nor less than gonorrhoea in the second or third stage, virulent as ever it was in the first stage, although the symptoms in the newly infected one may vary some from those of the initial stage of the disease; yet the infection from these gleety patients will produce secondary and tertiary symptoms, and are often just as virulent as the infection in the primary stage.

More will be said concerning the subject of gleet, as we will take up the subject again by itself. Besides these causes enumerated as aiding in the development of the tertiary stage, there are conditions arising that we wish to mention, as often assisting in bringing this thing about, for instance pregnancy. The sealing up of the uterus, and the turning of the physiological forces in another directon, will sometimes develop the third stage of Sycosis. It usually in this case makes its appearance in the form of some eruption, generally of a verrucous character (*verruca filiformis*) or as gouty states of the system, or as fibroid changes and growths. Occasionally mucous cysts and other conditions arise which we will mention later on. Again, operations prolonged fevers and injuries, are secondary or exciting causes for the developments of the tertiary stage of the disease, Sycosis. Of course, in all these conditions mentioned, we are to understand that unhomeopathic treatment and methods are employed, for, had the patient had true homeopathic treatment, we would expect no tertiary developments at all. After giving due consideration to all the above named causes by which the tertiary stage develops, we find, that secondary inflammations do run this course in a certain time, when as a natural result the tertiary stage follows. We see this in the gleety inflammations which later on become fibrous and there is no longer a discharge. Secondary inflammations sometimes undergo cystic degeneration; changes are met with in the form of gouty deposits, gouty concretions and even gouty inflammations, all of which are tertiary changes.

TERTIARY LESIONS

Usually the first tertiary lesions to manifest themselves are skin symptoms, and this is in agreement with Hahnemann's theory of disease, "that disease is evolved from above downwards, and from within outwards." This is the natural order of things, which is co-operative with the saving of life and the protection and relief of the internal organism. When tertiary developments do not come out as skin lesions malignancies are almost certain to follow, as there is no other way (except by reflexes through the nervous system) of preventing the centralization of the tertiary forces upon the internal organs. When I speak of malignancies I refer to cancer, carcinoma, lupus, epithelioma and a tendency toward diabetes mellitus, Bright's disease and tuberculosis; all of these may be developments from the sycotic taint, for fibrous changes are quite often malignant in their outcome, especially if internal organs like the uterus, kidneys, liver, or heart are involved.

The first skin lesions that we meet with are warty eruptions or warty growths. These appear in the form of *verruca filiformis, verruca vulgaris and verruca plana*. The acuminate form belongs to the condylomatous family, and therefore no doubt partake of both the venereal miasms, Syphilis and Sycosis.

Warts are of diagnostic value to us in distinguishing between the different stages of the disease. The *verruca vulgaris* is found in children who are suffering with hereditary Sycosis; they appear at or about the second dentition. The *verruca filiformis* comes as a tertiary lesion in an acquired form of sycosis. The *verruca plana juveniles* is another hereditary form found more or less upon the backs of the hands and faces of children and young people. They are usually pigmented, disseminated, and in irregular unilateral groups.

The filiform variety appears in adults, who have acquired Sycosis and who have had the disease suppressed in some way, although they may appear after secondary inflammations have subsided. I have met with them frequently after operations upon internal organs, especially after extirpation of organs such as the ovaries, or uterus. They are more apt to appear on and about the sexual organs, or on the trunk of the body, quite frequently in groups of a dozen or two, closely run together in fields or patches. They are small in diameter, often an eighth of an inch long, although frequently much shorter, slightly colored, brownish or greyish brown, pointed at the end with spindle-like attachments; when they appear in children or young people we find them about the eyelids and on the neck. Occasionally these disappear spontaneously and some other tertiary lesion takes their place. I recall now three cases where they made their appearance after operations. Case 1. May B., married, two children, was suffering with Sycosis for many years in the form of a secondary inflammation of the uterus. There was a marked subinvolution of the organ with severe catarrh of the cervix. The cervix was severely lacerated and it was thought best to repair it, which was done. The surgeon who performed the operation, curetted the uterus also. She got immediate relief from her womb troubles, but in about thirty days the whole trunk of her body was covered with little pendulous warts which were cured with Thuja.

Case 2. Mrs. R., age 31, was compelled to have the uterus removed at the fourth month of pregnancy on account of cystic growths and sycotic changes of a fibrous character. After recovery, or about the fourth week after the operation, the same warty eruption appeared. No treatment was given in her case and they disappeared in about one year. She died about five years later of diabetes.

Case 3. Mr. Chas. B., age 50, contracted gonorrhoea, which was treated with injections; within a year a sycotic eruption of warts appeared on the sexual organs and on different parts of the body. He was treated for them for over a year, before they disappeared.

I believe it may be said with some certainty that when a tertiary eruption makes its appearance, that a suppressed discharge, in other words, a suppressed gonorrhoea, cannot be reproduced, so that the disease Sycosis then becomes a slow and difficult thing to cure, just as we find is the case in the tertiary stage of Syphilis, which is so closely bonded with the life force and with Psora, that it becomes very difficult to separate. As long as the disease is suppressed in the primary or secondary stage, and has remained in a latent state, we have very little difficulty in reproducing the discharge. With the use of such remedies as Medorrhinum, Nux vomica, Psorinum, Sulphur, Calcarea carb, and others of that class, we have an armamentarium at our command, that makes the treatment of the disease comparatively easy, if taken in the first and second stages of suppression. Malignancies coming after suppression are easily managed, if we can reproduce the original gonorrhoeal discharge, but if we are unable to do this, our chances for a cure become very doubtful indeed. Often our only hope lies in reproducing the original disease, in order to cure any secondary disease, whether it be stomach trouble, indigestion, hemorrhoids, headaches, neuralgias, rheumatism or constipation. Even acute expressions of disease often depend on the same thing; for instance, it has been my experience in about fifty cases of acute arthritis, following speedily after the suppression of the sycotic discharge in the first stage of gonorrhoea not to be able to relieve the pain fully, or to arrest the progress of the disease, unless the suppressed discharge returned. These are the unfortunate cases that linger along for months and finally drift away from you and try all sorts of treatments in order to get relief—mineral baths, Hot Springs, mud baths, hot air baths, electricity, and local measures of all kinds. Indeed it becomes a search for a panacea of health. They often follow a blind hope throughout the remainder of their natural life.

The importance of these verrucal eruptions will be more fully dealt with, as we take up the treatment of them. Their removal by surgical, chemical, or electrical methods may be considered as a suppression, which is certain to be replaced by some other disturbance or manifestation of Sycosis. Occasionally, they reappear at the same point after removal, or appear in other parts. Such disturbances as headaches, neuralgia, rheumatism, stomach troubles, gouty states of the joints or organs, follow. We know that warts are a tertiary manifestation of Sycosis, and that all tertiary manifestations are the result of deep and profound action upon the organism. Although the secondary manifestations are more acute, and apparently more destructive in their immediate action, in the end we see that this is not so.

The tertiary manifestations of all the miasms, whether Psora, Syphilis, or Sycosis, though slower in action, often involve the more central organs, and the deeper structures of the organism. The malignancies arising from warts or warty growths are well known to the profession, more especially the flat smooth warty growth, known as the pearly papule, found frequently about the face and neck of patients having a tubercular or latent syphilitic taint and origin. Again, we notice this same condition, perhaps, in the ulcerating or degenerating wart, from which springs our epithelioma, or other malignancies. A sycotic element is found to be present in almost, if not every case. Accompanying the above mentioned form of warts upon the skin, and almost always present, whether hereditary or acquired, is the *red mole*, another tertiary symptom which appears more frequently upon the chest or anterior portion of the body, although they may occur anywhere, varying in size from that of a pin-head to that of a pea, There is no other eruption like it. It is smooth, round, shiny, often red as blood and of the appearance of a polka dot upon the skin.

This eruption is quite a positive sign that the one so affected has either acquired Sycosis, or their parents have acquired it. It seldom appears on exposed portions of the body as the face or hands, but occasionally they are found upon the neck. The *spider spot*, another specific sycotic lesion, is generally found upon the upper portion of the face, usually about half an inch below the lower eyelid or over the center of the maler bone; it consists of a little sprangle of dilated capillaries, resembling somewhat the meshes of a spider web. It is a little flag of distress, which the organism hangs out to tell that the enemy is within. It speaks volumes to those who understand it as a landmark. This is particularly a tertiary or hereditary lesion and is found in children about the period of second dentition, but may be there at birth. It increases in size up to puberty, when it remains stationary. At times it appears pale and bleached out, again it becomes quite red and prominent. How many times I have noticed it upon young girls at an early age, whose mothers have consulted me concerning it, thinking it was a birth mark or something of that nature. It requires two or three years to cure one of these cases and only the highest potencies have any effects upon it. I use Finck's, Skinner's and Swan's remedies in the highest potencies, cm, dmm, and cmm.

In these cases the father had invariably contracted gonorrhœa either before or during marriage, generally before, and the discharge was dried up and was followed by this eruption mentioned, the red mole. Later on in life they sometimes assume a warty nature, but generally they remain about the same all through the life of the patient. The red polka dot eruptions are met with more frequently upon the trunk of the body and anterior surfaces of the extremities. They are positively a diagnostic lesion, and when present, there should remain no doubt in your mind but that the patient has Sycosis either in the acquired or hereditary form. When you are in doubt about your diagnosis look for them and you are pretty certain to find them.

There is a form of *acne* that appears as large red angry-looking papules at about the menstrual period; they do not suppurate but are quite sore and sensitive to touch. They are unlike the small, pointed, itching papule of psora or the pustular and suppurating tubercular form of the disease. The chief feature of sycotic acne is the large, reddish, blunt-pointed, angry-looking lesion that is sore and sensitive to touch, non-suppurating and appears quite isolated and separate from each other and not in groups as is found in the psoric and tubercular forms; they are often found on girls at the menstrual period.

Lupus, whether of the erythematous or of the common form, belongs without doubt to the tubercular family of skin diseases, with a sycotic element present. My observation, extending back for many years, has been fully satisfied and convinced of this fact. The malignancies due to Syphilis and Psora are prone to develop about the age of 40, while that of Sycosis at any age. All three miasms, however, will be found in lupus patients, but Psora and Syphilis alone will not produce lupus. The proof of this fact, will readily be seen by a carefully-taken history of these cases, as to when the sycotic element entered the organism, and invariably the development of the lupus can be traced to some phase of Sycosis either suppressed or hereditary.

This truth is not altered in the least, by the fact that lupus often appears at an early age. A history of these cases will usually point to a suppression in the parent or to an imperfect cure. The reason why this disease is so difficult to cure can now be readily seen, knowing it is based upon a mixed miasm. The more miasms that are existant in your patient, the more complex, of course are the phenomena presented and the greater the difficulty in finding the similimum of the case. Here is a new field open for investigation in the treatment of lupus and other malignancies, which merit our research and earnest thought.

Many other forms of skin diseases might be enumerated as being of sycotic origin, such as *tinea sycosis* and *tinea barbae*. In fact all forms of facial skin diseases that are contracted in barber shops, with perhaps the exception of tinea favosa, are due to the sycotic taint or to a form of that miasm. Tinea circinata commonly met with, and mentioned by Dr. Burnett as having a tubercular origin, proves quite clearly to me this theory of the mixed miasm. In the scalp as well as in the beard we might mention another form, tinea circumscripta, which causes a form of alopecia and which responds readily to anti-sycotic treatment. In fact in all forms of ringworm, we see this specific sycotic element running all through the manifestations of these very mysterious lesions, of which so little is known. A suppression of ring-worm in any form means a suppression of Sycosis of a specific nature, and the invariable result of its suppression ill health, such as some form of rheumatism, or the development of chronic headaches, stomach troubles, chronic bronchitis, chronic coughs, melancholia, mania, hysteria in women and even malignancies. The suppression of ring-worm means a suppression of a specific form of Sycosis, usually upon a latent tubercular base, for tubercular patients are the ones who usually contract some of the many forms of tinia.

I question if rubeola and other similar exanthematous diseases have not a sycotic element as a predisposing cause. Variola, varicella in all their different forms have very marked characteristics of the sycotic element present, or of Syphilis and Sycosis combined. The serum of vaccination has without doubt both of these elements present. It can also be recognized in erythematous eczema, erysipelas, especially the phlegmonous variety, herpes, zoster, and impetigo contagiosa. Psoriasis has the gouty element so characteristic of Sycosis and this element has already been recognized. In reviewing Sajou's Annual and Cyclopedia of Medicine for

1896, '97, and '98, we find the statement that Psoriasis is dependent upon a blood state belonging to gout and rheumatism; the uric acid diathesis. Psoriasis, however, depends largely on Psora. The free indulgence in meat tends to aggravate these eruptions and vaccination is generally the exciting cause. Meat, alcoholic beverages, wines, and nitrogenous foods of all kinds aggravate both the gouty condition and the diseases based upon it.

Another disease to be considered, as positively of sycotic origin, is *gout* or the gouty diathesis. This disease of ancient origin has usually been associated with people of wealth, who live indolent lives, and who indulge in all sorts of luxuries and excesses in eating and drinking, but this is not strictly true. It is a well known fact that the excessive use of a rich diet, especially of a fatty and of a nitrogenous nature, the free use of wines and intoxicants, will develop a gouty diathesis. Sycosis, however, has the power to do this work without the aid of such foods or stimulants, although it is greatly accelerated by their use. Often, these people have a sycotic element in a latent form, and it is roused into action by their sedentary life and dietetic excesses. This gouty state of the system may present itself as a gouty rheumatism, or as it is commonly termed, rheumatic gout; all these conditions belong to the tertiary stage of Sycosis. When the joints are not affected or the gouty concretions are absent, we have another form of it, known as gouty liver, gout of the eyes, of the stomach, intestines, bladder, gout of the muscles. Gout of the heart and stomach are of such common occurrence today that sudden deaths from it are increasing greatly, especially in the higher walks of life, among the wealthy.

Examine these patients and we find all sorts of pathological changes, changes in the form or size of the organs, changes in the valves, hypertrophies, softening of the valves, dilitations and slow, soft, or intermittent pulse. In cardiac diseases they have no pain to speak of, occasionally a sharp thrust or a dull ache. Serious and dangerous conditions develop, while the patient is oblivious of the fact. How frequently do we hear of the sudden death of our great men, senators, business men, and those who lead a sedentary life, who take their spiced or imported wines and other intoxicants; wines in any form are more harmful to them, than any other of the stimulants or intoxicants. Those people are fond of aromatics, mustard, pepper, condiments of all kinds, rich and stimulating foods. Narcotics of all forms are the great excitants of a gouty diathesis. They meet with sudden death often from valvular diseases of the heart, from pneumonia, peritonitis, gastritis, or hepatitis. Many of them have dropsies, diabetes, Bright's disease of the kidneys, cirrhosis of the liver, congestion of the base of the brain, and even true insanity. They are subject to vertigo, dyspnoea, apoplexy, and hemiplegia. They have shortness of breath, puffing respiration with any over-exertion such as climbing a height. In acute diseases, especially where local inflammations or congestions are present, they snuff out like a candle. They can drink moderately of whisky all their lives with no special disturbance from it, but put them upon wines and stimulating foods and the luxuries of the rich, and soon they develop the gouty diathesis. We hear every day of sudden deaths in this class of patients. If you will watch the vital statistics of these people who consume much wine, and who eat a rich stimulating diet, especially where much meat is consumed, you will have your attention called to the frequency of sudden deaths. They die without warning from pneumonia, from congestions and from diseases of the heart, lungs, stomach, brain and intestinal tract.

Many of these patients suffer from prostatic and bladder troubles, and often the whole trouble seems located in the neck of the bladder, as frequently found in women as in men. Nothing seems to help these sufferers. The treatment does little more than palliate them, and many cases have come to me that nothing has helped. Then I found out the true history or cause, tracing it back many years to an early suppressed sycotic infection, which, although it had remained latent for a while, suddenly turned its whole force upon the bladder. Often these patients complain simply of a soreness along the urethral canal; occasionally felt when passing urine, more so when it becomes strongly acid. This may be the only symptom showing the disease is still there, but in a latent state. I recall now, one case in a young married man who came to me from St. Louis, who had complained of that symptom for fourteen years. A careful analysis of his case revealed Psorinum to be his remedy, which reproduced an old suppressed gonorrhœa, that was cured later on with Capsicum. His wife had suffered for years from hypertrophied uterus, and had had a number of physicians treat her with no permanent benefit. For the past two years of her life, she had received some relief from a change of climate and from mineral baths. In June, 1899, she began to take homeopathic treatment which was continued for ninety days, when she became pregnant and went through to full term. A male child was born, perfectly healthy, and as far as can be seen now, is free from any sycotic taint. The mother weighed only 95 pounds, but suffered scarcely any inconvenience during gestation; had an easy labor, and today is in the best of health. This history is one of an army of cases that find no relief until treated with homeopathy.

The coughs of these sycotic patients are usually bronchial. They are forever having bronchitis, hard, tight, dry racking coughs, frequently met with in early fall or winter. Not infrequently their troubles will begin with a coryza. There is much sneezing, with a profuse watery flow from the nose. In a few days it will pass down into the bronchii, and then they have a week, or ten days, or longer, of coughing spells. Expectoration is usually scanty. In the summer time they are usually free from it, but they are forever taking a cold in the head, on the least exposure to cold air or dampness (getting stuffy as they say). In fact, they can not, as a rule, breathe through the nose. If they should escape these troubles they have rheumatic pains or muscular rheumatism on the least exposure to wet or dampness or a chill. So sensitive are they to barometric changes that they make good weather prophets. They can foretell a change, it appears, days before. Sometimes these pains are of a transitory nature, again they may be localized and severe. Why should they be so subject to the elements, to a falling or rising barometer, or to planetary fluctuations? Because they have violated one of the Creator's laws, or by heredity have become subjects to the penalties of the broken precept. When we read in the Decalogue "Thou shalt not kill," or "Thou shalt not bear false witness," or "Thou shalt not commit adultery," we do not understand by this, that we are to become slaves to a principle, or that by the force of a Divine fiat we are to do this, or to do that. No. We understand that by a fulfilment of these principles, by a true recognition of these precepts, we are protected by all the power that is behind them. The principles so involved are the principles of power, and of life, and of God. It is an ascendency into the higher altitudes of a greater existence and of a larger life. To violate any of them, is to lose all the benefits of that power therein involved. The Decalogue is a divine gift to them, not a something that confines or coerces. It is a tree of life in our midst and he who eats thereof shall have life, but to violate any of its precepts means death in some form, for outside of them is no life. If through adultery we sin, that sin involves all that is lost in its violation, be it through heredity or be it acquired.

Thus it is with these sycotic patients. They have lost that power of resistance, that before their fall, was a genetic principle in the life force. If it rained they heeded it not; if the atmosphere was surcharged with moisture, it mattered not to them. The storm came and went; the winter and the summer passed but they suffered no special inconvenience. But what do we find is the case in our sycotically infected friend? He has lost all that which gave him protection, that which shielded, that which fortified him to them all, and now he becomes subservient to their influence and their power. When it rains he has pain; when the atmosphere is filled with moisture he suffers; when the elements clash, his organism is at war with itself; the rain, the snow, the cold, the barometer's rise and fall are his enemies. The planetary changes that before were his friends, his supporters in life, are now his peace disturbers, and his combatants. In health, his organism, his system was in harmony with the whole solar system and its countless changes, numberless variations, and infinite relationships. Now, like a slave, he cringes and writhes and whimpers under them, and we see him seeking relief or palliation in countless ways; from the use of drugs, sedatives, anodynes, palliatives of all kinds, hot fomentations, baths—thermal and electro-thermal, mineral, medicated and non-medicated.

All kinds of local measures are employed in the rheumatic and gouty individual. There is an army of them today at the numerous mineral springs of this country and of Europe. Sulphur and alkaline waters seem to palliate them, yet frequently they are only slightly or temporarily benefited. Again they receive, in some cases, much relief and benefit, and are tided over, as it were, until something else arises; some of the reasons that may be attributed to the relief they receive at mineral baths, are first, the prolonged or persistent use of heat, cabinet baths, hot mineral baths, such as those of White Sulphur Springs, Hot Springs, Mt. Clemens, Mich., or the mud baths of Mudlavia, Indiana—those of Europe, Carlsbad, etc. Secondly, the drinking of water in excess which is generally of the best and purest quality, often of an alkaline character, or of a lithic nature, neutralizes to some degree that excessively acid condition of the blood, from which the majority of these patients suffer—hence the great sale of lithia waters, such as Londonderry, Buffalo, etc., which today have been to some degree abandoned, and their place filled by the Lithia tablet, or the Vichy and Kissengen waters. Again, their excessive drinking of water at the mineral springs is a rule insisted upon by the medical advisers at these places, helps to flush out the kidneys, and throw into solution this excess of acid, and this excessive accumulation of the salts of the blood and lithic condition of the system. Thirdly, the change of diet and the rest, of course benefits them much. Such patients, especially those who have the necessary wealth, go up and down the earth, seeking relief. As the seasons change they suffer in multitudinous ways, especially from acute attacks of gout and rheumatism, which have a tendency to become more frequent or closer together with age. These are the sensitive, irritable patients, who have so stimulated and palliated the nervous system, that they are now super-sensitive to pain.

CHRONIC MIASMS

The question is often asked, is it necessary to know anything about the chronic miasms, in order to successfully treat those numberless chronic maladies that we meet in our every day practice? Let us see what relationship they bear to Homeopathic Therapeutics. Hahnemann has said, "The physician is likewise the guardian of health, when he knows what are the objects that disturb it, what produces and keeps up the disease, and what will remove it," etc. Sec. 4, Organon. The reverse of this would read like this, he who does not know what objects disturb the vital force or keep up the disease, is not a true guardian of health. In order to cure disease intelligently, we must regard the fundamental cause. I think I hear many say, are not the totality of the symptoms, all there is to disease? Yes, but to me it is necessary to know something of what is behind that grouping of the totality. If you do not know this you are prescribing for a Jack-in-the-box. You cannot follow the evolution of the curative process; you cannot even prescribe intelligently, the proper diet for a patient, unless you know the basic miasm. Of course, the diseases that are present will help you to some extent, but you have no surety unless you know the underlying basic disturber of the disordered life.

A psoric patient requires a diet altogether different from that of a tubercular patient, and the same thing may be said of those affected with Syphilis and Sycosis. A uric acid diathesis never lies behind a tubercular, syphilitic or psoric taint. So to know the basic miasm in each case helps us in many ways, besides that of being a therapeutic aid. It may form a basis not only of the patient's diet, but of occupation, mode of life, habits, social relations, sexual functions, and numerous other things. We cannot see the spiritual essence of disease, and it is not necessary that we should do so. But it is necessary to know what is behind each set of phenomena, and not to know, is ignorance. If you wish to say the patient took cold, or he over-worked, or became unduly tired, or it was indigestion, and a thousand other worn-out, threadbare excuses that are far from being scientific, you may follow out your old beaten path. That is just what men were doing before Hahnemann's time, and what they are doing today. The Allopathic school make but one bite of the proverbial cherry, when they write down germs as the cause of nearly every expression of sickness. We do not deal so with the acute miasms. No! We are very careful, and very diligent to find out with great certainty, the existing disturbing element, such as scarlet fevers, measles, smallpox, etc.

It becomes an offence to the state, if we do not know these things. Yet we may pass over a thousand cases of latent syphilis, tuberculosis, or sycosis, without offence, yet the state suffers more from our overlooking them, than from all the acute miasms put together. Not only does the state suffer but society suffers, our race suffers, humanity suffers untold agony, pain and distress; our jails and penal institutions are filled, and our insane hospitals increase in numbers all over the land.

"Totality of the symptoms is this image of the immediate essence of the malady, reflected externally." Sec. 7, Organon.

What do the symptoms represent? *The essence of the malady;* and what is the essence of the malady? *The chronic miasm.* Do you see why it is necessary to understand the phenomena of disease, and why certain symptoms persist and persist with no cessation? Organon II. "In disease this spontaneous and immaterial vital principle, pervading the physical organism, is primarily deranged by the dynamic influence of a *morbific agent*, which is inimical to life." Again in the 12th paragraph, the Organon says, "it is the morbidly disturbed vital principle which brings forth disease." What does Hahnemann mean by the *dynamic influence* of a morbific agent? He means that which causes all the morbid phenomena of disease to exist, he means Psora, Syphilis and Sycosis, or any intermingling or blending of the great triune. It is this morbific, dynamic influence which gives to the organism and life force its own nature, its own abnormal sensations, motions, mental and physical disturbances of all kinds and of every character, which we call disease. But in paragraph 18 it says, "that beyond the totality of the symptoms, there is nothing discoverable in disease." That is a great truth and we fully believe in it. It is not an understanding of the totality, that we are talking about; but an intelligent conception of the cause of the phenomena or totality.

We make no attack upon the law; no cure can be made outside of the law, for all law is fixed, eternal and unchangeable. But we do believe it is necessary to know whether the phenomena presented in a given case are of sycotic, syphilitic or tubercular origin; for the totality grouping must be about the symptoms of the active miasm. This is one reason why the peculiar or characteristic symptoms, when taken into consideration in making your prescriptions, gives us such wonderful results. Those brilliant cures that are occasionally made with the single remedy, occur where a single miasm lies behind the phenomena, but where the mixed miams are present, brilliant cures are not so made, and it is in those cases that it is so necessary to understand the order of their evolution.

This evolution, Hahnemann has portrayed clearly in the Organon, Sec. 38, when he says, "if the disease, which is dissimilar to the old, be more powerful than the latter it will then cause its suppression, until the new disease has either performed its own course, or is cured (removed by the indicated remedy), but then the old or former disease reappears." In this way the chronic miasms act; one is usually active, and holds the other in abeyance. For instance, Sycosis if present in any form or in any stage, usually takes the precedence. Suppose a case in which there is a marked pseudo-psoric condition, where perhaps a great many Calcarea symptoms are to be found. Now Calcarea is a basic remedy, and in it we find a perfect picture of the tubercular diathesis, but Calcarea will not meet the new order of things, even if it has the greater number of symptoms as far as you are able to enumerate them. But you cannot enumerate them, hence totality (if numbers alone count), does not fulfill the law of cure. No, it is the picture, the image of the active disturbing miasm that fulfils the demands of the law.

When the remedy of the first selection ceases to act or is found no longer to be curative, then a remedy may be selected from the grouping about the older miasm, the pseudo-psoric presentation, and the cure is complete. I have noticed many times men of good standing in the profession, prescribing Psorinum or Sulphur for the cure of an acute miasm, like Cuban Itch, Impetigo, and Scabies, when Sepia, Rhus tox, Rumex crispus, or some remedy that covered the acute miasm fully was all that was needed. True they found some symptoms calling for the remedies they selected, but these were found to greatly aggravate the case, much to their disappointment, by stirring up latent chronic miasms, and leaving the case worse than when they began. I have seen this kind of prescribing in cases that are incurable, such as organic heart trouble, tuberculosis, etc. In these cases it is a dangerous practice to prescribe deep acting anti-miasmatic remedies. It is a bad practice. We must follow not only the law of therapeutics, but the metamorphosis of disease, and understand the law governing it. Not infrequently in these cases of mixed miasms we are compelled to make one selection of the remedy from three to five symptoms, ignoring all others, and when this first remedy has brought the system to the proper condition, then all those symptoms that were rejected may be taken into consideration, and a second prescription made. This is especially true where suppressions are present, or where secondary processes develop from suppressions or from bad treatment, Organon, Sec. 50. "Even nature herself has no other Homeopathic agents at her command than miasmatic diseases." The more we study disease and the better we become acquainted with the law of cure, the more frequently we employ the nosodes or diseased substances.

Our Allopathic friends are following closely along the same lines, although their methods of preparing them are unscientific and in the end, harmful to the race. It is simply the application of natural diseases, as referred to in paragraph 80 of the Organon. Most of the Homeopathic treatment of today, like the regular school, is palliative in its nature, even with the single remedy and the potency. One reason for this, is a lack of knowledge of the chronic miasms, that lie behind the morbid phenomena with which we have to deal. Many of us know how to select a remedy, but we do not know how long to wait upon its action; in other words we do not understand the retrocession of each miasm, whether it be Syphilis, Psora or Sycosis. We have yet to learn their secondary and tertiary presentations, and the phenomena which attend each new setting of the disease. Again we have so little knowledge of them and are at sea when we find them blanketed and veiled by suppressive or palliative treatment.

Hahnemann makes but two classes of disease, and under this general head he classifies all forms and conditions of disease. "The first," he says, "are rapid operations of the vital power, departed from its natural condition, which terminates in a shorter or longer period of time, but are always of a moderate duration. These are the acute diseases." "The others," he says, "are less distinct, and often imperceptible on their first appearance." These diseases develop very slowly, and that force known as the vital power, cannot resist them. It is not strong enough to extinguish them, and in time they develop or grow, until they destroy the organism. These are known as chronic diseases and are produced by infection of a chronic miasm." We see by section 72, that Hahnemann had a clear and extensive knowledge of the chronic miasms, and we also know he wished his followers to become acquainted with them, and for that reason he wrote the first volume of Chronic Diseases, which is wholly given over to the study of the chronic miasms, Psora, Syphilis and Sycosis.

We have every reason to believe that after twelve silent years of study (as we see in Vol I. of Chronic Diseases), for he gave no knowledge of it to the world in all that time, he must have become very familiar with them. The sixty-four carefully written pages in volume one of Chronic Diseases, testify to that fact. In these pages he goes into detail and illustrates the subject by the many cases therein referred to. Not long ago a prominent physician said to me, "Hahnemann wrote the Organon after he wrote the Chronic Diseases." Yes, and he filled the Organon as well as the wonderful introduction to that valuable and indispensable book full of it. Besides, men like Charles J. Hemple, who translated The Chronic Diseases, and wrote its preface, believed and followed its teachings, and we have no less a light than Constantine Hering, who also wrote a preface found in Vol.I.

In this work Hahnemann not only gives us the character and nature of the chronic miasms, Syphilis. Psora, and Sycosis, but he tells us about the movements, the internal workings, and the law that governs their action, even that which governs the life force in the law of cure. Speaking of Psora, he says it is the fountain head of chronic ailments and is mother of all those numberless aiiments which we find enumerated in our pathological works, such as epistaxis, varices, hemorrhoids, hematemesis, menorrhagia, night-sweats, constipation, and all the host of names catalogued in our nomenclature. Again, he tells us of their disastrous results upon the whole human family throughout the age of plagues, and pestilences of which they were the father; of the millions, whose lives went out like the cutting off of the current from an electric bulb.

It is a fearful picture so dramatically drawn out in the first thirty or forty pages of Vol. I of Chronic Diseases, and Hahnemann meant the lesson for each of us to study carefully. He meant that we should become familiar with *his etiology* of *disease*, which in truth is the only true cause of disease worthy of our study. This brings all disease under a sin process, under transgression of law, "whose wages are death." He devotes pages to the history and data of many cases of suppression of chronic and acute miasms, giving the awful consequences and disastrous results of such suppression. In the ninety-seven cases to which he calls our attention, he presents a graphic picture of miasmatic suppressions with all their fatal endings, death processes and malignant ultimations. He pointed out these results as coming from the unscientific treatments that were unhomeopathic in each case.

Hahnemann again speaking of the lack of study, and attention given to the chronic miasms says, on page 50 in the old edition of Chronic Diseases, "that the circumstances relative to the cause of chronic diseases, deserve so much more to be noticed, as the common physicians, especially the modern, have from sheer blindness, overlooked it, although it was evidently the cause of all chronic diseases." On the same page he gives three rules we should follow in investigating the three chronic miasms. First, the period when infection took place; second, the period when the whole organism began to be tainted with the miasmatic poison, and third, the manifestations of the external expression, by means of which Nature indicates the complete development of the miasmatic disease of the internal organs.

Form these lines we learn that we are to become familiar with all the chronic miasms during their initial stages, their periods of invasion of the organism, and also when the secondary expressions appear upon the skin, which shows the completion of the miasmatic involvment. The third period is when Nature relieves the internal stress upon the organs, and a comparative equilibrium is established in the life force. This third process is frequently brought about during a course of treatment of the patient. You have all seen Sulphur or Psorinum, or perhaps some other remedy bring about these secondary expressions in the form of eruptions upon the skin, or perhaps by some discharge being reestablished or some former suffering renewed; often the mental sphere is relieved and the physical grows worse, or vice versa. One fact that Hahnemann brought to view very clearly in this connection, is, that the miasmatic infection becomes fully developed in the organism, before these eruptions appear upon the skin.

This is true of all the miams; they all produce

eruptions upon the skin in their secondary and tertiary stages. In Psora we have the papules, in Syphilis the polymorphic lesions, and in Sycosis, the great family of warts, moles and blotches that have already been mentioned in this work. "It is the same," Hahnemann says, "in the chronic miasms as in the acute, for after the internal disease is completed, the eruptions appear." It is a pathological law, that while the acute goes through its evolution within a few days or weeks, the chronic often take years. Not infrequently we lose sight of Syphilis for many years, when to our surprise it again appears as an eruption, upon the skin, or as some destructive ulceration. The acute disappears with a succession of rapid movements, often of a violent febrile nature, and the organism disposes of them quickly and forever, but we find it not so in the chronic miasms. Their evolution is slow, with pauses and rests, yet they are always present. Latent for years, they may give forth eruptive expressions of themselves in any of their cycles, which relieves the organism from great internal suffering.

The life force has no power to disengage itself from the chronic miasms, as they are not so self-limited as are the acute. This thought is splendidly illustrated by Hahnemann in page fifty-four of Chronic Diseases, Vol. I. In speaking of Syphilis, he says, "not till the internal disease is completely developed, does Nature try to alleviate or hush its sufferings, by forming a spot where the infection takes place, a local symptom as a substitute for an internal disease." The *contagiousness of the disease comes with this expression, and the power to convey, comes with and through the local manifestations, which did not appear until the whole organism* was thoroughly imbued with the miasmatic poison. "Only the vicarious chancre has the power of communicating to other persons the same miasm, which is the internal disease." All the chronic miasms, Psora, Syphilis, and Sycosis, take about the same period of time in the development of their first stages, which is from ten to seventeen days. "Psora," says Hahnemann, "takes from ten to fourteen days; the disease in all three makes its appearance at the point of infection and then develops secondary and tertiary processes."

Psora develops the itch vesicle or the itching papule, Syphilis, the virulent open ulcer, and Sycosis, the specific catarrhal discharge. All have a slight febrile disturbance and show signs and symptoms just before secondary infection. They all have malaise, functional disturbances and manifestations of specific poisons following the infection, and a little previous to the secondary expression of the disease. In acute diseases such as scarlet fever and measles we prescribe, as a rule, for the totality of the symptoms covering the malady, and why not so understand the chronic miasms, that we can do likewise? Paragraph 258 of the Organon, in speaking of this phase of the subject says: "We are to be careful not to entertain a prejudice aginst those remedies from which we may have experienced some check, because we had made a bad selection; and we should never lose sight of this great truth that of all the known remedies there is but one, that merits a preference before all others, namely, the one whose symptoms bear the closest resemblance to those which characterize the *malady*."

This *malady* I have found in every case to be the active miasm, and that active miasm is as frequently Sycosis as anything else, and the curative remedy will very often revolve about its symptomatology. In the same case, any prescriber could find a psoric grouping or perhaps a pseudo-psoric grouping, that appeared to be (to the student not acquainted with miasmatics) of great value. It is here I claim that majority of our failures occur in selecting the true simillimum. Thus a knowledge of the active miasm that lies behind the malady, assists us in grouping our remedies, whether they be anti-psoric, anti-syphilitic, or anti-sycotic. The second selection of the remedy will now, as a rule, cover that grouping that the first remedy covered by mistake. Then we conclude that the first selection of the remedy should culminate about the active miasm, and the second selection should cover the latent miasms, now disturbed or brought into action, by active miasm on which we based our first prescription.

To illustrate this, suppose we select Belladonna for scarlet fever, covering a splendid and positive totality. Behind this acute miasm (scarlet fever), we will say, lies a latent tubercular element (pseudo-psora), which becomes violently disturbed by the acute active miasm. Soon we notice the Belladonna group waning and the chronic miasmatic element advancing in all its fury, with an abscess perhaps of the middle ear, calling for Hepar, Mercury, or Arsenic. As this is the order things in the acute, so is it in the chronic. The difference is this, in the case of scarlet fever, it is easy to understand, for the phenomena are so prominent, and the symptoms so clear, but in the chronic blending, the symptoms are not prominent, not clear, and it requires much study and close observation to distinguish in the secondary or tertiary stages of chronic miasms, what is behind the existing malady, as referred to in paragraph 258 of the Organon.

Until I saw clearly that La Grippe was a sycotic disease, I often found it difficult to select a curative remedy that would wipe it out, without the necessity of a second or third selection; but now knowing what is behind the malady, I have seldom any trouble in securing such a remedy. As you study the disease, you will find the genus-epidemicus will, in over ninety per cent. of the cases, be an anti-sycotic one. We select our nosodes in that way and from just such knowledge. Yet I have seen Psorinum prescribed in an acute sycotic eruption, that was covered fully by Sepia, entirely on the symptom of itching. The genus-epidemicus is but another proof of this truth. The genus-epidemicus is the remedy that covers the totality of the existing malady, not all that symptoms of which are to be found in any one patient. Thus it is true of every other case. The disease forces combining with the life forces, produce or bring forth an inhibition, and about that inhibition is to be found a grouping of symptoms, that represent the similia of the existing malady, which is the phenomena of miasmatic action in every case. If you do not find this, your treatment is palliative and does not fulfill the law.

But you say, "it is so difficult to discern these things. How can we understand the symptomatology of the present active miasm?" We reply, "in the same manner as you study the drug picture, for drug pictures are but expressions of it." Gumma is an expression of a peculiarly disturbed life force with a syphilo-psoric basis. Rhus tox gives us a fine conception of a sycotic rheumatism; Benzoic acid of a gouty bladder, and of a gouty state of the system; Rheum and Chamomilla of a sycotic diarrhoea; Gelsemium of an acute state of La Grippe; Rhus tox, or Sepia, of a sycotic eruption, and so on through the whole list of remedies.

Here comes before some cases of Cuban itch. The patients are an old Homeopathic physician and his whole family. Their bodies are covered with the eruption, and they are fearful cases; they have suffered with it for five months. He has tried all the anti-psoric remedies, he said, with no relief; but "It is not a psoric disease," I said, "it is the army itch; a sycotic disease, pure and simple. What you need is an anti-sycotic remedy." Sepia, 1 m, was selected, which removed every sign of it in eight days. There was no itching to speak of after the fourth day, and much relief after the first twenty-four hours. Only four of five powders were given, and even less would have sufficed. "How did this happen?" you ask. It was a lack of knowledge of the element behind the malady; thus Sepia was overlooked.

The false teaching that has gone forth for years, that everything is Psora that is not Syphilis, has done much to harm the cause of Homeopathy. "But," you say, "Hahnemann taught that fact and made it prominent." Yes, and it was true then, but one hundred years have elapsed since that time, and things have changed. This new element Sycosis, has increased and multiplied ten thousand fold since that time. It was an uncommon disease in Hahnemann's time, and as a rule, was not considered very seriously, as we see on page 102 of Chronic Diseases, Vol. I. Yet he briefly describes the true or sycotic form in the three pages given to this subject. On page 113, he speaks of curing this form with Nitiric acid (meaning the form with the excrescences or condylomata which we now understand to be from a mixed miasm, or a form of Syphilis and Sycosis combined, for which Cinabaris, as well as Nitric acid are often indicated).

The other form is where these excrescences are not present, but where the common sycotic wart, verruca vulgaris, and the pendulous wart is present. In this form the symptoms were met with Thuja, and here Hahnemann gives the order of treatment, or the selection of the remedy as has been mentioned. He says, "If Allopathic treatment has so disturbed Psora or Syphilis, that may have been lying latent in the organism, so that they now become manifest and active, then the order of treatment is reversed, and we first annihilate the psoric miasm, by the subsequently indicated anti-psoric ; and then use the remedy indicated for the Sycosis." Do you follow those principles in your prescribing for your cases, in general practice, or do you keep pounding away at the Sycosis, and thus fail to cure your case ? You are weak right here where you ought to be strong, yet many of you are ready to oppose anyone who calls your attention to this important truth as laid down by the master.

I have no new truth for you, I make no claim to that ; I am simply "one crying in the wilderness, make the paths straight,"—follow the teachings of Hahnemann to the very letter, for if you disobey the law you are bringing it into disrepute, and thus injuring the cause of Homeopathy. The influence of chronic miasms upon endemic or epidemic diseases, is well known to those who are acquainted with the principles governing Homeopathy. (In this, of course I mean Hahnemannian Homeopathy, for there does exist in the world a system of medicine, so called Homeopathy, whose followers do not adhere to these principles, and thereby bring great disrepute and grievance to the cause of Hahnemann).

"This strikingly obstinate character of epidemic diseases," says Hahnemann, "is due to some psoric miasm," but, today we know it is not due alone to Psora, for Sycosis, as has been mentioned many times, plays frequently as great a part as Psora, and this is why cancer and the malignant diseases are increasing. A prominent medical writer of England says, "cancer, at the rate it is increasing will destroy all human life on the island in two hundred years." Malignancies increase and diseases multiply and are magnified by miasmatic blendings and suppressive treatment. I might say here, that in England there is not more cancer than in other countries, only in that country, the fact has been brought to light more fully. But we know diseases are multiplying in the earth ; we know that they are difficult to cure, more persistent and positive in their bond with the life force. The earth is full of sin, full of disease, suffering, death, and degeneracy of the human race. It is a veritable house of pestilence, and a hospital of the plague.

All kinds of false theories of cure are arising in the earth, and also false teachings as to the nature of disease and of life. Many of these false methods of treating disease have come into use within the past ten years, their name is legion. The majority of them are suppressive in their nature and palliative in their effects ; all complicate disease, stir up the chronic miasm, which of course increases malignancies and magnifies disease and the death processes. Again as we resume our subject in the study of the action of acute epidemics, like La-Grippe, upon the chronic latent miasms, we find that as soon as the acute disease passes away, and often before it leaves the organism, the disturbed chronic miasm will require special treatment. "Even," says Hahemann, "if our best remedies should have been employed against the acute miasms." Scarcely a case passes through our hands, that does not require at about the close of the acute epidemical disease, the selection of some deep acting anti-psoric or anti-sycotic remedy, before the patient is again restored to health. In this procedure lies the secret of success in the cure of disease. The same thing may be said of those acute diseases which intervene, called *"morbi intercurrentes,"* as Hahnemann calls them ; no acute disease ever arises (outside of contagious or infectious diseases) that is not an effort on a part of the life forces to throw the effects (internal disease or the internal workings of a chronic miasm) to the surface. When the life force fails to do this the disease centers upon some internal organ and we have pneumonia, bronchitis, or some other deep-seated disease process.

Not all medicines reach down to the miasmatic taint, hence Hahnemann called those that do so anti-psorics, anti-syphilitics, and anti-sycotics. In paragraph 251 of the Organon, he speaks of this fact, and in paragraph 252 he uses the word anti-psoric which he puts in brackets, saying "if when the (anti-psoric) remedy is given in the proper dose it does not produce an amendment, it is a sure sign that the cause which keeps up the disease, still exists and there is something either in the regimen or condition of the patient, that must be first altered before a permanent cure can be effected." There is a superficial setting in the therapeutic grouping of our remedies, and also a deep-seated one ; the first is palliative and the second curative ; both are necessary in the treatment of the sick, yet the first method of prescribing "is overworked," as is commonly expressed in slang phrase.

In this first form of prescribing, the remedy can be repeated frequently with good results, but in the second a frequent repetition will prove injurious to the patient and often entirely spoil the cure.

Again Hahnemann says in section 249 of the Organon, "every medicine which in the course of its operation produces new symptoms that do not pertain to the disease to be cured, and that are annoying, is incapable of procuring real amendment and cannot be considered as Homeopathically chosen." Herein lies one of the secrets of a cure. When we are not well versed in the nature and movements (progressive or evolutionary) of each of the chronic miasms, then we are unable to distinguish those symptoms which are drug provings from those which belong to miasmatic processes, or are due to the curative action of a well selected remedy, and of course we may have aggravations from supposedly well chosen remedies. Thus we flounder about in a labyrinth of symptoms, and are unable to disentangle the phenomena of each.

If, however, you are acquainted with the pauses and rests and the progressive movements of the miasms, you will know something of what is to be expected from a well chosen remedy and you will also know when the disease is eradicated wholly from the organism. It is what you see in disease and understand disease to be, that brings to your mind the importance of its treatment. If, for instance, you see only a circumscribed local inflammation, in an attack of gonorrhoea, you will at once try to extinguish (with a chemical fire extinguisher for that is what it is) that local fire (inffammation) ; but if you see in that circumscribed phenomenon of suffering the beginning of a deep miasmatic taint, with a long history of death dealing and destructive processes, a blasted life, a jail filling, prison building principle and a soul damning and life cursing medium, you will treat it from a miasmatic basis. Thus we see differently ; one sees a simple process that he vainly hopes to extinguish with his chemical fire hose ; he deems it local, self-limiting, capable of being destroyed in its acute process (as soon as the bacilli are killed) ; the other, having all the light Hahnemann has thrown upon disease, and his knowledge of its miasmatic origin, sees a prolonged and endless process, the wrecking of a life, and knows how to extinguish the venereal ulcer or discharge, by the natural process of the law with which he is a co-operator and a worker together in truth.

Hahnemann's "striking, singular, extraordinary, and peculiar symptoms" are basic miasmatic ones, always ; hence the wonderful curative effects produced, by remedies selected upon such symptoms ; they are capable of reaching down deep enough to extinguish, or what is a better term, to separate their miasmatic bond from the life forces. One of the translators of the Organon, speaking of a so-called homeopath who prescribes homeopathic remedies without a knowledge of the law governing their action, says, "but how will this careful and laborious process, by which the best cure of disease can be effected, please those gentlemen (sect), who while pluming themselves with the honorable title of homeopathists, for appearance sake, administer medicines in the form of homeopathists, that they have hastily snatched up (quicquid in buccam venit)." If it does not at once relieve the disease for which the remedy is given, they will impute the cause of the failure to the law, and not to their own insufficient knowledge of the law, and of that which disturbs the sick one, and produces the morbid phenomena.

The whole summing up of the matter is this ; The remedy that has the therapeutic power to produce an artificial disease closely resembling the natural disease, will subdue or destroy that natural disease, but in order to secure that grouping, that true picture which makes the selection of such a remedy possible, it is scientifically necessary to understand the phenomena that produce and keep up the natural disease. We do not say it cannot be done without this, but we do say, it is not scientific Homeopathy ; not the Homeopathy that Hahnemann endeavors to instill into the student of Homeopathy from every page of his writings. We further say, if new symptoms arise, the so called Homeopathy has no positive way to distinguish between them, whether they be drug proving or the retrograde metamorphosis of a latent miasm, coming forth in the order in which Hahnemann said they would. "The physician need not feel any uneasiness, when prescribing an anti-psoric remedy, if the ordinary symptoms of the disease, (Psora) is called out in a higher degree of intensity than they usually manifest themselves." This part of the law of cure is not looked into carefully enough, and it is so vital, so important, that we should understand it fully, for not to understand the symptoms of the re-appearing of the miasmatic process, is often to make a disastrous failure of our cure, and not only that, but to change all the physiological processes of elimination that are taking place under the curative action of your well-selected anti-miasmatic. It is this "calling out of symptoms," as Hahnemann calls the work of the curative remedy, that makes the splendid process of a cure. These called-out symptoms are the work of the law in its efforts to restore to normal the false processes due to disease changes in the organism.

We are not to select our remedy on the strength of the name of Psora, or Sycosis, or Syphilis. *No ! It is to be based upon the totality grouping of the disturbed or active miasm ; that grouping should be understood.* For the reasons given, and for a great many other reasons, we have not time or space in this article to enumerate. Hahnemann grouped his anti-psoric remedies, and from that grouping he made his selection ; his sycotic grouping was extremely limited largely confined to Thuja; this was of course due to his limited proving of remedies. Today we have almost as many anti-sycotics as we have anti-psorics, and we have also become quite familiar with the fact, that deep acting remedies like the metals, (I might mention Arsenicum) are curative and cover all the miasms, so deep and profound in their action upon the life forces. A thorough knowledge of these chronic miasms, makes plain the backward and forward movements of disease. It assists us in the selection, too, by the true grouping process of the anti-miasmatic remedies ; thus it helps us to watch the true progress of disease, and what to expect in the evolution of each miasm, until it has become completely extinguished or separated from its bond with the life. Besides, we are enabled to set aside these symptoms that are to a great degree, latent in the organism, and select a remedy based upon the active miasm, which when removed, may allow the other symptoms to come to the front so that they can be covered with a second selection. For instance a dose of Sulphur given a tubercular patient, and based upon an apparently good grouping of Sulphur symptoms, has so stirred up the tubercular element in a number of cases for me, as to require many months to repair the damage done to my patient.

It is also necessary for us to become familiar with the suppression of the chronic miasms, also to know those centers, or points around which each miasm centers itself. Many of these symptoms have already been given. Syphilis flies to the meninges of the brain and to the brain itself, to the larynx—throat in general—eyes, bones and periosteum. I have seen paralysis follow in two months, in a case of Syphilis in a man and his wife, when the first secondary expression of the disease which manifested itself on the forehead (roseola) was suppressed by a few applications of mercurial ointment. Psora spends its force when suppressed upon the nervous system largely, or upon nerve centers, often producing nervous and mental phenomena of a serious character ; but of course these are relieved when an eruption is thrown upon the skin. Sycosis attacks internal organs, especially the pelvic and sexual organs in the worst specific forms of inflammation, producing hypertrophies, abscesses, cystic degeneration, mucous cysts, etc., and when thrown upon the brain it produces headaches, severe acute mania, central insanity, moral degeneracy, dishonesty, etc. All these things ought to be familiar to the faithful guardian of the health or the true Homeopathic physician. As we study the chronic miasms, we notice that they are presented to us in a multitude of forms and modes. They present shadings as variable as the clouds in the heavens, and are as vacillating as the risings and fallings of the barometer in winter time ; here a forward movement and there a backward movement. In this way the contention between them and the life forces is kept up continually. As we look at the face of the sick one we have before us, a physiological mirror, reflecting their very presence, the degree of their disorderly action within, the indelible seal of their presence, stamped and impressed deeply by the life within, as with an oath. Here the clinician looks for signs of health or disease ; here he sees the pallor of exhaustion, the flush of fever, the hectic ring, the shadows of despondency, the mental rise and fall, the psoric papules, the syphilitic roseola, the sycotic spot. It is pale, flushed ashy, livid, grey, pigmented, sallow, muddy, bloodless, sunken, and anæmic; it has all the degrees and shadings that the practiced eye can conceive of ; all this we find mirrored upon this little field of our visage, the face. Again we look for them at fixed points, in well known centers, that the books on pathology have written so much about, and lastly we see them in the mental spheres, in the morals, and in the acts and very life of the human being.

We have written extensively upon the subject of the three chronic miasms—Psora, Syphilis and Sycosis—and their symptomatology as single miasms, but we have said but little about mixed miasms, except what has been said in Vol. 1 of this work. We cannot go deeply into this phase of the subject, but hope to later on. After the 3rd Vol. on the Chronic Miasm, Syphilis, has been written, we intend to write a work on the mixed miasms, of which pseudo-psora is one, so fully written on, in Vol. 1. Hering, in his introduction to the Organon, translated by Charles J. Hemple, says, "Hahnemann distinguishes the veneral miasms as Syphilis and Sycosis ; and also subdivides Psora with pseudo-Psora. The regular school has generally recognized the fact that tertiary Syphilis is not true Syphilis, and we know it is not, as we have to resort not infrequently to anti-psoric remedies to cure it."

We cannot take up this phase of the subject farther ; we simply wish to call your attention to the fact ; as it is these combinations with Psora that makes the practice of medicine and disease stubborn, intricate and difficult to understand. It is these combinations known as mixed miasms, from which our malignancies develop, such as cancer, lupus, burrowing abscesses, sinuses, tubercular infiltrations, growths and changes, and all the countless forms of malignancies. For instance, the specific secondary inflammation of Sycosis comes when Psora and pseudo-Psora blend fully with the sycotic element in the secondary stage. Again we see the fibrous changes in the kidneys, liver, etc., in the tertiary stage of that miasm Sycosis. The same may be said of the malignant tubercular changes of cancer and lupus. The condylomata are formed from the mixed veneral combination Syphilis and Sycosis, but the subject is so extensive and covers so much of pathology, that we cannot enter into it here.

In no instance should the mental phenomena of the miasms be overlooked in the selection of the remedy covering the case, for the mental should predominate over the physical always, and each of the chronic miasms has its own morbid mental peculiarity, all of which have been referred to in this work. Hahnemann has said that much care should be taken in watching the mental and moral symptoms in the progress of cure. "We should judge the degree of Homeopathic adaptation, existing between the remedy and the disease, by the improvement that take place in the moral condition." (Hering).

We should also notice that law of exchange between the mental and the physical in the care of disease, i. e., when the physical is $>$ and the mental grows $<$, and vice versa. How often through an external diseased process has the mental condition been relieved; insanity has disappeared by the appearance of an ulcer or an eruption upon the skin, or a vaginal discharge. We see the same law applied in the physical itself; a nose bleed has many times relieved a headache, an eruption a pain, a copious night sweat, which shows that the disease centered within, has not left its hiding place. A miasmatic grouping, however, covers all that is necessary to find the simillimum in curing the disease.

Let me quote Hahnemann again, and pardon me if I tire you with his quotations; speaking of the true etiology of disease, after having discovered Psora, he says, "This showed me that the Homeopathic practitioner ought not to treat diseases of this kind, as separate and completely developed maladies; nor ought he to expect such a permanent cure of these diseases, as would prevent them from appearing again in the system, either in their original or in a modified and often more disagreeable form. Why? We read further on, "This primitive disease evidently owed its existence to some chronic miasm." So we see clearly how Hahnemann looked upon disease, from a Miasmatic standpoint; and when he was prepared to make his slection of the remedy in chronic diseases, he based his prescription upon those symptoms that were centralized upon the existing, active, chronic miasm. How shall we become acquainted with Hahnemann's way of prescribing? By the study of his Organon of medicine and his work on chronic diseases. How shall we learn the symptoms of the miasms? By a study of each of the chronic miasms, Psora, Syphilis, and Sycosis, in all their stages, and in all their blendings.

Enough has been said in these two volumes to start you out well, and you have besides, your own observation from day to day in practice, and also the great principles of the law to govern and direct you, as set down in the Organon. Still farther you have your Materia Medica which is but the reflected image of the disease that is to be cured. You can see Psora in Sulphur and in Lycopodium, in Arsenic and Psorium; Syphilis in the Mercuries, in the Iodides, and in Nitric acid; Sycosis in Rhus, in Thuja, Kali Sulp, Capsicum, Medorrhium and a host of others, that will be tabulated at the end of this volume.

These cases of chronic trouble that do not receive the basic miasmatic remedy sometime in the course of their treatment are either palliated, or as Hahnemann says, "suspended for a time, only to return more grievous than before." Again the basic miasmic remedy fulfills all the requirements of the law; indeed the law is only satisfied or brought to its height of action against the contending forces of disease by an anti-miasmatic selection. In this way the vital energies are restored without loss and without hindrance, and their movements are continuous and progressive towards health; the functions are brought back to their normal rhythm; otherwise we abridge the process of the cure, and are apt to lead the perverted vital forces into greater dissipation.

Organon, Secs. 20 and 21, says in effect this, "we experience the hidden faculty of medicines, by observing their effects upon the human organism, when these medicines are well selected, based upon the *basic symptoms* of the disease." We see not only their curative action upon that disease, but we then disentagle the woven meshes of disease processes, fulfilling in every point the law of Homœopathy.

As we study the nature and action of the miasms, we are at the same time studying the true character of disease and the nature of sickness. It is not trying to establish a theory that the stomach, liver or the heart is a cause of the sickness, but that the phenomena of the perverted or disturbed life force, is the phenomena of a certain chronic miasm, whose character, we are to understand and which gives us the character and nature of the disease. We should know that these perversions in sickness are perversions in physiological law, due to some force or forces, the character of which is familiar to us, and its history and movements, even when suppressed, we should be very familiar with. "There is no such thing," says Dr. Kent, "as one organ making another organ sick or making the man sick." So if the blame cannot be put upon a part of the whole, where shall we place it?

We have learned that disease works from center to circumference, and that it is what starts the central wheels in motion, along lines contrary to law and in opposition to life and health, and to so persist as to include all there is in disease, even to the destruction and death of the organism. It is this power that we claim is the true etiology of disease; it is this power that we claim you become acquainted with when you become familiar with the character and origin of the chronic miasms.

"We ought to seek out the hidden and unknown interior of what is to be cured in disease and not depend upon exteriors alone." The remedy goes into the great power houses that control the forces of life and that cures permanently and promptly. Disease endings are found in its pathology, but its beginnings no man can see, except as he sees it through law and knowledge of the nature of the chronic miasms. *Physical* examinations give you a knowledge of the former, but only *dynamic* examinations give a knowledge of the latter.

"The needs of the patient," says the same author, (Dr. Kent), "are seen in the signs and symptoms," but a thorough knowledge of those signs and symptoms is only possible from a knowledge of the chronic miasms. A change of state, whether it be local or general, is due to some power acting or co-operating with the life force. Then let us become acquainted with that power, whose character will be seen in all its movements and in all its disease processes. One must know the pathways it takes and the phenomena it propagates.

Quoting Dr. Kent again: "If disease is cured from cause to effect, then it must remain cured ," we see that order only returns and remains when cause is hit hard with that power which annihilates it. To push it gently aside by a palliative remedy only causes its action to cease for a time, then to re-establish itself. Thus we recognize disease in its exterior manifestations and its interior manifestations are only the miasmatic forces switching about as they are influenced by suppressive measures or by bad treatment. We see the same thing taking place in latent diseases; such as the tubercular when roused into action by scarlet fever or other acute miasms, producing sequelæ. To understand this we must know something about the correlation of the forces and their transference from one part of the organism to another and the cause of these sudden transferences. The physician who uses local applications such as X Ray, the light or the electric current, can have no knowledge of these things; the disappearance of pathology is all that interests him. The pathology that returns, he calls recurrences, and their cause is a dead letter to him, as he has no knowledge of the law governing the interior forces. We know that all movement is governed by law, and this study from cause to effect is the inductive method of Hahnemann, out of which his knowledge of Homeopathy came to light. Sequelae and many of the dangers and malignant manifestations of disease, may be often charged to the physician who has no knowledge of the active character and movements of miasmatics. The constitition of each patient should be carefully studied, for his disease will be found to be dependent upon some miasmatic basis, and the physician who cannot detect the presence of Sycosis in his patient, without a history of gonorrhoea, has very little knowledge of miasmatics. Phthisis may be headed off before an abscess forms in the lung tissue, if we are familiar with the phenomena of its incipiency. The bond between two miasms can only be broken by a prescription that will meet the totality of the more active one. Each has its own phenomena of expression, its times, modalities and order of arrangement. The appearance of sequelae is an appearance of a chronic disease or rather an expression of one, dependent upon the miasmatic government within. Whatever has been sown in life, will blossom and bring forth fruit in the family tree. If you cannot find the insignia upon the surface of the body, voices from within will continue to cry out until it is removed. No secret sin can be hidden for all will and is made manifest or brought to light. "On making a prescription," says Dr. J. T. Kent, *"a great deal depends upon a physician's ability to perceive what constitutes a miasm. If he is dull of perception, he will intermingle symptoms that do not belong together."*

Dr. W. E. Reller of Council Bluffs, Iowa, speaking of Psora in an article to the Medical Advance in 1893, says, "none of the writings of Hahnemann have been so reviled and ridiculed as the teaching found in his works 'Chronic Diseases,' and yet any close observer, who will study his writings diligently and apply their teachings carefully and intelligently in practice, will soon be convinced of their genuineness. He further says, "the average Homeopathic physician does not live up to the privileges he might enjoy, by being fully grounded on the philosophy of Homeopathy."

The constitutional or chronic miasms may be either latent or active; they may be so latent that no symptoms may mark a deviation from health or show their presence even to one who is skilled in a knowledge of miasmatics. We observe this in growing children and in those of a robust nature in whom strong vitality predominates. The chronic miasms become active in the presence of acute diseases (such as the diseases of children), also at the decline of life, when the vitality of the individual diminishes. It is then we find tumors, malignant growths and all the pathology that comes through the mixed miasms at the age of decline, from forty years of age and upwards. Such is the history of disease in our works on practice and pathology; the cause always wrapped in mystery and obscurity. It was only after Hahnemann had spent twelve years of his life searching out his hidden mystery, that he set to work to find out the remedies that would cure them.

Quoting Dr. Reller again from the same article, he says, "I had opportunity in one family, to investigate and observe what has already been said to be true. Seven of the children in this family died before they were three years of age; all dying of gastro-intestinal difficulties, and nearly all had symptoms of hydrocephalus; those who did survive, suffered with chronic headaches. Three sisters on the maternal side, I found had died of tuberculosis and one was then in an insane hospital. On the paternal side, a grandfather and two sisters were insane. Is this not a terrible demonstration of Hahnemann's psoric theory?"

Two remedies may have the same symptoms as to external form, yet the rank of those remedies may differ widely, the one that corresponds to the active, basic miasms ranks the higher. Again, the remedy that acts from within outwards and from above downwards, is a basic remedy. There is still another rule; the remedy should meet the symptoms in the order in which they first made their appearance. In selecting a remedy we are then to arrange the symptoms according to their value, giving preference to those last appearing, for they are the symptoms of the active miasm, and classifying the remainder as belonging to the latent grouping. If these should continue after the first or active symptoms have disappeared, it may be necessary to study them for a new selection. Their order, their value and their latency or activity must be taken into careful consideration in the selection of a curative remedy. Of course if improvement ceases, a new examination must be made. Sometimes in this grouping, new symptoms appear, or old, latent and forgotten ones come to light. As in the first selection, so in the second, they must be considered according to their miasmatic rank. If an eruption appears upon the skin, an old sore re-opens or a discharge is reestablished, matters are often greatly simplified, and the cure follows the law of physiological progression.

A failure to recognize the underlying idiosyncrasy

or chronic miasmatic taint, even in the cure of acute diseases, may prove fatal to the patient; it is one of the difficulties of the therapeutic art. We must learn to read between the lines, for the symptoms that are often the most prominent and annoying to the patient, are not always the ones to base your prescription upon, and vice versa. Fifteen or twenty paragraphs of the Organon are devoted to the subject of Homeopathic prescribing, and in them, the foundation of the art is laid. How often have we given the acute remedies like Bryonia or Belladonna, repeated, or in their different potencies, with no results, when after a more careful analysis, we saw as we read between the lines, the deeper acting antipsoric, sycotic or pseudo-psoric remedies, to be the ones indicated.

An abnormal symptom is a sign, mark or indication of a disturbance in the vital force, and its clinical or pathogenetic value is the golden knowledge of the physician. Its real value rightly placed, brings forth the true results of the workings of the law. By the parrot-taught Materia Medicist, values are not given sufficient attention, due stress is not placed upon them, and the drug picture produced is correspondingly lacking. If possible, I begin with the mental symptoms and proceed outward to the physical; or from above downwards to the extremities. Pathology, outside of unavoidable surgery, should be an unknown quantity to the homeopathic prescriber, save that he should be able to trace it to its miasmatic source and know its miasmatic dynamis and origin. To Hahnemann, miasms were defiling, polluting, contaminating and soiling; he speaks of them as infectious noxes. Crude drugs, however, may be added to these noxes, for they are a part of the hydra-headed causes that make human beings sick.

Professor H. N. Guernsey, who is called the "father of the Keynote system of Materia Medica," says we "must be in harmony with the totality." "It seems like prescribing for single symptoms," says Dr. E. W. Berridge, "but it is not; it is only meant to state some strange characteristic symptom." It is these strong keynotes, these characteristic symptoms that denote the presence of the active miasm, and sometimes of the suppressed one, as has already been mentioned. We do not believe in prescribing for single symptoms, we believe in the totality of the existing active miasm, and not in making the "see the case at a glance" prescription.

I believe Hahnemann was the first to make the statement that Sycosis was a miasmatic disease, and no more self-limiting than Syphilis or Psora, running a similar course to Syphilis and having three distinctive stages, whose phenomena and pathology differ from each other as in other chronic miasmatic diseases. Hahnemann recognizes these different stages and further says, "that if the disease is not cured in its catarrhal stage or if its symptoms are suppressed by local means, the disease will become chronic." This is a history in brief that we have verified many times. We know that after suppression, there may follow an apparent interval of health, but on carefully and closely examining such a patient, we will find symptoms, too trifling, perhaps, to be complained of, but which show the existence of a condition not correspondent to the normal condition existing before the attack.

The slightest symptoms may remain stationary or may increase gradually, according to the stronger or weaker life force which holds them in abeyance. A time will come, however, when the life force loses its strength and tone and becomes undermined either by an acute attack of sickness or from some great mental disturbance, when the sycotic miasm will remain no longer latent, but breaks forth into some form of pathology, often of a malignant nature that promptly takes the life of the patient. The Vesuvius was silent, but a slight simmer and a trace of smoke showed it was only dormant, not extinct. But thanks for the gift of Homeopathy, it can silence it and remove every trace of its presence in the organism.

Before closing this article, I wish to say a few words about another mode of the entrance of the sycotic poison into the organism, and that is through the vicious method of vaccination, now in vogue. We believe this to be a form of Sycosis, indeed we have no longer a doubt of it. The frequent occurrence of all those acute disturbances, often assuming dangerous forms following the insertion of the virus into the system, cries out in the affirmative. Nevertheless it is but a modification, a potency plus the degenerative animal process it goes through in its preparation. Vaccination causes all the race to be sycotic, and is the father of a multitude of skin diseases such as erysipelas, impetigo, psoriasis, morbelliform rashes, some forms of gangrene, erythemas, roseola, papular and pustular eruptions of different forms, urticaria, eczema, dermatitis herpetiformis, pemphigus of one form, lupus vulgaris and many others that might be mentioned. All cry out "stop the death dealing process of vaccination or the whole race will soon become degenerated." We believe the people should rise up as one man, and with one voice demand this thing to cease. Every physician should be a zealous teacher, carrying these truths into every home and to every patient who employs him. Let compulsory vaccination cease and no longer let the people and especially the innocent child be led as a sheep to the slaughter.

We believe in prophylaxis in disease and the subject is of especial interest in such acute specific contagious diseases as smallpox, but let us not be confined to one stereotyped remedy as is now being forced upon the public by unjust laws (the crude bovine virus) that leaves its trail of death and disease behind it. It is especially dangerous to children, and most especially to the tuberculous child. "Away with it!" should be the cry.

TREATMENT

In the treatment of gonorrhoea, either of the simple or sycotic form, we, as Homeopaths, ought to learn a few things. Is the disease a local or constitutional one? If not local, then it cannot be reached by local means, as all local measures are circumscribed and directed to some local point. Therefore, the action of all local measures are from without inward, and are not eliminative, but suppressive in their action, and do not agree with any physiological process or law governing any form of life; besides, it is directly opposite to the homeopathic law of cure, "that disease is cured from within outward and from above downward," or through the natural evolution of the life processes. This is as true of a simple cell, as it is of an organism.

In this way all organic life grows or develops. If it be a cell, the evolution is from the nucleus, and if it be a biotic life, from the great central nervous centers. The true dynamis of the cell is from the nucleus, and the true dynamis of the organism is from the royal centers. What kind of an organism would it be if the twelve cranial nerves were absent? It would be no better than a worm of the dust that crawls upon the earth. The paralyzed arm that has lost its connection with a life center is dead to all its correspondents with that life; so is the ear that is deaf or the eye that is blind. The loss is not an outward but an inward failure. The inward power failed by virtue of some subversive change from within. Shall we whip it into action from without the walls by electricity, by the X-ray, by mechanical or chemical forces, or by any of the thousand and one methods and means now in vogue, or shall we send the help within the walls;

a selected force, a power that is governed by the same law by which the organism is governed in health? The physician who attempts to heal any disease by local means, either sets aside and ignores all the teaching of the sciences as revealed in physiology and the philosophy governing the laws of motion or of life, or else he is ignorant of them all. He evidently has not the spirit of Hahnemann, who not only has revealed to us a law governing the life force, but a law governing the action of our Therapeutics, out of which came the law of Similia or the law of cure.

Again, we must ask ourselves the question—is the curing of disease an eliminative process or a suppressive process? Which do you think will relieve the patient, and remove all the noxious influences of a sycotic gonorrhoeal poison from an infected organism—an astringent locally applied, or a remedy given internally through this law of cure of which we are so proud? We might press the question a little closer. Supposing you, fellow-healer, were that affected one, and you were about to marry a healthy, clean-bodied, refined young woman, through whom you had hopes of perpetuating your name and your race. I say, supposing this is the case, which treatment would you choose? Which do you think is the safest, shortest method of cure? You are aware of the danger; you know the history of such a relationship well; you have seen many of such cases and have heard that story often, a story full of grief, of suffering and of pathos.

If you want the ear-marks of a sycotic disease forever stamped upon your progeny simply suppress the disease in the parent and it will come. It never fails to appear in the new life. At its birth you will find it is labeled with the disease. Often we speak of the child having a birth mark. Where did it come from? I think I hear you say from some maternal impression, due to fear or perhaps fright or in other words a psychic effect. Yes, I know that is the old story of man reflecting the fault of his weakness upon his Creator, like Adam of old who said "the woman whom thou gavest to be with me, she gave me of the tree and I did eat," which is not true in this case, as if the all good and wise Creator subjected man to anything that would mar the organism or pervert the life. If we study carefully any form of noevus, whether of erythematous character or not, we can easily classify it among the sycotic skin lesions. In my study of skin lesions, I do not find it difficult to recognize their nature and to designate them as Sycotic, Psoric or Syphilitic, or even when they are of mixed origin. The lesions and manifestations of each miasm to a trained observer are so manifestly clear, that it is seldom a mistake need be made.

The true physician, who has any skill at all as a pathologist, can, by careful analysis, quickly recognize the presence of a specific disease in the organism of his patient. There is a mental aura about these patients, when the disease is acquired, that stands out strikingly prominent as we are taking down the case, that somehow tells its own story. Perhaps we may be unable to explain why, or give a reason for what we may feel, but nevertheless we know, by virtue of the fact that we are searching after the truth. But this gift comes not to the ignoramus, "for the truth is only made manifest by light," and we must first have the light within us, or the knowledge of the phenomena of these things, before the truth can be revealed; for, back of that inherent conception or intuition is the knowledge of research, whether it be our own or borrowed from another.

Therefore, in the treatment of this disease, Sycosis, in the multitude of forms in which it now presents itself, we must have the necessary knowledge in order to be able to detect its presence in the organism, even when it is hidden or veiled by suppression, or when disguised in new forms, which are but new vibrations and new perversions of the life force, due often to the attempt to cure by false methods, methods not in accordance with law. We know that all functions and all physiological processes in the organism are governed in health by physiological law, and that disease is nothing more nor less than a disturbance of that law, or rather a perversion of it, and that the disturbance is governed by physiological processes, plus the perverting element, whatever it may be. All disease must be first a disturbed or perverted function. There can be no pathology outside of traumatism or local causes, that does not come first through a functional change, originating in the false or abnormal molecular or cell movement. I am speaking now from an idiopathic standpoint. This might be illustrated by striking a key on the piano, say middle C, which gives us a revolving vibratory sound, thus MMM. It is the standard note in that instrument; and harmony is produced by tuning all the keys to that tone or pitch. So it is in the organism; the organs must be toned to the same vibratory note, as it were, and any slight variation from the standard will produce a discord. It is the same in the life force. A vibration similar to this XXX may produce a tumor or some abnormal growth, or it may produce a convulsion, or spasm, and even death. Thus, when the life force is vibrating normally, we can have no disease. Then it is the form or character of the vibration which gives us the expression or form of life, just as we see or note in a certain kind of light, heat, or sound. A slow vibration upon a musical instrument is but a grating sound, while a rapid vibration may give us a beautiful musical note.

The whole study of disease then resolves itself into a study, first of the action of the life force in health, as a normal standard, then a study of any deflection from that standard recognizable by our senses or by the feelings and sensations of our patients, such deflections being due to the workings in the organism of a certain order or subversive forces, as specified under the headings of Syphilis, Psora, and Sycosis.

The treatment of Sycosis at the present time has changed largely from local to constitutional measures in all schools, although there are yet many physicians foolhardy enough to persist in the use of local measures, knowing full well that in doing this they are damming up a reservoir of disease within that organism that at any time may break forth in all its violence, presenting itself in any one or more of the multiple forms before mentioned in this book. This will be clearly seen as we study the article on Suppression with the clinical cases given as examples, together with Beauchamp's Theory of the Origin of Bacteria. Occasionally the attending physican will volunteer the information that the patient may have some slight rheumatic difficulty, which is one of the probabilities that may follow a local suppression of the disease by such powerful crude drugs as silver nitrate, zinc sulphate or others that might be mentioned in common use today, given in the form of injections or as a douche.

Quite often a metastasis of the disease to internal organs is prevented by a continuance of a gleety discharge. A catarrhal discharge from almost any mucous surface relieves, to a great degree, and prevents the possibility of a pathological lesion in the organism. This fact should constantly be kept in mind, that a catarrhal discharge is a salutary and an eliminative process, and that it is very difficult thing to cure permanently any secondary or tertiary process that may arise from a suppression unless the discharge is re-established. And if the disease is in the tertiary stage, a true anti-psoric, such as Sulphur or Psorinum, may have to be given in order to re-establish it. Of course, it all depends upon the symptomatology of the case.

Only the higher potencies have proved satisfactory in these cases of suppression; the lower potencies seldom accomplishing the work, or have the desired effect. A suppressed disease seems to have such a complete bond with the life force, that only the higher potencies reach down deep enough to sever that bond. This truth cannot be given to another by word of mouth, it is only as we see the fact demonstrated in the sick organism through the processes of similia, that we can come to a true realization of it. A few trials will convince the most skeptical that the power in Similia is, to a great degree, in the potentiality of the remedy, as well as through the workings of the law. Dr. Swan's and Dr. Fincke's highest potencies are usually employed in these cases; although in some cases, especially in sensitive organisms or those easily effected, the lower potencies are to be used, such as the 30th, 200th, and the 1000th. As soon as an old gonorrhœal or gleety discharge is re-established, the other symptoms, whatever they may be (even of the severest type or character) usually subside. Thus headaches, neuralgias, rheumatic pains, whether of an inflammatory or non-inflammatory character, cease altogether or are greatly modified. Even schirrus, or abnormal growths, no longer increase in size; abscesses grow better, inflammatory processes, even of internal organs, get well, gouty states, and gouty concretions disappear; affected joints often greatly deformed-resume their normal condition, in short the disease disappears under the use of the higher potencies of the Homeopathic remedy.

The writer has seen all these things take place. Abscesses of the tubes have been cured frequently, nasal catarrh of a severe type is cured never to return; enlarged prostrates, bleeding hemorrhoids, rectal pockets and rectal abscesses, are readily cured by a careful selection of the right remedy in each case. The suppressed discharge cannot always be re-established, but then some other eliminative process may be brought forth, such as increased action of the kidneys, a pruritis ani, or of the vulva in woman, an eruption upon the skin in some form, quite often eczematous in its nature. We can never tell how the life force may re-act under the right remedy or the proper potency; that belongs to the mysterious law of action and reaction, and comes under the formula of Newton's third law of motion. The reaction will depend upon the nature and stage of suppression, upon the bond of the sycotic element, whether with Psora or when more than one miasm is present in the organism. The pre-existing miasm may be acting upon the ear or upon the eye in a latent form, or the patient may have Syphilis, which will change the whole aspect of this reaction in the life force.

I have just such a case now under treatment, and as the sycotic discharge lessens, the secondary eruption or the syphilitic roseolic flush becomes more prominent upon the chest. This is according to Hahnemann's teaching in the Organon, that in a mixed case as one miasm disappears or is cured, the latent one becomes suddenly active. So we have no right to speculate or hold in our minds any pre-conceived plan of action for the life forces to bring about a restoration of health in the organism, other than by the method nature takes for herself. The simpler the processes in the re-establishment of the patient to health, the better for all concerned.

Quite often we have seen or known physicians who were not familiar with the Hahnemannian homeopathic art of healing, attack these newly established processes (which are the only way by which nature can make a cure) by local medication, reflecting back upon the organism again the whole accursed disease-producing processes. How utterly empty these would-be-healers of the sick are of the knowledge of the true science and art of healing, and the nature and action of the disease, or in fact, of any process in nature or of physics in general. The law of action and reaction is in all motion, yes in everything. It is the key to motion; the key to the existence of the material and all created things. Therefore, the reaction set up in the organism by the homeopathic remedy is the curative action, and this curative action in the organism is equal to the diseased action. Should it become greater it amounts to an over-action, or what is known as an aggravation which is usually temporary, until the true curative, or equal action is established again. So we see that all we can know of disease, is what we know of the laws of action and reaction, of the laws of motion governing the life forces. It is solely a study of the phenomena of the functions of the organism in general. Perfect function is perfect health, and perverted function is disease in some form or other.

In the treatment of gonorrhoeal Sycosis, the patient should be fully made to understand the nature of his case; that such an infection is not a local affair, as many suppose, but a general infection of the whole organism, even to the last drop of blood in that organism. It is well for the attending physician to allow himself plenty of time for the cure of this very determined and stubborn disease. I usually say from six weeks to five months. Few cases have been prolonged over the five months, even where a chronic gleet was present. Many cases have been cured in six weeks, where the patient had not received free drug store advice, or where no local measures were in any way employed. Cases appearing for treatment in the late secondary stage may require one year's treatment, and even longer. On the other hand I have frequently seen cases clear up within two or three months. In the early tertiary period where warty eruptions appeared on the hands, sexual organs, and other parts of the body, they would dry up and dessicate, followed by no other symptom or sign of the disease. These cures were made in non-tubercular and not very psoric cases. Quite often, however, Sulphur, Calcarea carb., Psorinum, and some other anti-psoric remedies were employed to finish up the case.

The diet was usually modified, and if the disease was

in the tertiary stage, where gouty states were present, or where uric acid was in excess, meat was either greatly reduced or prohibited entirely. It seems to be pretty generally understood that the blood of sycotic patients is diminished in alkali, and the power to assimilate nitrogenous foods greatly diminished in most, if not all, cases.

Stimulants of all kinds are prohibited, as the results are invariably unfavorable, with tendencies to relapse or become complicated. The system should not be clogged in any way, but there should be a free and easy elimination in every organ. Water should always be taken freely, as it assists in diluting the excessive solids of the blood. Especially is this true of the kidneys. Patients taking treatment at mineral springs are requested to drink large quantities of the water, often from ten to twelve glasses in twenty-four hours. The result upon the system is soon seen, as the urine clears up, the bowels become more regular, the liver becomes more active—an organ that is generally dormant in Sycosis; the skin clears up, and the patient soon takes on all the health processes and the normal condition is again established. But this normal condition of things in gouty or rheumatic subjects is only temporary, unless they also receive careful homeopathic treatment which removes the miasm from the system.

The disease should disappear exactly in the reverse order in which it came. The discharge usually begins as a thin watery, gluey, or sticky fluid, glueing up the meatus, later becoming muco-purulent, and finally purulent; as the case progresses, it is reduced to a single drop, appearing in the morning, of a viscid, gluey nature, causing the lips of the meatus to stick together. Of course the pains if any and all other concomitant symptoms disappear also, before this last token of the disease. (This is, of course, in an acute case or primary disease). Should the case be a chronic one of a tertiary form, the patient cannot be said to be free from the disease so long as a warty growth, a red mole, or any such sycotic stigmata is present. The drying up or disappearance of the catarrhal discharge is not a certain sign of the cure of the disease, as long as any eruptive manifestation is present upon the skin. It is simply a step in the progress of the case. The parents in that state are capable of transmitting the disease to their offspring, even if the discharge is absent for twenty years. Should the child born to these parents be free, as far as could be seen or known at birth, from any manifestation of the disease, there will invariably appear at the period of second dentition, a warty eruption upon the hands or other parts of the body.

Now is the time to free the organism from this miasm, as children at this age or cycle are very amenable to treatment. Probably at no other age are we able to get better results from our potentized remedies. If one thing more than another ought to be impressed on the mind of the physician in his treatment of acute Sycosis, it is to give the indicated remedy, and wait on its action;

wait as long as there is any improvement. Then, when its action ceases, either repeat or change the remedy as the symptoms in the case demand. No special benefit is to be derived by a frequent repetition of the remedy. It invariably is bad practice, as it muddles the case and in many instances spoils the curative action, or produces aggravations of the symptoms which are liable to lead to a premature change of remedy. This is especially true where deep acting remedies are prescribed.

After the first stage has passed, and the disease has become a secondary condition, it is a loss of time to prescribe other than the deep acting anti-miasmatics, as the superficial remedies are only palliative and prolong the case, often leading to discouragement both of physician and patient. No other fact has been more deeply and more frequently impressed upon my mind than this: Sycosis is a profoundly acting miasm; it acts upon every cell of the human organism, even to the very depths of the physical being.

GONORRHOEA

The history of this disease or miasm shows it to be of ancient origin. Hippocrates records a number of cases, and farther down in the history of medicine we hear of it from Pliny, Juvenal, Celsus, Galen, and others. They all testify to the specific nature of the disease and its venereal origin. Few, however, speak of its secondary and tertiary effects or manifestations. None seems to have understood that it was a miasm or a continuous and permanent disease in the blood, and that the organism had no power within itself to throw it off. None knew of its progressive changes bringing forth new processes of disease, often with malignant aspect or running into chronic morbid states that often proved incurable to the most persistent treatment. There were, however, a few of the more studious minds that saw secondary and tertiary manifestations follow the suppression of the primary or seemingly harmless catarrhal discharge. Acute or sub-acute rheumatism and even gouty conditions followed in its wake. Not until our own day was this generally understood. Now the majority of well educated physicians understand to some degree at least, what is meant by gonorrhoeal infection and the complications that follow its suppression by local measures. Many physicians today no longer advocate the use of injections or douches to dry up, what was once thought to be a local disease, but prefer the slower method of setting up a drug urethritis by internal medication or use of crude drugs that act specifically upon the genito-urinary tract.

Finger, a great German authority on gonorrhoea, says, "Gonorrhoea of the male urethra is one of the most frequent diseases with which the practitioner has to deal." I cannot agree with Dr. Finger, if we understand him to mean the disease in the acute stage, but if he means the disease in all stages, including the hereditary forms, I am fully in accord with his statement. Noeggerath, speaking of the frequency with which it is met, says, "I do not know the statistics of other cities, but after carefully examining or questioning every patient who has come to me for the treatment of this disease in general, I am fully convinced that in New York City fully eight-tenths of all men are in some way afflicted with the disease." Others have given even a higher estimate. The same author further states that ninety per cent of these so affected human beings remain uncured. Think of a system of medicine whose leaders frankly admit the inefficiency of their methods of cure, when such an overwhelming majority turn away from even their best and most pronounced healers, uncured and often unhelped or in any way aided on the way to health. Not infrequently we find some of these helpless invalids wandering up and down the earth looking for the elixir of life. Nine-tenths of them have had the disease suppressed in the initial stage and have already a well advanced secondary inflammation or a tertiary process established in some organ or vital part, so as to be often past all power of restoration.

Noeggerath, Martineau, Hancock, Kollicker, Otis, Lydston, and a host of other equally prominent and high in authority, now fully recognize the fact, demonstrated by Hahnemann over one hundred years ago, that present day pelvic inflammations are generally secondary processes of gonorrhoeal infection. Thus they say metritis, endo-metritis, salpingitis, pyo and hydo-salpingitis, ovaritis, parametritis, pelvic peritonitis, sterility, and menstrual disorders, occur according to the age and severity of its toxic power. The same is known to every

THE CHRONIC MIASMS.   135

intelligent Homeopath, of the miasms Syphilis and Psora. We see by this that the best thinking and investigating minds in the Allopathic school are cognizant of the fact that gonorrhœa is, in the first place, not a self-limitimg disease, and in the second place it is not wholly a local process. We do not agree with any of these authors that the pelvic inflammations or any of the secondary processes develop by extension of the local inflammation, for we have seen destructive inflammations develop at remote points of the organism, quite separate anatomically from the genito-urinary tract. We have also noticed a systemic involvement to a greater or less degree with morbid mental accompaniment. As in Syphilis or Psora, all the miasms have their own fixed laws governing their evolutions and processes of development. When we recognize these governing principles, we recognize more easily their *modus operandi*.

As we become acquainted with these characteristics peculiar to each miasm, we readily classify all their pathology and the diseases that they propagate. All the various symptoms and phenomena belonging to a miasm are characterized by certain peculiarities belonging to that miasm and no other. To illustrate this, we might refer to Syphilis. We note the raw ham or copper color throughout all its cutaneous processes ; in Sycosis we must familiarize ourselves with its discharges, with their odor and color, with its pains, and with its climatic aggravations. This is the way to become acquainted with disease, to look into their death processes, to thus become familiar with their habitual movements, and their possible combinations with other miasms. For instance, cancer, lupus, tumors of all kinds, malignant inflammations, and processes are but blendings and combinations of the miasms.

Dr. Lydston very gallantly admits that the kidneys may become affected, and that even the whole renal tract may become involved. But we know that Sycosis is not a partial infection of the organism nor by any means confined to the pelvic field or genito-urinary path ; it is more, infinitely more ; it is an issue of the blood. When we come to understand that the life is in the blood, we readily see that this disease is an issue of the blood. Moses speaks of it in the fifteenth chapter of Leviticus, where he calls it an *issue* of the blood, or a running of the reins. We are to understand, however, that two forms of *issue* of the blood are mentioned in the same book, one a disease process, which we have every reason to believe was gonorrhœa, and the other a loss of the *seminal fluid*, commonly known today as nocturnal pollutions. But to return to our subject, this *issue* of the blood (as referred to in Holy Writ), only magnifies and verifies Hahnemann's theory of disease, that, "disease is a disturbance of the life force." We have already learned that the "life is in the blood," therefore this issue of the blood (gonorrhoea) involves every drop of blood in the human organism.

Thus far we agree with Noeggerath, that the infection can come at any stage of the disease, and that the symptomatology will correspond to the stage, when infection took place, modified as in Syphilis by the *constitutional dyscrasia* of the infected one. That is, the infection may occur when the disease is in its acute or inflammatory stage, or later on, when in a latent condition. For instance, if the disease is latent in a married man, there sometimes appears a similar latent infection in the wife. Therefore we must not expect to find the same set of phenomena in every case, nor the same specific acute action to its secondary or tertiary processes. An infection which if suppressed in its acute stage, might develop inflammations rapid and destructive in their character, would, if contracted in a latent or more chronic state develop the same processes in a greatly modified, less destructive, yet, nevertheless, equally persistent and difficult form. There will then be great liability to bring forth tertiary processes such as fibroids, cancer, lupus, or diabetes.

Sooner or later we find these patients suffering from some form of chronic or sub-acute inflammation. We have already given the pelvic inflammations in the female and we might also mention the more common secondary inflammations in the male. Beginning with the kidneys, we may mention nephritis, Bright's disease, anterior and posterior urethritis, buboes, prostatitis, cowperitis, orchitis, epididymitis, deferentitis, and seminal-vesiculitis, all involving the sexual and urinary organs. There are many other secondary inflammations that we might enumerate. As we survey this fearful array of symptoms of both male and female, we can readily see it vies with Syphilis and often produces greater suffering, and more speedily destroys life.

WAYS OF INFECTION

A few prominent writers on the subject of gonorrhoea have written extensively on the subject of innocent infection. As far as my investigation has gone, especially in clinical work (which has been quite extensive), I have found innocent infection in a very limited number of cases. I have met with one or two cases in women whom I had good reason to believe were infected through servants who were in their employ, and who were suffering with the disease in the acute form. Two or three cases of the disease in virgins came to my notice in private practice. I recall two severe cases, of innocent infection that were quite deplorable; one a case of gonorrhoeal ophthalmia in a young school girl, fifteen years of age, contracted from a brother, who carelessly left an infected towel in the bathroom. She lost an eye three days after infection. The case came into my hands too late to save the organ. The other eye showed symptoms of the disease, but was arrested promptly by the use of Argentum nit. 1m. The other case was that of a female child about three years of age, infected in some unknown way while under treatment in Cook County Hospital in

1906. There are many other cases on record of course, and doubtless many others that are not recorded.

These exceptional cases do not alter the fact that it is seldom contracted except by sexual congress, and no matter how persistently the patient may deny the fact, we, knowing what we do concerning infection, must either not accept his story as being true or else hold it for further testimony. Venereal patients are noted for their lying qualities and will refer the origin of their difficulties to a thousand and one improbable possibilities.

The infective field in this disease is so limited, that we could not expect it to be otherwise. We do great injustice, however, to those patients who give us a history of unknown source, without carefully going into the history of each case, as this disease that carries with it such a stigma, that great charity should be shown, and above all things justice, especially if the patient be a woman. We are all too hasty in forming a judgment in venereal diseases. Public bath-houses and public closet-seats are to be avoided when possible, and when it becomes impossible, great care should be taken to protect the mucous surfaces of the sexual organs.

The subject of the gonococcus in this disease, has received careful attention. Physicians both of this country and Europe, have rivalled each other in their efforts to search for the mite, not only in the gonorrhœal discharges, but also in all the morbid discharges. They have even carried their investigation to the gouty joint and have succeeded in finding the gonococcus there.

Neisser of Breslau made the discovery in 1879 and made his followers all happy in the fact that they had discovered the cause of gonorrhoea.

We find these little microscopic representations of gonorrhoea arranged in pairs and in colonies of ten to twenty, attached as a rule to the pus corpuscle. Owing to their arrangement in pairs, they are classified as a diplococcus. We might briefly describe the method of preparation for the microscope. A small drop of the pus is spread evenly on a glass slide and then dipped in methyl blue, the superfluous coloring matter is washed off with a stream of cold water; they are then mounted with Canada Balsam. A twelfth-inch oil-immersion objective which will give good results. In old long-standing cases it is difficult to find them in the discharges, they are found more readily in the acute stages of the disease.

But we know that the real cause of gonorrhoea has not been found in this minute organism, for every family of diseases and especially specific diseases are accompanied by their own peculiar micro-organisms, just as they are by their own peculiar phenomena and symptomatology. They are not the cause but the effect, and it is not necessary to have a single gonococcus present in the drop of sycotic pus that conveys the contagion from one to another. We leave this phase of the subject, however, for the present, and ask you to carefully investigate the late researches of the great French scientist Beauchamp in his exhaustive study of micro-organisms.

Much has been said with reference to the immunity produced by having once had the disease, but I believe this is not true. I make this statement after having examined many cases, and after having closely followed the history of a goodly number of patients, who had suffered from more than one attack. Of course as long as there is any trace of the disease Sycosis in the system, it prevents another acute attack in many patients. But again I have seen acute attacks that showed all the symptoms of a fresh attack of gonorrhoea, that had still in their organism traces of chronic Sycosis. This is especially true in tubercular patients or those who showed that diathesis in some degree at least. All perfectly cured cases of gonorrhoea and Sycosis we say are very liable to take the disease the second time.

SOURCE OF THE DISEASE

The main source of the disease in coitus with a woman so affected. That the disease cannot be contracted in any other way, is not true for a moment, for as has already been stated, it has many times been contracted in lavatories by the use of towels, clothing, and bed clothing. Gonorrhoea is generally classified by physicians as a "specific urethritis" in contradiction to a "simple urethritis," which is an inflammatory condition, simulating the specific form, yet having no secondary stage and being self-limited. There are many other ways of contracting the simple form, such as from injury, from diseased states of the system, from leucorrhœa or acrid, vaginal discharges.

The gonorrhoeal process, as has also been mentioned, may attack any mucous surface as the urethra, vagina, vulva, eye, conjunctiva, ear, nose, posterior or anterior nares, throat, anus, or rectum.

Scott, the author of the "Sexual Instinct," says gonorrhoea may attack individuals of either sex at any period of life, from infancy to extreme old age, if any of the poisonous substance is implanted upon a mucous surface in any way. We believe that the disease derived from such contact is of rare occurrence, yet is sometimes seen.

SYMPTOMS AND MODE OF ATTACK

Like all severe virulent processes, as that of scarlet fever, diphtheria, and smallpox, Sycosis has its period of incubation, invasion, advance, decline, and convalescence, but unlike scarlet fever, measles, etc., they do not disappear of themselves. It is only by careful and scientific treatment that they can be eradicated from the organism. Sycosis is often suppressed, and then it lies dormant in the organism like a sleeping volcano to set up later new processes more deadly and destructive than before. All cases go over some definite road, depending largely at what stage the disease is contracted, and the specific degree of the poison.

The patient in the beginning of the attack suffers with more or less chilliness ; a temperature is frequently present with loss of appetite, and there is mental depression, or an over anxionsness about their case. This latter symptom disturbs sleep ; dark circles are often seen under the eyes, and the complexion takes on a sallow hue. Sexual desire is morbidly increased or entirely lost. The desire to urinate increases in proportion to the intensity of the urethritis, and as the case advances, great suffering is experienced from the painful erections. For the two weeks following, the gonorrhoeal process increases unless modified by treatment. The acme is reached in a typical case, about the third week, after which the symptoms begin to decline. Of course, this case is supposed either to have no treatment, or unhomeopathic treatment, for all cases are modified and often cured in this time by skillful treatment. The majority of cases are accompanied with more or less pain, redness of the meatus, and swelling of the organ. In the first stage the discharge is mucous in character, in the second mucopurulent, and in the third stage it takes on a glutinous nature with an occasional drop of pus.

The redness at first is confined to the margin of the orifice of the urethra, but it soon spreads to the whole glans penis, and sometimes the whole organ becomes enormously swollen. Often, very early in the acute stage the lymphatic glands in the groin become swollen and tender ; sometimes this swelling can be traced from the penis to the groin. The inflammation begins usually in the anterior part of the urethra, and in about eighty per cent. travels down, until the whole length of the canal is involved. At this point the patient often experiences much suffering from the painful urination and chordee. The deeper structures of the urethra now become involved and the inflammatory products increase, until the canal is now pouring forth a thick, copious, creamy and sometimes blood tinged pus. The urinary passage which is normally the calibre of a lead pencil, is now almost occluded by inflammatory discharges. Hence we can form some idea of the suffering of the patient on urinating especially, which is now a matter of acute pain, even agony. The urine passes hot, often scalding in its sensation, and with great difficulty this is increased by the acidity of the urine, which becomes quite marked in the second stage of the disease. The pain sometimes becomes a spasm with even strangulation as the swelling and narrowing of the canal advances. Occasionally a catheter will have to be used in these neglected cases, but all instruments should be avoided if possible at all stages of the disease, even in gleet. They are, as a rule, always harmful, and in the end cause an increase of suffering and a tendency to produce scar tissue in the canal. Owing to this occluding process of the canal the stream of urine now becomes thin, is often passed in drops, dribbling away at times, or it becomes twisted and forked in its course.

The severity of the suffering varies greatly in the different temperaments and in the different constitutions. There is, however, always some pain, some burning, or difficulty in urination, with some kind of a discharge, either of a mucous or muco-purulent nature. The amount of pus or discharge is greater during the night, or at least it is noticed more, as the frequent urination during the daytime expels it, and so is not so noticeable as at night.

During the acute inflammatory stage, the patient should be confined to his bed, as rest assists much in a speedy cure. Many cases are prolonged and complicated on account of allowing the patient to continue at work; as walking, standing, lifting, or straining, not only keeps up the inflammation, but greatly aggravates all the symptoms. Should any secondary inflammation complicate a case, such as orchitis, rest in bed becomes the more necessary, and it should be demanded of the patient to keep quiet until the acute symptoms subside. All stimulating foods and the use of tobacco should be prohibited, as they retard the healing process and cure. *Make no sacrifice here in order to please the notions and fancies of your patient.* This is especially true if the lymphatics are involved, and where there is much backache with physical exhaustion. Even when the mental symptoms predominate, it is wisdom to keep your patient quiet and at rest. If the symptoms become worse at any stage of the cure, they become discouraged and are prone to change physicians, and you lose your case.

It is well to break away from the old customs of the past, and to use more common sense in the practice of medicine.

If such symptoms as backache, painful and swollen inguinal glands were induced by any other cause than from venereal diseases, we would not hesitate to put them to bed at once and keep them there until well. Often they have temperature but we do not use a thermometer to take it. They have chills, fever, backache, are worried, anxious, fretful, due largely to their occupation. Many of the symptoms disappear when they become rested and quiet. These patients should sleep on a bed which is not too soft, nor too springy, and the room should be kept cool, as warmth and the night hours often aggravate the symptoms; especially the sexual centers, which are of course, greatly excited in this disease, and abnormally disturbed. Chordee is also increased by the heat of the room and the warmth of the bed. Often this chordee is the most disturbing symptom of the disease. Cooling applications of water are very grateful to many cases, while others are relieved by hot fomentations, in the acute stage of the inflammation.

There is also great congestion in the corpus cavernosum and corpus spongiosum, owing to a spasm of the longitudinal fibers. If the patient is allowed to work during the day, he suffers for it at night. Sometimes the amount of pus or mucus discharged is very small, again it may be copious. In one patient the disease can be readily recognized, and in another, the patient might not be certain that he had an attack of gonorrhoea. In addition to the worst symptoms already spoken of, we may have involuntary pollutions, gonorrhoeal rheumatism, gonorrhoeal ophthalmia, or conjunctivitis, or an inflammation of the brain or heart, ending fatally.

Always keep in mind that the mildest and simplest inflammation may prove exceedingly severe by spreading to the deeper portions of the urethra, causing many complications, or if others are infected by the virus, the most virulent case may develop. The virus does not affect two people alike; all depends on the constitutional dyscrasia and the sensitiveness of the patient. Occasionally fibrous threads and numerous little rice-like bodies pass away with the urine from the beginning of the disease until its close. These are found very plentifully in severe cases. As long as these are present, the disease is still virulent and it is exceedingly dangerous to cohabit. Too many physicians allow these infected patients to pass out of their hands too soon; often even before the discharge has fully disappeared.

Some physicians are foolhardy enough to think, that when the disease is in the gleety stage, there is no longer any danger of infection. No greater blunder was ever made than this. I have seen as disastrous effects from an infection at this chronic stage of the disease, as at any other. Even when the discharge has entirely disappeared, being dried up by the use of injections, it is still dangerous to cohabit, or to bring forth children into the world, as they will show, in a greater or less degree, manifestations of the disease. This disease can be transmitted through the semen as in syphilis, and gonorrhoea will often leave its marks as definitely as syphilis. We can never know how gonorrhoea becomes latent in the organism. Often for years it lies dormant accompanied with but very few annoying or distressing symptoms, and yet it may be reproduced with the aid of Medorrhinum or the indicated homeopathic remedy administered in a high potency. I have reproduced the discharge many times, when the disease had been suppressed from one month to even ten years. I have in mind the case of a man, 41 years of age, who had been suffering with a chronic lumbago for five years and who had a history of a gonorrhoeal suppression. The discharge was reproduced with Medorrhinum in Swans' D.M.M. potency. I will go a little farther into the treatment of this case, I will first mention that he had had the urine tested a number of times, fearing some lesions of the kidneys, but none was found yet a test for pus always showed its presence although its origin had not been located. I gave Rhus tox, in a high potency with marked palliative results for one week, then the symptoms returned as severe as ever. The peculiar mental anxiety of this patient called my attention to Medorrhinum. These sycotic patients are prone to get their minds fixed upon the affected point. No matter how simple the disease may be, it is a serious matter to them, and this is not due to the persistence of the symptoms, but it is a mental characteristic of this miasm. Another symptom was, on the approach of a storm he would have irritability of the bladder, frequent desire to urinate, and some burning. He had many sycotic moles on his body. He had been to many physicians and was discouraged. A dose of Medorrhinum relieved this patient at once and at the end of a week he was free from pain and the stiffness and soreness of the muscles of the back had entirely disappeared. These sufferers drift from one physician to another and become victims of all kinds of treatment, yet fail to get relief, simply because the doctor is not acquainted with the etiology of the disease, and has no knowledge of the disturbing element that is hidden within the organism.

But new symptoms or rather old ones began to reappear; they were burning at the meatus, and very acid and hot urine. In two weeks, a mucous discharge appeared from the urethra, and was accompanied with symptoms of a mild attack of gonorrhœa. Of course it is needless to say the lumbago did not appear again. Homeopathy is such a wonderful system of medicine, and there is so much to it, that it is impossible for us to become acquainted with it in more than a limited degree, in the short period of life in which it is ours to work and investigate these deep and mysterious movements of disease. We can boldly say, however, that homeopaths alone understand the etiology of disease. This wisdom was given to Hahnemann in the beginning; but so few of us treat our patients from this standpoint. We are prone to follow the teachings of the nominal school, and to associate and center our remedies about a pathological state or name, as had been done in the case of lumbago. In taking the pathogenesis of any case, we must give the miasmatic symptoms prominence, and especially so when we find a history of suppression.

Recovery is usually rapid when the proper rest, diet, and surroundings are given due consideration and the remedy selected carefully and in the highest potencies. The highest can be given with the best results, and seldom leave any trace of the disease behind. If the proper remedy is exhibited in the early symptoms or stage of the disease, a cure ought to be made in from six to eight weeks ; but in neglected and unhomeopathically treated cases it will be necessary to take five months. When they are cured with the homeopathic remedy in the higher potencies, they will not and cannot transmit the disease. This cannot be said of any other system of medicine.

Repeated attacks or infections are often more severe than single attacks. They are liable to run into the sub-acute form and run from one sequela into another, sometimes with fatal results. Gonorrhœal rheumatism, gouty conditions of the heart, stomach, and liver bring about fatal endings. It is well to remember that it is never a local disease ; therefore, any complication may arise at any time, in any part of the body, no matter how strongly it appears to be a local disease. A specific virus like gonorrhoea with a history of sequelae and profound complications, can never be a local disease. Then, when we add to it, the fact that it is one of the miasms, and not self-limited in any sense of the word, its importance can be seen. It is never cured without medical assistance; I mean the true sycotic form. None of the chronic miasms are self-limiting, and this is one of them. All abortive methods of cure are bad, unscientific, suppressive, and unprofessional. Even one of the best authorities in the Allopathic school, says abortive methods are unjustifiable. "The severity of the disease is often enhanced by the use of abortive measures," says one writer. We should not lightly assume the responsibility of treating so serious a disease, without the exercise of care and good judgment.

It is of great importance to let these patients early understand that gonorrhoea is a serious disease, and that the outcome, if not treated scientifically, is dangerous not only to their life, but to the life of others, and may blot the life and prospects of many. Many cases through these abortive methods are changed from an acute into a chronic state much earlier than in the natural course of the disease. Others renew the attack in some form of secondary inflammation, as for instance, orchitis in the male, or some form of salpingitis in the female. Still others when suppressed show no secondary inflammation, but slowly run into a chronic tertiary process, in which the physician loses sight of the disease Sycosis entirely, seeing no connection between the two processes. I feel that I am quite safe in saying, that fully eighty per cent. of the physicians come under this enumeration. This is where the great danger lies in the use of local means in the cure of severe acute diseases, and especially is this true of serotherapy. I have found that in many cases of gonorrhœa, nervous or hysterical symptoms often develop, due to worry or caused by loss of strength and worry in those who have to work constantly to make a living, and who get or little or no rest. There are cases which become easily discouraged and change from one physician to another, so that the case not being properly managed, goes on from bad to worse. The prognosis in this disease may be considered good when the proper rest, regulation of diet, sexual hygiene, and the continuation of the treatment are ensured until all the symptoms of the disease have been eradicated from the system.

GONORRHOEA OF FEMALES

The diagnosis can be made easily in the male, owing to the painful and distinctly marked symptoms, but in the female we do not have such extremely painful and distinctly local symptoms. Occasionally urinary symptoms of quite a severe character are present, which call our attention to the presence of the disease in the acute stage. In the more chronic or later stages of the disease, the leucorrhoeal discharges and the pruritus are quite diagnostic, especially if the pruritus is induced by the acidity of the discharge. Some women are so accustomed to vaginal discharges of some kind that they seldom seek medical help in good time, therefore the disease is apt to be chronic before they begin treatment. Often, however, the severity of the pruritus, or perhaps a severe vulvitis will drive them early to the physician, thus we seldom get an acute stage of gonorrhoea in women to treat and especially in married women.

Often when these patients come to their physician for relief, they have previously fallen into the hands of men who do not understand the treatment of this disease, or the importance of avoiding suppressive measures in its treatment, and so great damage is done by suppression of leucorrhoeal discharges, by strong medicated lotions. Secondary processes are brought on in some of the pelvic organs (secondary inflammations) and the patient's sufferings are increased from day to day, often with alarming symptoms. It would have been better had she not applied for assistance from her physician in the first place, but had suffered with the disease in its original state, or in the sub-acute condition.

Gonorrhoea in women is, of course, rendered more grave by the direct communication with the pelvic organs; the disease being fanned into renewed activity at each menstrual nisus. It is also greatly magnified if she become pregnant, as abortion is so liable to take place at any intermediate period, and is followed by a general infection and general pelvic invasion of the disease. Where the disease is contracted in a chronic or latent form, the women cannot fix any date; often she may never be aware of the cause of her illness. Many times we see women who have suffered untold misery from the disease, contracted from their husbands in a latent state, and finally died within a few years with a complication of diseases. It is certainly the duty of every man who has had gonorrhœa to abstain from marriage until he has had permission from a physician who understand all these phases of the disease, and can give him intelligent advice.

Not infrequently, when we are called to see a woman suffering from gonorrhoea, the young life is already wrecked; the fires are not just lighted, but are a smoldering heap. We see the furred tongue, the foul breath, the fever, the misery, the suffering, and the pain; we see surgical cases, the removal of organs, death processes with their organic changes in the pelvis, bad mental states, and all the untold story of its chamber of horrors.

The favorite sites of gonorrhoea in women are the urethra, vagina, Bartholin's glands, the uterus, Fallopian tubes, ovaries, and peritoneal cavity. It causes sterility, even to a greater degree than Syphilis. Not infrequently sterility follows after the first birth, but if a mild or latent form of the disease be present it may not follow until the birth of the second child. In twenty-four per cent. of the French marriages no children are born, and in twenty percent. only one child was born, and for this condition Syphilis is given as the cause. If these statistics are true, and we have no reason to doubt them, then is it astounding? This together with the sterility due to Sycosis, and annual abortion, has put the birth rate of France down until it is lower perhaps than any other country in the world. The cause of complete sterility lies more frequently, I think, with husbands, who have had repeated attacks of gonorrhœa previous to marriage, than with the wives. "Stricture," says Scott, "is chronic gonorrhœa, and it is not to be treated as single symptom, as implied in the word stricture; it is not to be dilated with bougies, cut open with instruments or treated with medicated lotions." No! It is to be treated as chronic gonorrhœa; knowing that to remove by mechanical or chemical methods this offending lesion, is to suppress the disease which is sure to appear in some form, usually a tertiary one. Such treatment causes us to become the fathers of disease and the perpetrators of crime. Sir Henry Thompson has given us a few statistics, showing the development of strictures in different patients out of 164 cases. The development was as follows: "Ten cases of stricture acquired during the acute state, seventy during the first year, forty-one from three to four years, twenty-two from seven to eight, and twenty from twenty to twenty-five years." So you see stricture comes not alike to all; the time required for the disease, gonorrhoea to form a bond with Psora, varies and is modified, of course, by the character of the treatment, the constitutional dyscrasia and the natural resistance of the life force in each case. It is when the patient is on the downward track, that complications develop, and the life force begins to suffer from the effects of suppression, and new processes begin to show themselves. We notice by a close study of gonorrhoea that a systemic involvement takes place during the pause period that elapses after infection, know as the period of incubation (seen also in Syphilis). Still farther, remember that gonorrhœa is not a self-limiting disease as taught in our works on pathology. True, the acute phenomena are self-limiting, but the systemic or constitutional involvement never leaves the organism unless removed by the law of similia. No other treatment will remove it; this I say without hesitation or reserve. James Foster Scott in his work, "Sexual Instinct," says on page 336, "Chronic Gonorrhœa is often spoken of as synonymous with gleet, but the former term is more correct." This is true, gleet is but a symptom, yet a very positive and sure one, of the disease after it has relapsed into a chronic state. Relapses occur when we change the remedy too soon, or fail to select the proper one. Seldom have I attributed relapses to any other source.

Every author will tell you that the gonococci lie dormant or in other words remain latent in the organism for years. But this is only a term, and done to uphold the germ theory of disease; we understand the disease to be latent, and, that the gonococci are but the result of the degenerate or death process of all disease. There are thousands today of both sexes who are suffering with some latent form or expression of gonorrhoea that physicians do not recognize. They do not see the connecting link due, to either and imperfectly cured or suppressed case of gonorrhœa. Ricord's admission concerning the obstinacy of gleet is decidedly pat. In his writings he speaks of having a dream (which will illustrate very clearly the allopathic physicians' conception of this disease, and their inability to cure it) of being dead and of having been sent to Purgatory. When asked what sort of a place it was he replied: "Pleasant enough, except for the fact that the whole troop of male specters about him pointed each the ghastly finger of scorn and exclaimed: 'Ricord! Ricord! You could not cure the gleet.'" (G. Frank Lydsten, M. D., Gonorrhoea and Its Treatment. Page 79).

Those who succeed in suppressing chronic gleet, can never truthfully say that they have made a cure; they have simply driven the disease in upon the organism, to manifest itself sooner or later in some other form, or to be brought to light in their wives or children. We must not look upon gleet as a local lesion or local inflammation, but as a smoldering amber of latent internal fire. Sir Henry Thompson puts before us, a few statistics of the time of development of gleet. Out of 164 cases the record was as follows: In 10 cases, the disease developed during the acute stage of gonorrhoea; 71 during the first year; 41 within three years; 22 within eight years, and 20 did not develop until between the twentieth and twenty-fifth year. Do you recognize the value of these statistics? Does it not show you the chronicity of the disease, as well as the evolution of the processes in each individual? It shows besides that it is not a self-limiting disease as is supposed by most authors.

This writer says further, and here he agrees with the teachings of Hahnemann, "That the tissues of man in the prime of life, resist disease, and the repair and waste processes keep an approximately parallel course but when he begins to go down hill, and turns his face towards the evening of life, then the balance between repair and waste is discovered in favor of the latter." Nothing will start these retrograde processes or degenerative actions in the organism like a suppressed disease in its acute or malignant aspect. Too much cannot be said on this subject or suppression, when we see the degeneration and destruction of the race follow in the wake of the prevalent suppressive treatments. We must bring this subject to a close, however as we cannot afford the space in this work to give clearer light upon it.

To sum up the symptoms of gonorrhoea briefly, there is a period of incubation of from three to five days' duration, in which but few if any symptoms of the disease can be recognized. This is followed by a prodromal period of about three days' duration, in which the first evidence of the disease makes its appearance. It reaches its acme during the second or third week; the acute stage begins to modify at the close of the second or beginning of the third week; at the end of the third week, with careful homeopathic treatment, the symptoms in a mild case, will begin to disappear, and at the end of the fifth week even a severe case of gonorrhoea should show marked signs of improvement; a perfect and complete cure should be made in from six to eight weeks.

But when cases come to us that have received no constitutional treatment, nothing but local measures, we may consider ourselves fortunate to cure them in from three to five months. In chronic neglected, or badly treated cases, it may take a year or even years to make a complete and perfect cure; this is especially true in chronic cases involving the pelvic organs of women. As recovery begins, the discharge becomes less profuse, less greenish or pus-like, more thin and watery, and eventually a greyish mucus appears which stains the linen yellow and glues the meatus together as it did in the beginning of the attack. If, however, the acute or secondary stage is allowed to drag along from eight to ten weeks, the probability is that the case will be slow and difficult to cure.

Relapses will occur when the patient is allowed to indulge in excesses of eating, or from the partaking of stimulants, even from overwork or from taking cold. I do not agree with some authors, who say that the disease is self-limiting, for we know if it is the sycotic form of gonorrhoea of whch Hahnemann speaks, that the organism is unable to throw off the disease. It is a chronic miasm, and chronic miasm is only cured by and through the law of similia. This error has arisen from a number of causes, first that in many cases it can be suppressed by astringent injections, and secondly it is time slowly dwindles or disappears into a chronic gleet, scarcely noticed by some patients and which is considered by many physicians as being only a point of local irritation in the canal, and having little, if any relation to the original disease, which they think can be cured by mechanical measures. But knowing that Hahnemann has said that no manner of treatment can cure a single case of these chronic miasms, except through the law of cure, we can readily see that all so-named cures are either suppressions or the disease modified by suppressive measures until it manifests itself in a mild and latent state.

This, however, we do know, that following allopathic or unhomeopathic treatment of gonorrhoea, there follows a host of chronic diseases such as gout, gouty rheumatism, muscular or arthritic rheumatism, of a subacute or chronic nature. These gouty states of the system or any form of the rheumatic element, are apt to develop into heart lesions, such as endo or pericarditis with a fatal ending. This is the history of unhomeopathic treatment of gonorrhoea today, and it has been its history for a thousand years, and will continue to be throughout the years to come unless the thick scales fall from the eyes of these creators of disease. Words cannot tell the endless disease processes that develop through the suppressive measures, and the thoughts of man cannot paint in words, the manifold sufferings of humanity that follows the development of these gouty and rheumatic processes alone, to say nothing of those involving the different organs, such as the stomach, liver, intestines, kidneys, bladder, brain, nose, throat and lungs. Of the moral degeneration, the insanity, and the train of mental and moral perversions that we see arising on the earth, and multiplying as a great oriental plague, we can only refer to them in a work like this. But it must in time bring disastrous results to the human race.

Dr. P.P. Wells, speaking of suppressed diseases at a meeting held at Brooklyn, in 1887, said: "One of the objects of getting upon my feet, first, to speak of the discussion of this paper, is to impress upon this company and all my associates, that a suppressed gonorrhoea is a suppressed inferno; and to me the characteristics which our old school associates annually recommend, are simply the result and not the disease at all; not any more than what you gather in a handkerchief in influenza, is influenza. You have simply shut up the exit of the ventilation of the organism of disease, there to work the work of destruction. We must be successful navigators; we must know where the rocks are steer our vessel clear of them, and land our patient upon the shore of health, and not upon the hidden rocks where the breakers grind and crash." I here add to the above testimony, a few reported cases due to suppression.

Case 1. A young man given to much dissipation, was found suffering with intestinal colic; it had been temporarily relieved with brandy, ginger and a hot water bag. Nux relieved the pain in thirty minutes, but the attacks were renewed many times, yet always relieved by Nux vomica 1m. The history of the case was, that he had contracted gonorrhoea, which was suppressed in a few days; the treatment of which he greatly praised. Medorrhinum was given in the 1m potency, and the gonorrhœa returned within a few days, with greater severity than in the first place, but no further history of colic, although two years elapsed.—J. S. Hayne, M. D. 1905.

Case 2. Mr. E. E. P. was lying very low with neuralgia of the bowels (so called by the regular school). At the end of three weeks of suffering, I was called and finding Pulsatilla to be his remedy, gave it to him in the 200th potency. Three days later the bowel symptoms had disappeared, but a copious gonorrhoeal discharge had been established, which had been suppressed with medical injections.—Dr. E.P. Gregory.

BACTERIA, THEIR ORIGIN

Probably no greater mystery has ever worried or puzzled the mind of the medical profession, than has the subject of the above heading, the origin of Bacteria, the micro-organisms of disease. Theories have been advanced by many minds and the subject has been given serious attention by the profession all over the earth, yet nothing positive or certain has come to us, so that we can feel with any assurance that the mystery had been solved. It seemed to be held back by a mighty hand, only to be given as a gift to Beauchamp to disclose this secret of life. Beauchamp's writings have not been, I believe, translated into our language as yet; and few of us have become acquainted with his master mind or know the depth of his love for the sciences pertaining to the healing art. We are pleased to note, however, that his zeal has not carried him away into the speculative, for we find him too practical and too earnest to indulge in the speculative, especially in this critical and earnest period of the world's history and progress.

Like all great physicians, there was no science or no secret of any science, that bore any relation to medicine, but what he was interested in it. His chemical investigations and researches are far beyond those of Pasteur or Koch, or any of his predecessors; indeed, he stands alone in this special field of investigation. *The march of the human mind is slow, but it is unceasing, vigilant, eternal; and its goal is upward, onward, towards, a solution of the infinite mind, and the uncovering of the unknown.*

We find many of these characteristics in the mind of Beauchamp. He began his investigations a number of years ago, and his discoveries of microzymas in chalk (microzymas, "living points") opened the door to a secret of life that heretofore had been hidden from the mind of man. Where there was thought to be no life, he found life in its lowest state, it was a part of the inorganic deposit, and the mighty changes which it had undergone had not been able to completely obliterate its vitality. These investigations make truly interesting reading, if we are at all interested along these lines of thought. "When the cells of the living organisn are diseased," says Beauchamp, "it means the microzymas are diseased, and they give rise to what is erroneously called pathogenic bacteria." Thus we see the pathogenic bacteria or micro-organisms are not the cause of morbid conditions, but the results thereof. This has been the bone of contention between the two schools of pathologists; those who believe in micro-organisms as the cause of disease and those who do not. In Dr. Beauchamp's work, "Du Sang et Soutioisienu Element Anatom, que," he explains why both free and functional microzymas exist in the blood, and are invisible under ordinary conditions. They are in a sense imperishable, although they can be destroyed by acids or burnt by fire. At a meeting at Nantes in 1875, he exhibited the microzymas in their relation to fermentation, and illustrated the subject with drawings, showing the evolution of the microzymas into bacteria and into cellules.

Some were seen in the process of formation, and others had already assumed the form of true micro-organisms like the *bacteria* of disease. He particularly points out how the microzymas, according to the solution in which they were placed, evolved either cellule or bacteria, and according as they evolve bacteria or cellules, they produced lactic acid or alcohol. During the process of fermentation, the microzymas disappeared as such, developing into bacteria. This was shown when a clot of fresh blood was confined in a vessel that was practically air tight, although in time, air did slowly penetrate, effecting the outer portion of the clot, and a process of fermentation followed. The microzymas died and bacteria made their appearance about the margin of the clot, while in the center of the clot the microzymas were found perfect.

It would be necessary to go fully into the details of the various manipulations and numerous processes through which he carried forward his many experiments, in order to fully understand how he produced the different forms of bacteria. So carefully and thoroughly were these experiments made, employing both animal and vegetable matter and even the inorganic, that we feel firm in our opinion, that he has clearly solved the mystery of the origin of bacteria. He quite clearly proves the fact, that bacteria evolve from a life process, through the influence of some death or degenerative process working in the organism, such as acute or chronic miasms.

THERAPEUTICS OF GONORRHOEA

ACONITE

In the early stage of the disease, when there is fever, thirst, a hot, dry skin, much restlessness with burning in the neck of the bladder when not urinating; urine scanty, dark; feels hot when passing. Painful, anxious urging; gonorrhoeal discharge of a thin, transparent, or white mucus; acute gonorrhoeal orchitis; testicles hot, hard, swollen; much fear; great restlessness and anxiety of mind.

AGARICUS

Indicated sometimes in old chronic gonorrhoea or gleet; organs cold, shrunken, relaxed; chordee very painful; itching and tingling along the urethra; urine flows slowly or dribbles, and is often milky; a single drop of the discharge appears in the morning (like Sepia). Loss of sexual power even to complete impotency. Indicated in old sycotics, who are a mental wreck from over-indulgence, and sexual debauchees; (Agnus castus), genitals cold, shrunken; suffers from spinal irritation, from self abuse; violent sexual excitement with chordee, chronic gonorrhoea or gleet, where all kinds of local treatment have been used. Discharge of white mucus, or bloody discharge with itching and tingling in the urethra; a single drop often appearing in the morning (Medorr., Sepia). Twitching and trembling of the limbs; awkward movements; paralytic heaviness and weariness in the lower extremities; burning and tingling in spine.

ALUMINA

Chronic gleet in old men who are debilitated with the disease, as well as with old age; urine bloody or having a clay-like deposit; the urine is very slow to start, and he urinates better while standing. Discharge yellowish, painless, bland, gleety; discharge always yellow or pus-like; prostatic enlargement; feeling of fullness in the perineum; great weakness of the sexual sphere; voice low and weak; skin dry, no perspiration.

APIS

Indicated in all stages and especially in the pseudo-psoric diathesis. Burning and stinging when urinating; frequent hurried calls to urinate; cannot wait a minute; sometimes the desire is incessant; urine colorless, or dark and smoky-colored; violent burning, scalding, stinging; frequent emissions of small quantities of colorless urine; urination slow, must wait and strain a long time; great irritation with burning and stinging in the neck of the bladder; strangulation with stricture; urine copper colored, smoky or bloody; great swelling of the fore skin; discharge copious, thin mucus, with burning and stinging pains; great œdema of the scrotum or prepuce; tissues greatly swollen, pale, translucent erysipelatous-like swelling of the penis with much œdema.

ASPARAGUS

Sexual excitement very marked; urine very offensive; sticking pains in the urethra or sides of the penis; fine stinging in the meatus, with a sensation after urination as if something was still passing; lithic or greasy deposits on sides of vessel. Frequent but scanty discharge, with a sensation as if something was sticking in the urethra; swelling of the penis, with erections and urging to urinate; urine of a stinking odor; cutting in the urethra.

ARMORACEA

Dysuria, inflammatory stage of gonorrhoea. Frequent desire to urinate, with smarting, burning, tenderness and general inflammatory condition, as seen in the first stage of the disease; copious or scanty white mucous discharge, with burning, cutting, smarting and tenderness while urinating. Compare with Cap. and Canth.

AMMONIUM CARBONICUM

Pain in testicles, and spermatic cords; violent erections, worse in the morning; urine excoriates the parts passed over, causing biting and itching; it has an ammoniacal odor (Benz: ac.) Gonorrhoeal discharge thin, scanty, acrid, producing itching, swelling, and burning of parts passed over.

AMMONIUM MURIATICUM

Much tenesmus on passing urine, (Like Nux or Cantharis), confined to neck of bladder; the urine copious, strong smelling, moldy, musty, or ammoniacal, discharge like white of egg, or brownish and slimy; worse after urination.

ARSENICUM ALBUM

Indicated in all stages of the disease, especially in tubercular patients, and when complicated with chancroid or suppurating bubo; frequently indicated in these cases. Discharge thin, white, acrid; producing erythema on the parts over which it passes. Gonorrhoeal cachexia well marked; face pale; puffiness about the eyes, face and lips; mouth dry; thirst for frequent but small drinks of water; rapid loss of strength and failing of the vital forces; fear of death, with great anxiety; <at 1 P. M.

ARGENTUM NITRICUM

When mental symptoms predominate as result of suppression. Gonorrhoea in young boys who look prematurely old. Impotency after repeated attacks of the disease (Agnus castus); tendency to sycotic growths, warts, and polypi; meatus very red, raw, puffy (Medor). Discharge copious, yellowish-green, bland, (like Puls.), turns green when exposed to air; bleeding of the urethra; erections very painful, severe; urine often passes unconsciously; desire for sugar or sweets which aggravate; craves fresh air; chilly when uncovered; urine passes too slowly.

Patient feels tired and exhausted; sensitive; easily confused; no desire to talk; forgets the words he should use (Sycosis); gonorrhoeal discharge, thick, copious, greenish-yellow; epidymitis or orchitis following a suppression; much pain, hardness, swelling, with burning and stinging; gleety discharge, thin, light yellow, follows the copious, thick, bland, greenish-yellow discharge of gonorrhoea, bearing down or dragging sensation in testicles; chest and voice weak, hoarse; rheumatism worse in damp or changeable weather.

ANGUSTURA

Urine copious, frequent and light or orange colored. Voluptuous itching of the tip of the glans, causing rubbing; much itching of the scrotum; drawing pain in the left spermatic cord; papular eruption on the genitals, which burn and itch (Rhus tox); a bruised pain when urinating with tenesmus.

ANANTHERUM

Pressing and burning pain in the bladder, with urging to urinate every minute; sensation as if the kidneys and bladder were full; bladder can hold only a small quantity of urine. (Calad.) Retention of urine, with retraction of the canal; urine discharged in drops or in little spurts, thick and full of mucus; catarrh of the bladder; strong odor to urine, with an iridescent pelicle. Gonorrhœal discharge, white mucus in the beginning of the disease, but later on it becomes thick, yellowish green, with burning in the urethra; burning and deep seated pains in scrotum and testicles; during coitus sufferings relieved, but greatly increased afterwards. Venereal appetite greatly increased while patient has gonorrhoea. Aggravated in the morning, with change of weather, wine and coitus.

BORAX

Dark blue spots about the orifice of the urethra, with

biting pain when urinating. The discharge agglutinates the orifice, with smarting pain on urinating or burning and tension in the glans penis; severe urging and even after urinating urging continues; screams when urine is passed as it is hot as fire (in children and young people). Gonorrhœal discharge white mucus and pasty.

BENZOIC ACID

Gouty symptoms following a suppression, gout of the bladder, especially in children who have the sycotic taint from their parents; urine very offensive, foul smelling, pungent like ammonia; dark brown strong like beer, and very offensive, smelling like hartshorn. Indicated often in the tertiary stage of Sycosis, asthma alternating with gouty or rheumatic complaints. Indicated principally in women and children with the sycotic taint well marked. Gouty concretions and nodes are found in the joints with the above described urinary symptoms.

BERBERIS

Sickly looking pale-faced individuals with blue circles about the eyes, stabbing or shooting pains in the kidneys, with much distress in the renal region after suppression of the discharge; enlarged prostate after suppression; sensation as of a lump or pressure in the perineum; much soreness and aching in the lumber region after suppression; bladder very irritable with pain on urination; aching in the spermatic cord and testicles or a burning sensation along the cord; thick, dark, copious reddish sediment in the urine.

BRYONIA

A wonderful remedy for the symptoms that follow the suppression of the gonorrhœal discharge. The symptoms and diseases following are often sub-acute. Gonorrhœal arthritis; many cases are cured. Orchitis worse on the right side always. It is indicated usually in fibrous-tissue inflammations, in those of the serous membranes and in the ligaments of the joints. Pneumonia following suppression. Pains are sharp, shooting or dull pressing; parts always feel too heavy, as of a dead weight; motion aggravated greatly, also heat. Patient very thirsty for cold water; drinks large quantities; frontal headache. Patient morose, irritable, with constipation; stools large, hard and dry. Craves things yet has an aversion to them when obtained; craves acid drinks. Stitches in right testicles and spermatic cord; gleet with greenish discharge and some burning. Suppressed discharge usually followed with rheumatism, acute orchitis or sub-acute rheumatism. Testicles swollen very large; marked induration, worse on right side; urine diminished, hot and dark colored.

BALSAM OF PERU

Sticking pains in the urethra when not urinating;

frequent urination during the night; urine clear but scanty; with a peculiar resinous odor; drawing pains in the right tibia and severe pains in the arch of the palate and avula.

BONDONNEAN
(A Mineral Water)

Urine has a strong odor; pricking in the urethra when urinating; much mucous discharge from penis with itching; gonorrhoeal discharge copious white mucus; frequent morning erections; great and continual hunger, with abundant saliva from the mouth; taste clammy and sour.

CALCAREA CARB

Chronic gonorrhoea in a marked pseudo-psoric diathesis. Calcarea cures fig warts that have the typical herring-brine odor. Chronic gleet in lymphatic individuals that perspire profusely about the face and head, who have cold feet or perspire in the palms of the hands on the least physical or mental effort. Calcarea has excessive sexual desire and lascivious fancies; cutting in the urethra with burning at the meatus at night; burning before urinating and a cutting pain while urinating; worse while drinking. Induration of the testicles, with general Calcarea symptoms; scrotum hangs relaxed. Sterility from the pseudo-psoric diathesis or from long suppressed gonorrhoea. Discharge bland and light yellow, of a stinking odor; warts round, soft at the base, same color as the skin; itch and bleed easily.

CANTHARIS

Inflammatory gonorrhoea with intense sexual erythism, strangury and intense vesical irritation, discharge mucous or bloody with urging and straining to urinate, frequently only passes a drop at a time with much pain and suffering. Irritation of the neck of the bladder from suppression; intolerable tenesmus of the bladder with violent cutting and burning at the neck. Chordee violent and painful. Sits and strains but gets no relief. Urine burns like fire; screams or groans on passing urine. The penis is very much inflamed and painful, sometimes with fever, violent delirium and sexual frenzy.

CAPSICUM

Indicated in the beginning of the second stage. Quite often the remedy in those having a tubercular taint, especially indicated in light haired, blue eyed, red faced, plump, plethoric individuals, who are chilly and sensitive to cold; prepuce swollen; meatuis red and puffy; often pain in the prostate gland; discharge thick, yellow, copious, and of a creamy consistency, coldness of testicles is sometimes present. Burning and biting after urinating, or a hot peppery feeling at the meatus, or itching at the urethra; burning pain with urging to urinate.

CANNABIS INDICA

Indicated in the early stage of the disease; symptom acute, painful, inflammatory; sexual desire greatly increased even to satyriasis; violent chordee, worse when moving or walking. Forgets what he intended to say, (sycotic), thoughts crowd on brain. Sharp, pricking, like needles in the urethra; slight burning on urination; discharge yellowish-white, profuse; strains to urinate the last drop, bladder will not fully empty itself; has to wait before urine flows. Uneasy sensation in urethra with frequent calls to urinate.

CANNABIS SATIVA

Indicated in the first stage and beginning of the second; symptoms painful, inflammatory (Cann. ind., Canth.), copious, mucous discharge. Dark redness of the glans penis. Later in the disease the discharge is thick, yellow, purulent; urethra very sore, sensitive to touch, walks with limbs wide apart; sticking, shooting pains from the orifice upwards in all directions. Spasms of the urethra; urine ceases to flow at times. Sticking and jabbing pains when urinating; much swelling of the urethra and orifice, gland covered with bright red spots. Sticking pains with burning at the meatus when not urinating; urine turbid, red and full of fibre (Canth., Caps., Gels., Petros., Cann. ind.); coldness of the genitals with warmth of the rest of the body. The whole penis is swollen, painful as if burned and worse when walking.

CARBOLIC ACID

Burning and itching in the urethra; strains to pass urine, urine dark, olive-green; discharge white or purulent, acrid, offensive, corrosive, produces erythema of parts touched, longs for stimulants, especially whisky, desire relieved by drinking lemonade.

CEDRON

Anti-sycotic. A good remedy to give in a high potency after allopathic doping with crude drugs; nervous excitement followed by depression; languid, heavy, and depressed. He complains of a heavy pain in the region of the kidneys, frequent ineffectual desire to urinate (Nux); discharge thin, whitish, gleety, with a feeling as of a drop were passing from the urethra (Kali bich., Medorr., Thuja).

CLEMATIS

Urination very severe at the commencement, a few drops pass with much pain then the spasm subsides and he urinates with comparative ease; stream interrupted. Discharge suppressed with orchitis; testicles painful, hard, swollen, inflamed, tender to touch, with drawing and shooting pains extending up the spermatic cord. Swelling and induration after suppression (Bry., Puls.).

< at night; discharge gleety, or thick yellow pus; urine turbid, milky; the last drop causes much pain and burning (Sarsa); urine dribbles drop by drop in severe cases. If the gonorrhœal discharge is suppressed, the disease involves the testicles, neck of the bladder, and spermatic cords.

COPAIBA

Violent emotions and sexual desire constant; urethra sore, swollen, painful, with biting, burning and itching on urination, indicated in an early stage. Discharge yellow, purulent, or muco-purulent; urine foamy, turbid, with odor of violets. Frequent calls to urinate with tenesmus and pressure on the bladder; tickling sensation at the orifice of the urethra. Stream thin, twisted (Cann. sat., Medorr.); antidote for its abuse nux vomica. It is often the Aconite of gonorrhœa; think of it in connection with Gelsemium.

CUBEBA

Sensation of constriction and cutting in the urethra. Indicated in the early stage of the disease; discharge copious, white, mucous or tinged with blood; scalding or cutting pains or sensation of heat in the urethra. Later on in the disease the discharge is profuse, pus-like, and glutinous; and still later in the disease it is thick, yellowish-green, obstructing the flow of urine. Ropy mucus escapes from the urethra as the last drop of the urine is voided. After urination a sensation in the bladder, as if all the urine were not passed. A nettle rash often accompanies the gonorrhœa.

CHIMAPHILA UMBELLATA

Urging to urinate even after voiding urine (Nux., Mer. cor., Canth.); cutting and scalding pain while urinating; passes in drops or the stream is forked and thin; urinates better standing with limbs wide apart. Gonorrhœal or catarrhal discharge copious, muco-purulent, even ropy and bloody; gleet with stricture and strangury; lithic diathesis very marked; smarting pain in the neck of bladder, extending the whole length of the urethra.

CALADIUM

Urinary Organs. A sensation of fullness in the bladder is a constant symptom in both sexes; full to bursting it seems, yet only a small quantity passes; fullness with very little desire to urinate, or fullness with urging. Region of the bladder sensitive to touch. Urine offensive, and burns like hot water when passing or drawing from bladder to penis. Impotence in the male.

Gonorrhoea with the *corona glandis* covered with very red points or spots (Thuja, Medorrhinum); glans dry, red and itching; erection painful, or perhaps imperfect, with no sexual desire. In the female violent itching on the external genitals, often inducing onanism.

Complementary to Nitric acid.

DIGITALIS

Great irritation of the neck of the bladder with strangury and frequent urging to urinate; urethra much inflamed with severe burning; discharge thick, bright yellow and purulent. Copious secretions of thick pus over the glans penis (Farrington), chordee with violent and prolonged erection; slow pulse, intermittent, with sensation as if the heart would stop beating.

DULCAMARA

Its rheumatic element and sensitiveness to climatic changes are indicative of Sycosis in the third or chronic stage. All its symptoms are greatly aggravated by a falling barometer, kidney troubles that are induced by Sycosis may need this remedy, sometime during the treatment. Gonorrhœal discharge muco-purulent, yellowish-white and copious. Mucous discharge may be bloody and offensive in renal difficulties; urine scanty, turbid, offensive; worse in damp weather.

DORYPHORA
(Colorado Potato Bug)

The whole body has a feeling as if swollen; great weariness and heaviness with desire to lie down; a feeling of heaviness in the rectum; difficult urination, with retention. Dark, dirty, red colored urine, voided with much pain. Glans penis swollen and bluish red ; itching and burning in the glans. Desire to urinate but cannot pass urine ; pain in the back and lumbar region with trembling of the extremities ; aggravation from eating, drinking and smoking. Dysuria with burning and stinging pains (Canth, Apis.). General dropsy, but it does not "pit." The face has a besotted look as if the patient had imbibed freely of intoxicants. He is very irritable as in Nux.

EUPATORIUM PURPUREUM

Deep, dull or cutting pain in the kidneys, passing urine every ten minutes, with aching in the bladder ; gonorrhœal smarting and burning in bladder and urethra, very marked when urinating, stream very small ; chronic forms of catarrh of bladder from various causes.

ERYNGIUM AQUATICUM

Gonorrhœa in the acute stage ; acute inflammatory ; frequent desire to urinate, passing a drop at a time (Canth., Cann., sat., Mer. cor., Nux vom.) ; stinging pains on urinating, in the urethra and behind the glans penis ; tired feeling in the lumbar region ; sexual desire greatly depressed; heavy pain in left groin and testicle ; thick yellowish, tenacious mucous discharge ; intense itching of the skin.

ERECHTHITES
(Fire Weed)

Urine quite scanty and painful in passing ; scalding and burning at the meatus on passing urine ; specific gravity very high ; urine very acid in its reaction, smoky colored, scanty, dark and often mixed with blood ; hemorrhage from kidneys or bladder ; urine has a milky appearance on standing ; aching tenderness and swelling of the right testicle in suppressed gonorrhœa ; dull aching in the small of the back ; erection with dreams and emissions toward morning, similar to Cubeba.

EPIGEA REPENS

Acute gonorrhœa (inflammatory) with much tenesmus of the bladder ; burning in the neck of the bladder when urinating ; urine pale or with a bloody sediment ; gonorrhœal discharge with much mucus and pus.

ERIGERON CANADENSIS

Dysura in teething children ; the child cries when urinating ; urine of a very strong color, and it irritates and inflames the parts passed over. Gonorrhœa ; urging to urinate with but a few drops ; sharp, stinging pains in the region of the left kidney ; pain in the right kidney, extending down to the testicle ; much distress in the bladder with frequent urination. Symptoms all worse in rainy weather.

EUPHORBIA PILULIFERA

Burning pain on urination in gonorrhœa; obliged to sit down and keep quiet; violent desire to urinate (Cann., Canth.).

FLUORIC ACID

Urine scanty, pungent, fetid with burning after urinating and aching in the bladder; strong sexual desire at night with a violent desire for coition. Gonorrhœa in old men with greatly increased sexual desire; penis swollen, with pain in the spermatic cord; chronic or subacute gonorrhœa when but a single yellow drop appears in the morning. (Sep., Medorrh.)

FAGOPYRUM ESCULENTUM
(Buckwheat)

Acute gonorrhœa in early stage; dysurea with great difficulty in voiding the last drop; cutting like a knife at the close of urination or during urination; (Sarsa.) pain in bowels after urinating; much lassitude and weariness with yawning and stretching; ameliorated by motion, eating and open air; aggravated in afternoon and evening.

GELSEMIUM

Acute inflammatory gonorrhœa with fever, general aching, headache, and backache. Headache relieved by passing large quantities of urine; much relaxation and prostration of the muscular system, very irritable, nervous, sensitive, with trembling of the extremities, with desire to lie down. In its febrile stage, he is torpid, drowsy and hates to move. Dull pain in the back with a basilar headache and fever (acute state). Heavy, flushed, besotted appearance of the face. Gonorrhœal discharge of white mucus, scanty, with heat, smarting, and redness at the meatus, and slight burning; gonorrhœa suppressed soon after the appearance of the discharge with threatened orchitis. Gonorrhœa at the beginning of the attack, with slight burning on urination, fever with drowsiness and general aching of the limbs and back. Gonorrhœa suppressed with medicated injections; high fever, pain and much swelling in the testicles; no discharge; urine copious and painful; very nervous, trembles when he attempts to move. Face flushed, pulse slow, soft; confined to his bed. Many other expressions of this valuable remedy might be given, but what has been given is sufficient to see its action in gonorrhœa.

GNAPHALIUM POLYCEPHALUM
(Cud Weed)

Sensation of fullness in bladder even after having

emptied it (Calad.); sexual desire very great on awakening; severe pain in the prostrate gland or an intense pain along the right sciatic nerve with a feeling of numbness; dull heavy expression of the countenance; face appears bloated; vertigo on rising with dull pain in back of the head. (Nux vom.)

HYDRASTIS

Acute or chronic gonorrhœa with very little pain or soreness in the urethra; discharge, copious, thick, viscid, ropy, yellowish or greenish yellow mucus; indicated in old sinners who are addicted to alcoholics or other stimulants; much debility and general nervousness; chancroid and gonorrhœal ulcers, with indolent granulations and yellowish discharges; ulcers bleed easily and the discharge is copious, thick, yellow and painless, with dragging in the groins and testicles and a cachetic expression of the face; urine has a decomposed smell. Gonorrhœa in the second stage after the acute inflammatory condition has subsided; discharge thick, yellow, fibrinous or ropy at times; gleet with thick yellow discharge; tongue coated a dirty yellow color; constipation similar to Nux.

KALI MURIATICUM

Gonorrhœa in the acute inflammatory stage or mixed with chancroid and soft bubo; acute orchitis after suppression by injections. Discharge thick, white, slimy mucus. Induration of the left testicle after suppression; chronic catarrh of the bladder with a copious discharge of white mucus; chordee very severe; fibrous exudations with glandular infiltrations and indurations.

KALI IODATUM

Indicated in the mixed venereal diseases like Syphilis and Sycosis, or Sycosis with a syphilitic taint, although it may be indicated in Sycosis with a tubercular taint, or where there is a glandular involvment. Burning pain in kidneys with a bruised pain in the small of the back; sexual desire diminished; testes atrophied or enormously swollen and indurated. Penis greatly swollen with constant semi-erection. Gonorrhœal discharge muco-purulent or bloody with burning in the urethra. Gonorrhœa in old chronic cases with a syphilitic history; thick, greenish discharge with no pain and very little soreness. Chancroid with gangrene, accompanied with gonorrhœa. Bubo abscesses with fistulous openings and with an offensive, bloody, ichorous, corrosive discharge. Curdy discharges.

KALI BICHROMICUM

This remedy is indicated quite often in mixed venereal diseases. In Syphilis and gonorrhœa or chancroid and gonorrhœa; discharge is in tough strings, ropy, adherent; can be drawn out in long mucous strings; ulcers deep with a punched-out edge; irregular with a yellow base, pressure at root of nose. Frequently indicated in Sycosis or Syphilis of the nose. This is another remedy where the patient is addicted to stimulants, developing gastric ulcers, etc. ; vomits blood and thick, ropy mucus ; hawks up much ropy mucus, indicated more frequently at the close of second stage, when there is a scanty, ropy, gleety discharge. After urination, a sensation as if a few drops remained or if a drop were passing. Gouty states follow catarrhal suppression. Tongue smooth, dry, red, sometimes cracked. Difficulty in expelling the last few drops of urine. Diphtheritic forms of gonorrhœa, adapted to fat, fair haired people, who are relieved by cool weather.

KALI SULPHURICUM

Indicated in second stage, discharge yellow, or yellowish-green, (Puls.), sometimes slimy or sticky. Gonorrhœal ophthalmia ; painless, thick, yellow discharge ; no urinary symptoms ; a slight soreness only in urethra ; sycotic metastases to lungs or to testicles following suppression ; < in damp weather, and from rest. "Loose cough with soreness and pain in left chest" (Nash). I have found it useful in chronic cases of long standing where Pulsatilla seems to be indicated and fails. It comes in between Pulsatilla and Capsicum. Scrotum and prepuce oedematous and much swollen after suppressive measures have been used. It is also useful in the tertiary stage, in mixed venereal difficulties, when warts and condylomata or gout of feet, follow suppression or bad treatment (to be compared with thuja). The warts are all about anus or sexual organs, also on face and around the eyes; vesicles containing a yellowish fluid are met with about the hands. (complimentary to Thuja). Sycosis engrafted upon a tubercular base, (Caps).

LITHIUM CARBONICUM

The bladder symptoms are very marked. Before urinating, flashes of pain appear in the region of the bladder, $<$ on the right side; after urinating the pain runs up the left spermatic cord. Gonorrhœa with much soreness in the bladder and sharp stinging pains in the neck; urine dark, with reddish brown, brick dust deposits. (Sep., Phos., Lyc.) Gonorrhœal discharge, greenish, profuse, thick and purulent, indicated in sub-acute or chronic cases, tenesmus strong, with pain in the neck of the bladder and along the urethra; indicated often in the tertiary stage of gonorrhœa, when the lithic diathesis develops.

LAC CANINUM

This remedy is one that will sometimes be called for in mixed venereal diseases, or gonorrhœa and Syphilis or gonorrhœa and chancroid. Chancroid with large fungus-like ulcers on dorsum of the penis, ulcers deep with sharp clean cut edges with a glistening or slimy appearance, no pain. Chancroids of the prepuce, that bleed easily and profusely. Gonorrhœa with severe intermittent pains in the middle of urethra, or in penis ; constant desire to urinate with intense pain ; urine dark, scanty ; sexual organs very sensitive to touch ; dreams of snakes, death, and dark water ; no desire to live ; disgusted with life ; discharge whitish and thin, odor fetid.

LACHESIS

Indicated in mixed venereal difficulties with chancroid or gonorrhœa or chancre and gonorrhœa. Gonorrhœa with intense sexual excitement ; constant erections at night with night sweats ; chancroid or syphilitic ulcers on foreskin of a dark blue color ; scrotum or penis greatly swollen. Gangrene or phagedenic ulcers of the sexual organs. Buboes with fistulous openings ; hectic fever and a general septic condition ; urine dark, even black, and scanty with albumen in it. A feeling as if a ball were rolling in the bladder ; gonorrhœal discharge offensive or bloody mucus ; parts very sensitive to touch ; violent burning while passing urine ; symptoms $<$ on the left side, and also $<$ after sleep ; great physical exhaustion with trembling and fear of death in phagedenic and septic conditions.

LYCOPODIUM

Gonorrhœa with urging to urinate but has to wait a long time before it will pass ; strangury ; urine scanty, dark, muddy, with red sediment like brick dust; penis cold and relaxed. Much flatulence and distension of the colon with gastric disturbances; face sallow, sickly, cachetic-looking; gonorrhœa in the second stage; chronic symptoms < on right side and at 4 P.M. Mucous membrane of urethra greatly swollen; discharge milky or yellowish-green, thick, and offensive. It is a splendid remedy where chancroid is present in gonorrhœa.

MERCURIUS SOL

Useful in the mixed disease; I have cured a number of cases of gonorrhœa where syphilis was also present. It is an easy matter to suppress the disease with this remedy even in the potency. (Symptoms syphilitic). Discharge thick, yellow, green, or purulent, sometimes bloody, offensive; < at night; urine often bloody, and is passed with burning and smarting. Ulcers in throat and on sexual organs with syphilitic skin eruptions, ulcers, flat with a lardaceous base; seldom if ever indicated in a simple case of gonorrhœa.

MEDORRHINUM

Urine may be either pale or dark in color; the stream is usually small and is passed slowly; it may be forked or twisted; chilly after urination; much uneasiness and pressure in the bladder; urinate frequently at night, and this symptom, if found in young men, is a strong indication for this remedy ; frequent calls to urinate at night, long after gonorrhœa has been suppressed ; there may or may not be any pain or burning or uneasy feeling at the neck of the bladder, with these frequent calls to urinate. (Chronic) Gonorrhœa, with acute burning upon urinating ; discharge transparent or of a gummy consistency ; staining the linen yellow. Gonorrhœal discharge thin, white, mucous, profuse or scanty with intense and frequent erections day or night, but usually < at night. Gonorrhœal discharges have been cured with this remedy after it had remained a chronic gleet for from five to twenty years. It is especially called for in suppression, when no other remedy seems indicated. In the majority of cases, however, it will reproduce the discharge while the constitutional symptoms will all subside.

Chronic cystitis where the urine passes very slowly with loss of propulsive power ; when he becomes warm in bed or the body becomes warm generally, he urinates readily. Gonorrhœa with burning at the meatus on urinating ; the orifice is red, puffy, swollen, with great soreness along the whole urethra ; very little tenderness but just dull soreness. Discharge mucous or yellowish-green, offensive and generally scanty, but profuse in patients of a tubercular diathesis ; a sensation as if something remained after urinating or as of something passing from the urethra. (Thuja, Kali. bich.)

Gleet, chronic or sub-acute, painless or with pain ; only a drop appears in the morning (Sep.,) ; orifice is gummed up every morning ; color of discharge yellowish green (Thuja) ; discharge always < in the morning. It is increased for three days after every dose ; cannot retain urine at night ; often no pain or burning, but the neck of the bladder is so irritable that urine is not retained long. Aggravation in damp weather, cold, at night, also < at 10 a.m. and after 12 p.m. ; heat of bed aggravates the bladder ; > on motion ; lying on stomach or face downwards ; near the seashore ; in dry atmosphere and in medium altitudes in summer.

NUX VOMICA

This remedy may be used at any time in the early stage of gonorrhœa, where there has been much allopathic drugging, especially where Copaiva, Cubebs, Cedron, Cathartics and medicated injections have been used. I usually find the nux headache present in such cases. It may be given for a few days in those cases before the curative remedy is selected, and it cures many cases without the aid of other help. Irritable, quarrelsome, cross, fretful ; easily angered ; over-sensitive to light, noise and other impressions ; tongue coated dirty brown ; breath offensive ; taste bad ; feels dull, sleepy and drowsy when sitting or reading. Patient often chilly with backache ; < when lying down, tenesmus with urging to urinate (Mer. cor.). He is very nervous and business annoys him very much ; wishes to be alone. Sometimes he is broken down and exhausted sexually and craves stimulants and condiments of all kinds ; after straining to urinate, the urine dribbles away. Discharge copious, white, mucous. He feels $<$ in the morning and is better from quiet and heat.

Case a. Mr. B., age 30, rigid fiber; dark brown hair and blue eyes, has had gonorrhœa for two weeks, suppressed by medicated injections. He was very irritable with dull headache in the temples; tongue foully coated, with loss of appetite and bad taste in the mouth. Nux 1m relieved the headache at once, re-established the discharge and sweetened his disposition very much. In four or five days I gave him Medorrhinum which cured him.

Case b. Mr. J. G., age 37, tall, dark complexion; a laboring man. He had taken oil of cedron until his stomach was in a bad state; urine very scanty and is passed with much straining; has a desire to stool also; when he urinated he used much profanity and is very irritable. Nux 1m cured in a short time. The discharge was re-established at once and his abnormal mental symptoms all disappeared.

Case c. Frank L., age 26, a machinist; has taken all sorts of cures from his druggist; is much discouraged and is very nervous; his face looks drawn and has a distressed look; complains of being chilly, with loss of appetite and of desire for tobacco, which he uses to excess; the tongue has a heavy brown coating and the breath is offensive. He craves beer; wants either pepper, mustard, or horse-radish on his food; there is a copious muco-purulent discharge and some straining when he urinates. Nux c. m. relieved all his symptoms except a gleety discharge which was cured by another remedy.

NATRUM CARBONICUM

Urine dark yellow ; fetid and sour, with pressure in the region of the bladder ; burning in the urethra during and after urination ; straining and tenesmus in the bladder due to prostatic enlargement ; heavy, bruised feeling with a drawing sensation in the testicles.

NATRUM MURIATICUM

Gonorrhœa in pseudo-psoric people ; discharge transparent, watery, or light yellow, with cutting and scalding sensations on urination ; no pain later on with the gleety stage. Discharge leaves thin, transparent spots on the linen. In women the discharge turns green on exposure to the air ; urine starts slowly, has to wait for it. The mucous membranes feel dry ; urine dribbles, with a sensation as if more remained in the bladder. Indicated in mild, chronic cases, especially in the gleety stage.

NITRIC ACID

Gonorrhœa with Syphilis or a syphilitic taint ; much pain and tenderness in the testicles. Genital ulcers that are deep, bleed easily and have false granulations with sticking pains in the ulcers. Discharge like dirty water, slightly bloody with fish-brine odor. Discharge may be greenish with a tinge of yellow and very thin, acrid, and offensive ; urine very offensive, dark brown, smells like horse's urine ; at times feels cold when it passes. Seldom do we find yellow or pus-like discharges in Nitric acid. Warts and sycotic eruptions appear frequently about mucous openings ; moist, oozing ; bleeding easily on being touched ; sticking pains like splinters.

NITRATE OF URANIUM

This is said to be a good remedy in Bright's disease or in diabetes mellitus. The patient passes large quantities of sugar and albumen ; urine pale or milky colored, with night sweats and great debility ; sexual organs cold, relaxed and sweaty ; pain in the lumbar region, with weariness and heaviness in the legs ; constipation with increased hunger and thirst; pain in left scapula on taking a deep inspiration ; urine smells fishy. I can readily see this will prove a good remedy in organic diseases of the kidneys, that are induced by suppressed gonorrhœa, or for many of the severe tertiary expressions upon the urinary tract.

PETROSELINUM

Indicated in the first stages of gonorrhœa, (Cann., Canth., Medorrh.). The sudden seizure or urgent desire to urinate being the keynote (Apis) ; cries out or jumps up and down with pain, if he has no opportunity to urinate when the desire comes. It is also suitable in bladder troubles of old people, or in gonorrhœa where the neck of the bladder is involved ; when a stasis of the disease to the neck of the bladder is induced by injections, this remedy is the one ; voluptuous tingling and burning in the whole urethra tickling in the fossa navicularis, biting and itching in the urethra, with a thin, whitish and scanty discharge.

PALLADIUM

Pressing pains in the region of the kidneys, as if retaining urine too long ; < when sitting ; pressure in the bladder as if over full ; frequent desire to urinate with aching in the bladder. Sub-acute gonorrhœa with a full feeling in the bladder as if too full of urine, yet there is not much there ; stitching pains running through urethra to glans ; urine turbid ; heaviness in sexual organs or an unpleasant sensation with painful weakness ; fleeting, transient pains all over the body; sensation as if the body was growing larger and taller or as if something dreadful was going to happen.

PIPER NICRUM

Bladder feels full and swollen ; frequent inclination to urinate ; burning pain in bladder as from live coals ; much inflammation and swelling of the penis ; excessive priapism, with burning pain. Discharge greenish and offensive.

PRUNUS SPINOSA

Cramps and much tenesmus with burning and biting in bladder, urine hot and corrosive, stream forked; when urine reaches glans penis it causes violent pain and spasms. Discharge white or bloody mucus. Dry heat in genital organs.

PULSATILLA

Indicated in patients with blond complexion, of a mild, gentle disposition (Nat. sulph.) In gonorrhœa the face is often sallow. There is a tendency to orchitis, for which it becomes the remedy next in frequency to Bryonia. Symptoms are itching and burning on inner side of prepuce, with a bland, thick yellow or yellowish-green discharge. The patient feels >moving about and in the open air. The nose is often stopped up in a warm room and his symptoms are all< in the evening. The face has a sickly look and is often mottled and puffy looking. There is no thirst, but a desire for sour, refreshing things, and an aggravation from fats and greasy foods of any kind. The tongue has a loose, pasty, white coating, and the saliva is cottony with a slimy taste. The urine is scanty and is passed often with burning and smarting, and the bladder symptoms are aggravated by lying on the back. The chordee may be severe, long lasting and accompanied with backache. Often the foreskin has a dropsical appearance like Apis, and the gonorrhœal inflammation is prone to attack the prostrate and testicles, with a cutting pain along the cord. Even in this gleety stage the discharge is thick, yellowish-green and bland.

SACCHARUM LACTIS

Much soreness in the urethra when urinating. Thin yellow discharge after urination, with cutting pains running up the urethra.

SANICULA

Indicated occasionally in chronic gonorrhœa and gleet, but more apt to be indicated in the beginning of the tertiary stage. There is a cramp-like pain along the left ureter when trying to retain urine. Gonorrhœal discharge smells like fish-brine (Medorr., Thuja, Teuc.) Leucorrhœa smells like stale fish or fish-brine (Medorr.); cold, clammy sweat about the scrotum. Fig warts about the sexual organs. See general symptoms of Sanicula (Clarke). Symptoms constantly changing (Puls).

SENECIO AURENS

Indicated occasionally in the third stage of gonorrhœa, when the prostate gland is enlarged, is hard and has a swollen feeling. Dull heavy pains in the left, spermatic cord extending down to the testicles ; lascivious dreams with pollution ; renal congestion after gonorrhœa with fever ; severe pains in the lumbar region ; motion increases the pain. (Bry.) Severe pain in the right kidney which is extreme on urination ; urine reddish colored, hot and acrid ; smarting in the fossa navicularis ; great weariness in the lower limbs ; a tendency to hemorrhages from kidneys and bladder with congestion in right kidney ; discharge greenish, especially in women.

SENEGA

Great irritability of the bladder, < at night while in bed; urging and scalding before and after urination ; sub-acute and chronic catarrh of the bladder. Discharge, mucous filiments with greenish tinge.

SEPIA

Urine often turbid, dark, high colored with a clay-like or reddish sediment ; sensation as if bladder was full and a feeling of pressure. Gonorrhœa ; urging to urinate with pressure in the bladder ; urine passes slowly ; buring after urinating, < in evening and morning. Discharge, mucous or muco-purulent, scanty ; sub-acute or chronic cases having only a drop of yellowish green pus in the morning with much soreness along the urethra ; increased sexual desire with great weakness of the genitals ; perspiration of the scrotum with much itching of the parts ; itching of the prepuce ; indicated often in the gleety stages of gonorrhœa, where a single drop of yellowish green pus appears in the morning, staining the linen yellow ; no pain or burning when urinating, but bright red, round herpetic spots on glans penis.

SARSAPARILLA

Painful constriction of the bladder with urging and burning ; tenderness and distension over the region of the bladder ; frequent urination at night (chronic) ; scanty discharge and burning; cutting pain on urinating, which is < at the close or completion ; severe pain at the close causing him to cry out. Gonorrhœal discharge, white, mucous or muco-purulent and acrid.

STAPHISAGRIA

Urine scanty, dark and heavily loaded with urates, urging to urinate, yet only passes about a teaspoonful, with burning before and after. Irritability of the bladder after sexual excesses ; chronic gonorrhœal prostatitis after suppression or from sexual excesses ; urine dribbles away ; testicles swollen and greatly inflamed with burning, stinging, pressing or drawing pains in the cord ; sensations as if compressed ; great atrophy after sexual excesses or onanism. Indicated in mixed venereal diseases. Great sexual excitement ; very nervous and melancholic ; despondent after sexual excesses or losses ; great dullness of the mind ; easily angered and suffers much after it.

STILLINGIA

Stillingia has dull pain in the right kidney or across the back in that region ; urine thick and milky with foam which forms bubbles. Gonorrhœa, with violent smarting pain through the entire course of the urethra, and while urinating a sharp pain in the glans extending up the urethra ; much urethral irritation and chordee. We may have scalding, burning and smarting on urination with sticking or shooting-like pains like in Cann. sat.

SILICA

Tenesmus of the bladder and anus ; continuous urging with scanty discharge ; nightly incontinence of urine ; profuse urination relieves the headache (Gel.) ; slight soreness and burning on urination ; discharge of prostatic fluid on straining at stool. Gonorrhœal discharge, pus like or bloody pus, often shreddy ; gonorrhœa with supperating buboes, with fistulous opening ; offensive foot sweats , want of vital heat ; great weariness and sense of exhaustion where suppuration is present ; < early in the morning, by covering up warm, by hot applications to the diseased parts ; sour night sweats which are debilitating ; diseased parts hard, swollen and bluish.

THUJA

Sycotic pure and simple. Seldom indicated in early stage, it is usually preceded by Medorrhinum; it follows this remedy later in the disease; do not think of giving it for acute gonorrhœa. Loss of power to expel urine; sensation as if urine or some fluid were passing from urethra when not urinating. Sense of constriction in urethra, wants to pass water but cannot. The inclination is frequent with burning. Impotence after gonorrhœa (Staph., Agnus castus), sub-acute or chronic gonorrhœa with a dark watery yellowish-green discharge. Gonorrhœa checked by injections or prostatitis, following the use of suppressive measures; red spots and excrescences on glans penis or on prepuce. The discharge in Thuja smells like herring brine or at least it has a pungent, strong odor. The warts are fan-shaped or they are large, seedy, often sensitive and pedunculated—found on the sexual organs or on hairy parts. He sweats on uncovered parts, which ceases when he sleeps. (Reverse of Samb.) Sweat is fetid and sour smelling. The nails are brittle and corrugated. Skin looks dirty, (Sulph.). Thuja does not bear the same relation to Sycosis that Mercury does to Syphilis, as has been said by the old writers; it seldom cures a case of Sycosis in the first and secondary stage, but it does cure the tertiary expressions of Sycosis, that is, when the warty eruptions and warty excresences appear at the close of the secondary stage; this is its place in Sycosis. Rheumatism following a suppression.

TEREBINTHINUM

Violent burning in urethra while urinating, urinates every few minutes with relief of the pain. Tenesmus and violent burning on urinating with scanty flow of urine; acute stage of gonorrhœa (Canth.). Gonorrhœa with severe cystitis and pressure in the region of the bladder; strangury, and retention of urine. Gonorrhœa where the force of the disease is thrown upon the kidneys, (Berber.), with burning pain in small of back; urine cloudy or smoky colored, yet often bloody, or pure blood passes from the bladder; coffee grounds sediment, gonorrhœa with tenesmus, strangury and frequent painful urination; discharge greenish or bloody pus. He gets relief from urination. Urine smells like violets.

MATERIA MEDICA OF THE URINARY TRACT AND SEXUAL SPHERE
ACONITE

Aconite is seldom indicated outside of psoric or pseudo-psoric states, yet I have used it a number of times in febrile conditions in young people in the beginning of the disease, where there was high fever, hot dry skin, dry mouth, much thirst, great restlessness and mental anxiety. Burning in the neck of the bladder when not urinating; urine scanty, dark, feeling hot as it passes. Painful anxious urging with passing of dark, scanty, hot urine; acute gonorrhœal orchitis; testicles hot, hard and swollen.

CASE 1. Mr. L., age 18, had gonorrhœa for four or five days ; discharge suppressed by medicated lotions. I found him suffering with a high temperature, skin dry, hot ; great restlessness with much tossing about the bed with active delirium ; much thirst ; frequent, painful urging to urinate, passing only a few drops of bloody urine, with much suffering. Temperature passed away during the night and the gonorrhœal discharge was re-established, and a case of acute cystitis avoided.

AGARICUS

This is another remedy which has cold shrunken organs in the male. It has many special reflexes due to sexual excesses. It acts also in the cure of old chronic gleet or gonorrhœa. The erections and the organs are painful, often violent chordee. In Dr. Kent's Materia Medica we find this symptom, constant itching and tingling along the urethra. It has the last drop of the discharge prolonged like Sepia. Like Nux vomica or Medorrhinum, it is often the remedy to follow much local treatment. The urinary flow is intermittent or dribbling after urinating. It is occasionally milky, with burning in the urethra after urinating and much itching in the hairy parts.

Case 1. John C., age 50, tall, spare of flesh, despondent, low spirited, fears death ; has had gonorrhœa for six months; discharge yellowish, mucous, with aching along the spermatic cord ; complete impotence ; penis relaxed, small ; organs generally cold and flaccid. He has seminal emissions twice a week ; fears he will die or that he is incurable. Cured by this remedy.

AMMONIUM MURIATICUM

Urinary organs. In this remedy we have almost the tenesmus of Nux, Mer. and Canth ; indeed it is not far behind Cantharis in its tenesmus, although it has not the strangury of that remedy, great urging while but a few drops pass. This tenesmus is confined principally to the neck of the bladder.

Urine. Copious, strong smelling, moldy, musty, ammoniacal.

Gonorrhœal or leucorrhœal discharge like the whites of eggs, or brownish or slimy ; worse after urination ; colicky or griping pains accompanies the discharge in the female.

ASPARAGUS OFFICINALIS

Urinary Organs. Nephritic colic ; urging to urinate ; urine has strong odor (Nit., ac. Benz, ac.) ; discharge frequent, scanty, with sensation as if something were sticking in the urethra, with slight burning. Frequent urinations with fine stinging in the meatus. Urine scanty, straw-colored, offensive, followed by cutting and burning in the urethra, < from 6 to 8 A.M., sensation as if something was still passing after urination ; red lithic deposits on side of vessel (Sep.) or a greasy deposit.

Male Organs. Sexual excitement, with stitches on side of penis, with urging to urinate, swelling and erection.

ALUMINA

This is a remedy for chronic gleet in men who are debilitated both with old age and with the disease. While it is not very frequently indicated, it does good work when the symptoms call for it.

Urine. The urine is passed frequently and in small quantities, often bloody or mixed with clay-like deposit. Alumina may be thought of as a remedy in the tertiary stage of the disease, especially when Bright's disease or diabetes has developed from suppression and the symptoms point to this remedy. The urine is very slow to start in this remedy, urinates > in a standing position. The vaso-motor paralysis is seen all throughout the action of its proving.

Male Sexual Organs. Gonorrhœal discharge yellowish, painless, and bland. The gleety discharges are yellow, never becoming white as in other remedies. Other symptoms might be mentioned as prostatic irritation, and enlargement ; sensation of fullness in the perineum ; paralytic weakness or paresis of the sexual sphere in general ; voice weak, low, feeble ; skin dry ; no perspiration.

ARUNDO MAURITANICA

Urinary Organs. Nephritic pains. Pricking in bladder.

Urine red with sand like sediment Phos. Lyc, Kali phos. Sep.) Red sand (compare with Lyc.).

After urination, weight, burning, itching, in uretha.

Male Sexual Organs. Sexual desire ; increased lascivious ideas ; frequent erections.

Coition ; pain in spermatic cord after.

ANTIMONIUM CRUDUM

Urinary Organs. Cutting pain in the urethra while urinating, and backache during the emission of the urine, are quite positive symptoms of this remedy. The majority of the symptoms center, as we know, about the stomach and digestive tract. It is a much prized remedy when we come to sycotic gastric disturbances and marked gouty states of the system. It is also to be used in the sycotic snuffles of infants, that are aggravated when the room becomes warm, like Puls. The gonorrhœal discharge is copious, thick mucus resembling Nux vom.

AMMONIUM CARB

The ammoniums are seldom indicated in sycotic troubles. Occasionally we find symptoms calling for this form of the drug in women who have a weak heart, with a marked tendency to faint. This is more marked in elderly women or in old maids. They have usually a tubercular diathesis with a hemorrhagic tendency. The blood will not coagulate and is very dark. The heart symptoms are aggravated in a warm room or by overexertion. It may be considered before Lachesis in hysterical affections.

Urine. Pressure in bladder especially at night. The urine excoriates the parts it comes in contact with, producing biting and itching.

Male Organs. Pain in testicles and seminal cords, violent sexual desire without erection ; < in the morning.

Gonorrhœal discharges in women, thin, acrid, scanty or profuse, producing itching, swelling and burning of the pudenda or perineum. This remedy like Puls. is ameliorated by lying on the stomach and its aggravations are similar to Rhus. tox., namely, wet weather, washing, and during menses. Sometimes the discharge has an ammonical odor.

ARGENTUM METALLICUM

Like all minerals this is a deep acting remedy. It is found very useful in both sycotic and psoric diseases. It is said to act more especially upon the nerves and cartilages, but we may safely say it affects every cell and fiber of the organism. The patient grows more emaciated as he grows more nervous. Argentum patients look careworn, tired, pale, and sickly.

Urinary Organs. Urine pale, fetid, often of a sweetish odor ; often very profuse in nervous patients ; nervous conditions relieved by passing large quantities of urine. The nervousness passes off in that way. (Ignatia has this symptom also.)

Sexual Organs ; chronic Orchitis with much infiltration and hardness of the testicle, after gonorrhœa. The pain is spoken of as if the parts were being crushed. Urine diabetic.

The gonorrhœal discharge is yellowish-green and thick even in old chronic cases. This is an unusual symptom as the discharge usually grows thinner as the disease grows chronic and painless. In women it is apt to be purulent, ichorous, bloody, accompanied with more or less pain in the left ovary and a bearing down sensation in the inner parts. It differs largely from Argentum nitrate in its nervous symptoms.

The cachexia of Sycosis is often very marked in this remedy. The face is pale or bluish, cheeks sunken, sallow, dirty looking, and prematurely old.

Urinary Organs. An ulcerative or splinter-like pain along the center of the urethra is peculiar to this remedy ; urine burns when passing ; passage feels swollen with a sensation as if a drop remained behind. (Thuja, Kali, iod. Medorrhinum). Urine dark or dark yellow in color. Quick urging to pass urine ; passes frequently and a little at a time ; orifice quite sensitive ; orifice swollen, puffy, in which it resembles Medorrhinum. In fact it resembles Medorrhinum in many ways in its action upon the urinary organs.

Male Organs. Chordee with bloody urine ; contusive pain in the testicles with enlargement and hardness. Discharge in gonorrhœa, copious, yellowish, green mucus. In fact all the discharges of this remedy, the diarrhœas, leucorrhœas, gonorrhœas, and catarrhal difficulties have that same copious, dirty-greenish, or yellowish green mucus. Its ophthalmia is a type of this remedy. The diseased mucous surface is always red, puffy, swollen and covered with this peculiar discharge. The discharges have a musty, old hay or stale fish odor. The gonorrhœal discharges of Medorrhinum are more scant, but they are of a similar odor and consistency. Often we find strings of mucus in its discharges. It excoriates and produces erythema as it passes over healthy skin or mucous membrane. The fact that this remedy in the crude state is a powerful suppressive agent in the hands of the old school proves to us how efficient it becomes as a curative agent in gonorrhœa.

ANTHROKOKALI

Urinary Organs. Copious evacuations of pale, colorless urine, with no sediment, of alkaline reaction. Itching, slight burning and tickling at the orifice when urinating.

Male Organs. Long lasting, painful erections; skin eruptions, and many symptoms increased by sweating. Diarrhœa, with increased secretions of urine, an unusual symptom. A more complete proving of this remedy should be made.

BARYTA CARB

Urinary Organs. Irritation of the bladder, increases at night; constant irritation cannot retain the urine (old people.) Urine clear, abundant; before urination, great desire; during, burning in the urethra; after, renewed straining with dribbling.

Male Organs. Impotence, diminished sexual desire, penis relaxed, erections only in the morning. Prostate gland hypertrophied. Gleet or gonorrhœal discharge, purulent with pain in the fossa navicularis on pressure; sweat about the scrotum with soreness.

Female Organs. During menses pinching colic with cutting in the abdomen; feeling of weight over the pubic region; bruised pain in the small of the back; lameness, weight and heaviness in the small of the back. Flow of a bloody, mucous nature. Leucorrhœa, bloody, mucus-like, with tearing in the pudendum, attended with anxiety and palpitation of the heart, found in obese elderly women, or weak, dwarfish, undeveloped young girls.

BENZOIC ACID

Benzoic acid has many symptoms of Sycosis in the hereditary and tertiary stages of the disease. Like Lycopodium, Lithia carb., Nitric acid and other sycotic remedies, it meets especially well the urinary symptoms and the uric acid diathesis. It has the true gouty and the lithic constitution, which as we all know is one of the persistent sycotic states so difficult to cure. We have frequent recourse to this remedy to relieve the acute lithic expressions of chronic Sycosis. When these gouty waves reach their maximum, the offending debris is eliminated or thrown off through the urine, and are made manifest in the urinary secretions.

Its symptoms are spasmodic and changeable. Just as these gouty states are influenced by the course of living, diet and weather changes.

Urinary Organs. Urine suddenly changes from a clear to a dark beer color. When the urine is scanty, the patient suffers with gouty secretions in the joints, or gouty states of the heart, liver, stomach and intestinal tract. As soon as the urine becomes profuse, the suffering is relieved. Urine strong-smelling, like horse's urine; urine scanty, dark, full of a brick-like or red pepper deposit and very offensive smelling. Dr. Kent very wisely says we are not to check the excessive output of the kidneys, for it would be as harmful to the patient as suppressing any other discharge. When the urine is full of these lithic deposits the patient feels well and vice versa. The urine is often of such a strange pungent odor, that it meets your nostrils as soon as you enter the patient's room. We find this often in children or even infants whose parents have acquired Sycosis. (Nitric acid., Ammon., mur.) The body and clothing of these children has a urinous odor.

Discharge muco-purulent; urine dark, often of a deep red color.

Sexual Organs. Sexual desire depressed both in men and women, often completely gone in women; great prostration after coition; cutting pains after sexual intercourse; great excitability and weakness in the morning after coition. Burning in the urethra after coition, or burning pain in the spermatic cord extending to testicles in the male.

Gonorrhœa. Penis hard, contracted around upper surface. Burning in the glans of the penis in kidney troubles; cold sensation in the prepuce and glans of the penis. Great weakness in the parts is noticed after urination. Constant urging to urinate with pain in neck of bladder, or pains extending to hips and thighs.

BERBERIS

Urinary Organs. This remedy may be studied and carefully compared with Benzoic acid and Lithium carb. in its action upon the urinary tract. It has its gouty and lithic phenomena like these remedies. Dr. Kent says "it is indicated in anæmic, feeble constitutions, especially in elderly people who are pale, sickly and constantly chilly." Urine is either very scanty or profuse, clear in color or full of lithic deposits. It has red sandy deposits like Lyc., Sep., and Phos. This is more apt to come from the left kidney. The pains are sharp, sticking, the majority of which radiate about the region of the kidneys or from the kidneys.

Bladder. Crampy contraction, or aching pain in the

bladder, whether full or empty. Cutting pains, deeply seated ; violent, sticking pains in bladder, with desire to urinate ; great urging, with pain in the neck of the bladder, burning with scanty urination. These cutting pains are invariably $<$ in the left side of the bladder or pelvis. Chronic sycotic catarrhal troubles of the bladder of long standing, (similar to Thuja or Sarsa.), with pains shooting about the loins, or pelvis. Pains in the hips and thighs before urinating ; $>$ by urinating. These pains awaken the patient about every two hours during the night, relieved by urinating ; went to sleep as soon as she urinated and pains ceased. Cutting and burning in the urethra, $<$ when urinating ; violent burning and shooting pain in the orifice of the urethra. Urine often blood red; urine filled with a copious, grayish-white or reddish sediment, yellowish-red crystals, small calculi. Sometimes urine flows very slowly, with much pain and pressure in the bladder; violent urging, $<$ in the morning, accompanied with pain in the loins and hips. In gouty conditions there are pains in the spermatic cords and testicles. These pains may be stitching or burning, and are $<$ in the left cord with sexual weakness. Pain in spermatic cord extending into the abdominal ring or into the testicles. Drawing from the left testicle to the spermatic cord. Sexual organs cold ; shrunken with shooting or burning pains in spermatic cord.

CANNABIS SATIVA

Urinary Organs. Very painful swellings of the penis

with painful erections ; shooting or cutting pains on urinating ; sexual desire greatly increased during an attack of gonorrhœa. Its action is quite similar to Cann. ind., Canth., and Petros. Burning, smarting in the urethra ; it feels sore and inflamed the whole length of the canal; during erection, a tensive drawing pain as if urethra were drawn up in knots. Pains extending from orifice of urethra back to the neck of the bladder ; painful spasmodic closing of the sphincter, with urging to stool when urinating. (Nux. vom.) Pain $<$ at the close of urination. (Sarsa.)

Male Sexual Organs. Priapism with copious, mucous discharge in acute gonorrhœa. Urination accompained with shooting pains (Cann. ind.); penis swollen ; prepuce dark red ; red, lentil-sized spots on the glans of the penis ; indicated in the acute inflammatory stage of gonorrhœa, where the inflammation is deep seated. Gonorrhœa acute, with stitching pains on urinating ; frequent prolonged erections with shooting, stitching pains ; much swelling of the prepuce ; when walking, penis feels very sore ; walks with legs wide apart.

CAPSICUM

The aromatics and the peppers are all good anti-sycotic remedies. They all, as a rule aggravate the disease in any stage when employed as seasoning in food. The allopathic school is very exacting in prohibiting their use, to all patients afflicted with this disease ; often as much so as they are in prohibiting the use of stimulants, for the same reason that they aggravate the discharge and prevent or hinder to a very great degree the suppression of the disease. Strange to note, however, these same remedies are given in powerful doses internally to assist the local measures in their so-called cures of gonorrhœa. Cubebs, Copaiba, oil of cedron, and other anti-sycotics are commonly used and they are all profound irritants of the urinary tract. Even the use of tea, coffee, pepper, tobacco, are also taken away from these patients, as soon as it is discovered that they are victims of the disease.

For the reasons above mentioned Capsicum proves a valuable remedy in this complaint. Mental symptoms—Tormented with thoughts of suicide ; does not want to take his own life, but the thoughts are *persistent and never leave him*. If he does commit suicide it is because of these strong impulses. Sycosis produces suicidal symptoms more than any other miasm. Capsicum is adapted to rosy, red-faced, clear skined, blond individuals who are fond of beer or stimulating food, and aromatics. They are as a rule quite plethoric, easily tired and have slow and sluggish reaction.

Urinary Organs—Burning in the bladder is given in Herings' Guiding Symptoms as a marked symptom, but I have not verified this symptom. Burning at the meatus or at the orifice is a strong symptom of the remedy in gonorrhoea ; a burning as of fire. It is a burning, peppery, urine hot as it passes the orifice and the burning continues for some time after urination. Burning, biting, cutting, smarting, scalding with tenesmus and chordee after urinating. Urine reddish or even bloody.

Male Organs. Gonorrhœa with painful erections, and a thick cream-like discharge with a slight, greenish tinge to it (Nat. sulp). Chordee relieved by cold bathing. Bland, thick, cream-like gonorrhœal discharge with no pain (second stage); meatus swollen, puffy and red like Medorrh.; coldness of the scrotum; prostatic pains; sensation as of pepper sprinkled on the parts, worse on the skin of the affected parts.

Compare the gonorrhœal discharge with Puls., Nat. sul. Aggravated by touch, ameliorated by bathing in cool water. It is frequently indicated in the tertiary stage or in the characteristic gouty states of this remedy. It is followed often by Sul., Sil., and Nat mur.

Case 1. Mr. Charles L., age 21, light complexion, blue eyes; face flushes easily; the tubercular element is well marked in every feature of his face; indeed his whole make up, even to his fingers show the tubercular diathesis. He has had gonorrhœa for three weeks. The urine feels hot on passing and is accompanied with a cutting, smarting and burning pain. The orifice is red, puffy and swollen. The discharge is thick and cream-like and resembles the tubercular pus. Capsicum 1m given, a few powders and in ten days followed by the c. m. potency. Cured in four weeks.

Case 2. John S., age 26, light complexion, blue eyes, inclined to be fleshy and has no desire to work. Is constantly condemning himself for having caught the disease; has been taking gels., but the discharge has suddenly become thick and pus like. Capsicum in a few doses 1m in ten days has decreased it to a thin, scanty and watery discharge. Case retaken when Silica was given which cured the gleety discharge.

CHAMOMILLA

This too is a true antisycotic remedy. Its action in hereditary Sycosis or in the sycotic child is known to every physician; although we may not have known that the majority of these little sufferers were sycotic, and were born of sycotic parents, who themselves had acquired gonorrhœal Sycosis. We see this in their mental irritability, in their oversensitiveness as to being looked at or spoken to, in their inability to endure pain, in their colicky pains and in the green slimy stools (as we see also in Rheum); we see it in their relief from motion, from being carried or rocked, which are common ameliorations in sycotic diseases.

Urinary Organs. The pains of this remedy are of a sticking character about the neck of the bladder, often worse when not urinating; urine passes without force; urine hot, yellowish with a flaky sediment, turbid or claycolored soon after passing.

Male Sexual Organs. Violent erections and excited sexual desire in gonorrhœa. Swelling, soreness and much redness of the prepuce.

GAMBOGIA

Urinary Organs. Urine passes intermittently. The scanty flow ceases entirely, but finally returns with burning at the meatus. Urine smells like onions.

Male Sexual Organs. Gleety discharges, agglutinating the orifice in chronic gonorrhœa (Graph.).

General biting as from ants on the sexual organs. Aphthæ about the labia during the menses, with agglutination of the parts in the morning. It is also indicated frequently in the dark, green, sycotic stools of infants and young children, or in Sycosis of the gastro-intestinal tract (Borax. Cham., Arg., nit ; Rheum Crocus sat., Mag. carb.).

CARBO-VEGETABILIS

The whole mental and physical state of this remedy is slow and sluggish. Capillaries and veins are full ; circulation is sluggish ; veins are congested all over body ; hands and face are puffed ; the part feels full and enlarged ; the skin is dusky ; and the parts remote from the center of circulation cold. It is often indicated in old people with devitalized bodies ; when every disease affecting the patient is deep acting and profound, threatening often the life.

Urinary Organs. Soreness at neck of bladder ; urging to urinate frequent ; anxious day and night ; pain on urinating cutting and sharp. Urine is offensive, turbid, scanty, sometimes bloody mucus only ; dribbling of urine in old men ; urine stale, dirty brown or yellowish.

Gonorrhœa in old men, with broken down chronic conditions, brought on by sexual excesses ; old chronic catarrhal conditions of the bladder in old men or in old people, with coldness of the extremities and general debility. Organs relaxed, and hang down ; bathed with cold perspiration, and with dribbling of the urine.

CANNABIS INDICA

Urinary Organs. Frequent urination with a burning pain ; acute gonorrhœa, < in the evening ; urine flows slowly, has to force out the last few drops ; dribbling of the urine after urination ; great urging to urinate, with much straining, but cannot pass a drop (Canth., Nux., Mer. cor. Con., Bell.). There is also scalding and burning in the urethra before and after urination.

Male Sexual Organs. Erections violent, painful; worse when walking or sitting, better when lying down. Sexual desire excessively increased even to satyriasis ; sharp pricking pains in urethra, with burning on urinating ; acute inflammatory gonorrhœa, with a copious, yellowish-white discharge ; mucous discharge often glossy.

CINNABARIS

The red sulphuret of mercury is no exception to other forms of mercury in its strong, anti-syphilitic action. It, however, spends its force more especially on what might be called mixed Syphilis, or on a syco-psoric-syphilitic individual, if I may be privileged to express it in that way. It affects every tissue in the body, and includes every lesion from a papule to a wart, and from an ulcer to that of an exostosis. It partakes of sulphur which gives us its psoric phase, and of the mixed Syphilis or Sycosis and Syphilis in its tertiary stage or when the disease follow soon after birth ; it meets morbid growths especially condylomata about the orifices of the body, which make their appearance in the form of a coxcomb, cauliflower excrescence, papillary or blackberry-like growths. These growths appear after birth or after badly treated cases of mixed venereal diseases. Like Nux, Medorrhinum or Psorinum it will often restore a suppressed gonorrhœal discharge. It has great soreness and tenderness along the urethra which disappears on the re-appearance of the gonorrhœal discharge. Warts and condylomata appear when the discharge is suppressed or when Syphilis is suppressed with over does of mercury.

Its discharges are copious, thick, dirty, greenish, or yellowish pus ; bleeding easily from diseased surfaces is a very common symptom. (Nit. ac.). The discharges are generally offensive like decayed meat, or of a stale or dead fish odor. Bone pains and periosteal neuralgia with exostosis are always to be looked for. Many of its symptoms are worse from heat and always $<$ at night, and from lying on the back and during the summer time. Better in a medium temperature.

CHIMAPHILA

Acute prostatitis following gonorrhœal suppression with dysuria and retention. Sensation in perineum as if sitting on a ball; urine fetid, copious, thick; sensation as if there were a swelling in the perineum.

CAUSTICUM

The action of this remedy upon the bladder and urinary organs is very interesting. We find paralysis of the sphincter vesicae and also of the expulsive power of that organ. The sphincters relax and the urine cannot be retained or when it is retained it cannot be expelled. The urine passes without his notice, and he is unconscious of it. He has to examine his garments to see if they are moist or not from the passing urine. This symptom is found in both sexes and often in children. They wet the bed without being conscious of it. In women, the urine escapes involuntarily from coughing, laughing, sneezing. Paresis from long retention of the urine or after child birth is also a symptom to be remembered. It vies with Opium in that respect. Rhus often follows this remedy after straining of the bladder. Painful retention of urine from taking cold; prostatic troubles cause many chronic bladder troubles in this remedy, due to pressure, dribbling of the urine, spasm of the neck of the bladder. The spasm often extends to the neck or to rectum, urging to urinate when suffering with enlarged prostate;

urging to urinate without being able to pass a drop. Has to wait a long time before he urinates, (Puls.). We have the two extremes in this, urging to urinate with a spasm of the bladder and involuntary urination, unconscious of it. The paralytic symptom usually show itself in some degree in both, sooner or later (Sarsa).

Urine. Dark brown, turbid on standing, deposits a yeasty sediment or oxalate of lime.

Male Sexual Organs. Bloody semen; burning in urethra after coition; erections feeble. Gonorrhœal discharge not marked, must depend on general symptoms, especially of the bladder. Leucorrhœa profuse; flows like the menses; color is dark and excoriates the vulva. Sometimes it is ropy but clear. Complexion very sallow, and sickly looking. Leucorrhœa often < at night; weariness in the thighs; pulling pains and lameness in small of back; has an aversion to sweets and fresh meats; appetite vanishes as soon as they begin to eat. Aphonia, weekness of the voice.

DULCAMARA

We have in Dulcamara, a remedy closely related to all the stages of sycotic disease from the first symptom of it, until it has demonstrated upon the organism, every expression of its progressive proving. It is more especially adapted to the second and third stages, or the chronic diseases of mucous membranes and its rheumatic element; often no more perfect picture of a sycotically diseased mucous membrane can be found than under this remedy. No other remedy except perhaps Rhus tox, is more sensitive to climatic or barometric changes than the bittersweet. It has the sycotic stools and catarrhal condition of the bowels so marked in children in their autumnal dysenteries, induced by chilling of the solar plexus when the nights are cold, following hot days during the summer or fall months. In this it is like Ars., Aloes, Croton tig., Cham., and others. It touches more specifically the rheumatic affections that appear in the third stages of Sycosis and that are brought on by getting wet, or due to suppressed perspiration, induced by changing from a high to a low temperature, or from cold to hot weather. It is the great autumnal remedy for sycotic patients.

Mental Symptoms. Forgets words or cannot find the right word (Med.), cannot concentrate his thoughts, therefore there is much confusion in his mind. He is restless, impatient, easily angered, quarrelsome, and anxious about his future. All these symptoms are greatly aggravated by lowering barometer or change of weather. Psorinum is always cold, Mercury is better by cold, and Medorrhinum worse in cold or wet weather; dampness and falling barometer greatly aggravate all sycotic patients.

Urinary Organs. Kidney difficulties induced by Sycosis, exposure to cold and dampness; Bright's disease also from these causes, especially in the acute stages of the disease, or Bright's disease following scarlet or malarial fevers; swelling of the lower extremities with a waxy appearance of the skin like Apis.

Urination. Constant desire to urinate felt deep in abdomen. This constant urging often comes from getting wet or taking cold or when the body becomes chilled. Better on becoming warm.

Gonorrhœa. Burning in the meatus while urinating. Painful pressure in bladder; urine scanty, offensive, turbid, with much mucus. Catarrh of bladder from taking cold; all the bladder symptoms are worse in cold, damp weather; when body becomes chilled, has urging and frequent desire to urinate.

Male Sexual Organs. Gonorrhœal discharges, mucopus, yellowish-white, copious, offensive, catarrhal. Sometimes during the acute stage the discharge is bloody. Herpes preputialis painful, red or pale red, round, small and scaly. Urticaria often accompanies the disease in which Dulcamara is indicated. It appears in large red or white wheals which burn and itch; they are worse from chilling the body or from a cold in any form. Often these patients have rheumatism alternating with diarrhœas or sore and inflamed eyes. All the constitutional symptoms are worse in cold or damp weather. Colds, coryza, sore and inflamed eyelids, rheumatism, and diarrhœas follow taking cold or dampness.

Aggravations. Evening, wet, cold and damp weather.

Ameliorations. Warmth, dry air, dry weather and motion.

Concomitants. Much restlessness and very impatient, easily angered and desires to scold during menses. Cannot find the right word in talking. Sleep uneasy and full of dreams. The urine, during menses is often fetid and turbid with constant desire to urinate.

Rheumatism. The proving of this great anti-sycotic remedy has shown forth the rheumatic element very clearly. It is full of pains and aches. The joints become suddenly inflamed red, sore, swollen and sensitive to touch. They come on from suppression of the perspiration or from working in water, getting wet and the pains are bettered by changing positions like Rhus tox.

EUPHRASIA

This is a very valuable remedy in the hay-fever expressions of Sycosis. It also palliates or relieves greatly, those tubercular expressions of hay-fever that come on about August the 10th or from the 10th to the 20th. These syco-tubercular expressions of hay-fever have a marked periodicity about them. I have frequently noticed that they would return annually on the very same day. On closely examining the tubercular make-up of the patient, you will readily see that there is blended in, a sycotic element. Now if you will closely question these patients, you will find that in their youth they had some experience with gonorrhœa, that was treated in the old orthodox way. If the patient is a child, you will find other marks of heredity. I now recall the case of a young school girl that I treated during the hay-fever period for three years, when she no longer had any symptoms. Of course, she had still many symptoms of Sycosis, but the hay-fever outbursts were manifest for two years with symptoms of this remedy, but the third year she received Pulsatilla, which finished the cure. One dose of Euphrasia would usually relieve her when given in the c. m. potency.

The symptoms of Euphrasia are more particularly those of the head, eye, and nose, although it has in some cases marked laryngeal symptoms, and meets those cases described in the beginning of this work, where it was claimed that the colds of Sycosis began in the nose with a fluent mucous discharge, lasting a few days and followed by a laryngeal cough and sometimes asthmatic symptoms. Euphrasia follows this law, often to the letter. First, headaches, blurring of the vision, stitching pains in the head, photophobia, then a profuse watery discharge from the nose and eyes, with sneezing, smarting and burning. The discharge is watery and acrid, causing burning of the septum of the nose, with a sensation as of dust or sand in the eyes, much itching with desire to rub them.

All the mucous surfaces about the throat, nose and eyes are involved; we have a copious lacrymation and coryza. Sometimes the discharge from the nose is bland, however, in the majority of cases the disease extends to the larynx and is followed with a severe cough and sometimes accompanied with asthma. The symptoms of this remedy are clear cut, fluent coryza, chilliness and fever, often alternating with photophobia, burning, but tears sneezing, headaches; sometimes a rash similar to measles will break out during an attack. The patients always complain of strange odors, as of pus or sweet odors, or odors which they cannot describe.

Aggravations. Morning, open air, cool air, the least draft, or moving about.

Amelioration. Warmth, being in the house, lying down, or keeping still.

FLUORIC ACID

Urinary Organs. Urine scanty, pungent, fetid, often alkaline. Burning before and after urinating, with aching in the bladder. Urging, frequent and ineffectual; pain on the vertex after ineffectual efforts to urinate.

Male Sexual Organs. Satyriasis, strong sexual desire at night; violent desire to cohabit. Gonorrhœa in old men with increased sexual desire, or sudden loss of sexual power. Penis curved, greatly swollen, with fullness and pain in the spermatic cords. Chronic gonorrhœa, when only a single yellow drop appears in the morning (like Sepia).

Female Sexual Organs. Indicated in old women in deep seated chronic cases. Mind buoyant, self satisfied, fears nothing. Menses too soon, copious, thick, coagulated. Leucorrhœa yellowish, corrosive.

General. Syphilis and Sycosis combined, chronic cases when Silica fails (Pruritis ani. Sycosis of the nose) ; passage always obstructed. Posterior nose feels expanded. Chronic, fluent, watery coryza. Chronic sycotic rhinitis. Mental symptoms; aversion to one's own family, forgetful, loss of memory, feeling as if something dreadful would happen, dullness in the forehead.

GELSEMIUM

This remedy may be considered the Aconite of gonorrhœa. It is often called for in the acute or early stage of the disease, especially where there is much pain or inflammation accompanied by fever. The fever comes on slowly and is accompanied with a slow, soft pulse, general malaise, muscular prostration, chilliness, no thirst, muscular soreness, general aching and drowsiness; pain at base of brain, and throughout the body. The aching and pains may be absent in gonorrhœa, but the febrile state of this remedy is often met with. It frequently aborts a case, if given early enough. It loses its effects in a few days, however, and has to be followed by some other remedy.

Urinary Organs. Pain, heat, redness and burning at the meatus; frequent urging with scanty omission of urine, and with more or less tenderness of the bladder. Other symptoms are trembling of the hands, despondency, muscular prostration, with a dragging sensation in the testicles. Gonorrhœal discharge whitish, mucous, scanty in the febrile stage; copious after fever subsides. Urination often relieves the headache. Similar to Nux. vom. in its mucous discharge.

Case 1. Arthur B., age 20, light complexion, was

taken suddenly ill, without any apparent cause; temperature 103; face flushed slightly; generally prostrated with some aching in the extremities, and a dull headache at the base of the brain; he is irritable when spoken to, drowsy, wants to sleep; much burning at the meatus when urinating, which comes on about every hour. Acute symptoms were all relieved by this remedy. I learned within a day or so that he had taken a medicated injection which caused the discharge to cease. There was a copious mucous flow a few hours after taking the remedy.

Case 2. Wm. L., age 32, dark complexion, has been taking oil of sandal for nearly a week; symptoms, fever, general aching, headache, drowsiness, stupid, wishes to be left alone; urinates every few minutes when on his feet; better lying down; much prostrated and is chilly; pulse soft and slow as compared with the temperature which is 102. Discharge is scanty, like starch-water which was greatly increased after ceasing the use of the sandal oil. Case was cured in one week with no change of remedy.

KALI NITRICUM

Urinary Organs. Stitches in the region of the prostate gland while urinating; frequent urging with at first only a few drops, then the stream becomes natural (T. F. Allen). Gonorrhœa with stitches in the orifice of the urethra when urinating; burning, biting or a tickling sensation in the orifice when urinating. When the urine begins to pass it causes a shiver to pass over the patient as if he were chilly; burning at the close of urination; swelling of the testicles and especially the epididymus after suppression; testicles drawn up and sensitive; discharge, white mucus.

LACHESIS

In these days of strenuous living and of stress and strain, we frequently need such a remedy as Lachesis. We need any of such remedies to restore harmony to the abused and overworked nerve centers of our patients. How many of its symptoms correspond to the symptoms of Sycosis as do those of Rhus. tox., Gels., Lac., can. and Thuja. Remember in Lachesis we have the quick, comprehensive, supersensitive patient, or we may have great dullness of intellect with bodily weakness to correspond with the low state of mind. They are often sad, melancholic, whimsical, suspicious, distrustful and above all jealous. The face looks anxious, distressed and uneasy. The discharges are all dark foul-smelling, thin and watery. The lesions are malignant or semi-malignant, supersentive or hyperesthetic and are aggravated by heat, touch, warm bathing and after sleep. Selfconsciousness stands out boldly at all times, and no pressure or weight can be endured on any of the nerve centres of the body. This is peculiar to Lachesis in all its provings and clinical work. In insanity they think they have superhuman power or control and are oversensitive to impressions or touch, all the faculties being oversensitive and intense. Yet strange as it may seem, hard, firm pressure will often relieve. The face in this disease is of a purple color or mottled in severe cases, with hemorrhages of dark, thin watery blood. Again the face may be puffed, livid, besotted, sallow and œdematous.

Urinary Organs. There are stitching pains in the kidneys extending downward through the ureters. In cystitis there is a feeling as of a ball in the bladder or in the abdomen when turning over. There is ineffectual urging with much burning when the urine passes. Again, the urine may be scanty, and very dark, and cause violent burning. The urine is strong, dark brown, offensive in fevers, or it is black and foamy, and it may be as if mixed with coffee grounds, as in scarlatina. Then, again, it may be black and albuminous in that disease.

Male Sexual Organs. Great sexual excitement and sexual desire is manifested in this disease. A jealous mania or epilepsy often follows sexual excesses in this remedy. There is excessive sexual desire with continuous erections at night or after first sleep; the semen has a pungent smell. On the sexual organs you will often find sycotic eruptions or ulcers of a dark, bluish color. The scrotum is greatly swollen, of a dark color; there is threatened gangrene of the sexual organs; chancres or chancroid ulcers, dark in color and phagedenic in character; buboes of a dark color, very sensitive to touch, and with fistulous openings.

LAC DEFLORATUM

We are only beginning to understand the use of the

milk remedies, and we are greatly indebted to Dr. Swan and Dr. Laura Morgan for what we know of this remedy. It shows clearly, that we ought not to stop in selecting from nature's storehouse, remedial agents for the cure of the sick. Strange and peculiar are the symptoms that develop from the animal fluids and excretions, deep and profound are their action; they go down into the innermost chambers of life, in their work upon the vital force.

Mind Symptoms. Depression of spirits; listlessness, with disinclination to either bodily or mental labour, seems to be quite a constant symptom. Headache with great depressions of spirits. It cures (like Natrum) a headache found in very anæmic, tubercular patients especially in women who are run down in health and very anæmic. Their residual supply of nerve energy is very low, therefore they faint easily or have fainting spells. The headache of these patients is often worse lying down; when they get out of bed and get on their feet, it induces fainting or a faint feeling, as in China and Ammon. carb. The pain is usually in the forehead just above the eyes; occasionally it reaches to the occiput. The pain is often unbearable, intense, and lasts for days. Nat. mur. and Tuberculinum have a similar headache. When the pain gets very severe, nausea and vomiting is often induced, they have a great dread of light, noise and motion. It is relieved by copious urination. The inner edge of the right eyebrow is favorite spot for the headache of this remedy to begin. It is called the "American" sick headache

Chronic constipation with these sick headaches is not infrequent; stools are dry, large and hard, causing the patient to strain much, and often the stool lacerates the anus.

Urinary Organs. In women the urine is pale, copious, and retained with difficulty. There is pain in the region of the kidneys, that passes around towards the bladder like berberis, or the pain goes from the kidneys down the back to the thighs. Sometimes the urine passes in a great gush and like hot water.

LAC CANINUM

Dr. J. T. Kent says that milk remedies are animal products and foods of animal life, and therefore correspond to our innermost physical nature. True it is often necessary to select from some of these milk products, in order to find a remedy that will reach down deep enough into the life and remove the potent, disturbing element. Lac. caninum is one of these remedies for consideration and study. It has many mental and nervous symptoms peculiar to Sycosis. In the crude state it was used three thousand years ago for the expulsion of the dead foetus and as an antidote for poisons. Its symptoms are as follows: The mind is very forgetful, in writing, uses too many words, and not the right ones, forgets words and sentences (Medorrhinum). Its mental symptoms remain long with the patient and are very distressing.

A few of the more marked sycotic diseases might be mentioned, that are curable by this strange remedy. Hysteria, acute or subacute mania from suppressed gonorrhœa, or mental conditions following operations in sycotic diseases in women, such as removal of the ovaries, uterus and tubes. The mania is similar to Lachesis, so are the dreams and hallucinations; the dreams are of horible diseased states of the body; foul ulcers, as if her body was so diseased she could not touch it. They are constantly washing or scrubbing the body to get it clean. Is this not true of Sycosis more than any other miasm? Psora is afraid of water and it usually aggravates all its symptoms. Like Lachesis, Lac caninum is worse after sleep; as soon as the eyes close she sees snakes, dark or black water, and horrible sights that make a lasting impression on her mind. One case that I now recall would not shake hands with her friends or touch anything for fear of polluting herself. There is no desire to live; in this we have another suicidal remedy. Her mania is often of a violent nature like Bell., Stram., Verat alb. The diphtheritic symptoms show the malignancy of the sycotic element present. All the discharges are putrid and offensive; it has ulcers, sore throat, pustules, and eruptive diseases of all kinds.

Urinary Organs. Constant desire to urinate with intense pain; urine scanty, dark, high colored, excoriating external genitals; urine often coffee colored, loaded with mucus or albumen. Urine suppressed with no desire to urinate whatever (Opium).

Male Sexual Organs. Syphilitic ulceration of penis; fungoid chancre on glans penis; chancre shiny; odor from ulcer fearfully offensive, malignant looking; buboes, with much pain.

Gonorrhœa with intermittant pains in the middle or posterior part of urethra. Mixed venereal diseases; chancre with gonorrhœa, or chancroid and gonorrhœa, malignant types of venereal diseases; diphtheritic-looking chancres or chancroid ulcers, with much pain, great sensitiveness and nervousness. Ulcers round usually, greyish white or shiny, glistening in appearance.

Aggravation—touch, motion, standing, being alone.

Amelioration—menses, during flow.

A single dose should be given, not under the thirtieth potency; if it is necessary to repeat give at the same time of the day. Suitable to tall, slim, dark-haired people of a marked nervous temperament.

MANGANUM

We have but few symptoms so far in the proving of this remedy that bear upon the urinary tract or the sexual sphere, but it is such a profound tissue remedy and has such power to break down the blood corpuscle, that it will probably prove itself to be a wonderful curative agent in all sycotic patients, especially for those that have a marked pseudo-psoric basis. It acts upon every tissue of the body. It produces nearly all the skin lesions and breaks down such tissues as bones and lung tissue. It may be classified with Sil., Tub., Cal. C, Cal. phos. and Hepar.

These pseudo-psoric patients are the ones who have least resistance to venereal diseases, and when they do become affected, they experience the worst forms and are the most difficult cases to cure.

Mental Symptoms. Great fear with anxiety. Very apprehensive and anxious about their condition; fears something awful is going to happen. Let this patient become affected with Sycosis with all its train of mental phenomena, and we can readily see what a disturbed mental state would result. Women with this profound tubercular taint when affected with Sycosis, especially in the second stage, are inconsolable. They are sad, despondent, weep easily and find no peace of mind. Dr. Kent says this remedy in its mental symptoms is similar to Argentum nit., Phos., Graph., Sulph., and we may add Tuberculinum.

Urinary Organs. Frequent urging to urinate, with cutting all along the urethral canal. Darting pain in uterus when passing flatus. Urinary sediment earthy, or violet colored.

Male Sexual Organs. Urging to urinate with pain in cord. General sensation of weakness in the organs with pain in the spermatic cord. Discharge copious, greenish-yellow, offensive and tubercular like.

NUX VOMICA

Urinary Organs. Frequent, scanty urination with urging, yet he cannot empty the bladder. Urging to stool and to urinate at the same time; full feeling in the region of the bladder with urging. Suppressed gonorrhœa with cystitis from suppressed discharges. Discharge suppressed with strong drugs, such as Copaiba, Cubebs and any of the vegetable or mineral poisons. Gonorrhœa aggravated by over-eating, from rich food, wines, beer or liquors of any kind, sexual excesses or excesses of any kind. Straining and painful urging; urine passes in drops (Canth.). Strong, acid urine after debauches, increasing at night or upon lying down. Burning and tearing in the neck while urinating, or burning about the meatus; constipation with urging to stool (Mer. cor.).

Male Sexual Organs. Painful erections increasing in morning. Very excitable but power weak. Gonorrhœa, with burning and urging to urinate, with desire to stool. Discharges copious, mucous with swelling of the testicles. He is cross, irritable, peevish, becoming better by warmth and after breakfast or as the day proceeds. Discharges, slimy, mucous, or tenacious and purulent.

Orchitis. Left testicle hard and swollen, with drawing or tearing pain along the spermatic cord. Constipation, irritable; sleepy; drowsy when sitting or reading; dirty-brown, coated tongue; bad taste in the mouth.

Female Sexual Organs. Menses dark, profuse and scanty, quite often irregular. Constipation with urging to stool. Stool scanty, dark, often with nausea and vomiting and marked gastric disturbance.

Leucorrhœa. Fetid, staining linen yellow; weight and heaviness in the uterus with stinging and burning in the vagina. Very irritable; wishes to be alone and close to the radiator or stove; feels better when warm; feels < in the morning, by cold and after eating; improves towards noon, by warmth, rest, or when not performing any mental labor.

Case 1. C. E., age 20. Gonorrhœa suppressed, with swelling of the left testicle; feels chilly all the time, decreases when warm; is constipated with loss of appetite. Patient is cross, irritable and disgusted with himself. Pain in testicle and spermatic cord relieved by heat. Speaks in a short, snappish way to his friends. Discharge suppressed ten days. Reproduced within twenty-four hours, with relief of all his symptoms.

Case 2. N. B., age 35. Swarthy complexion, dark hair and eyes. Contracted gonorrhœa two months before, had taken Copaiba, and the usual remedies given in that disease by the regular school, with injection of zinc sulphate, which suppressed the discharge within twenty-four hours. One week later he had sexual intercourse with his wife, to whom he conveyed the disease, although there was no discharge to be seen for four or five days. The patient then complained of left-sided temporal headaches, was chilly all the time and had a desire to sit near the radiator. Sleepy in the evenings, yet could not sleep at night. If he did sleep he awakened early and could not go to sleep again; was very much constipated, very irritable and cross in the morning; wished to be left alone. No discharge since the use of the zinc. Three days later there was a slight mucous discharge from the urethra. General symptoms better. Four days later severe chordee and pain on urinating, with desire to stool, when a profuse muco-purulent gonorrhœal discharge was established; mental symptoms first improved, then the gastro-intestinal and finally the discharge ceased.

PAPAYA VULGARIS

(Pawpaw)

Tearing pains on the bladder with a constant desire to urinate; desire to urinate irresistable on hearing the sound of running water; burning in the urethra before and after urinating; pain running from perineum to middle portion of the penis, or a sharp pain in the testicle awakening him at nights; discharge, jelly like or glairy mucus.

PAREIRA BRAVA

Urinary Organs. This remedy produces a severe form of nephritic colic; pain shooting down the ureter, especially the left, with violent tenesmus, accompanied with nausea and bilious vomiting. Urine passes drop by drop and only when kneeling or with head pressed against some hard substance. Dreadful pain with straining. Patient screams out with pain (Canth.), shooting or burning pains at or in the orifice or urethra.

Male Sexual Organs. Constant ineffectual urging when urine passes in drops, burning hot in the urethra. Severe urethritis with prostatic complications. Perspiration breaks out when urinating. Discharge thick white mucus; indicated in the first and second stages of a severe spasmodic form of gonorrhœa.

PETROSELINUM

Urinary Organs. Desire to urinate frequent, caused by a crawling stitch-like pain in the navicular fossa (T.F. Allen). After urination, cutting and biting. Burning in the navicular fossa when urinating; better when standing or sitting.

Male Sexual Organs. Priapism without curvature of penis; voluptuos tingling in navicular fossa.

Gonorrhœa with stranguary and irresistable desire to urinate with crawling in the navicular fossa. Acute cystitis following the use of medicated injections in gonorrhœa (Canth., Nux v., Pareira brava, Medorrh.) Discharge is milky, albuminous, and sometimes yellow.

PULSATILLA

Urinary Organs. Bladder; tenesmus very great with stinging in the neck; frequent desire to urinate with sharp cutting pains in the region of the bladder; burning in the neck with chilliness; better by gentle motion, walking slowly about. The urging and straining to urinate in this remedy is similar to Nux. vom. All the bladder symptoms are worse lying on the back; better lying upon the sides, especially the left. In Pulsatilla we have involuntary urination in women while coughing or sneezing. Like Broyonia or Causticum, the child has involuntary urination as soon as it goes to sleep (Sep). Dribbling of the urine in women (old men Carbo. veg.)

Male Sexual Organs. Seminal emissions worse in the morning; orchitis with aching and burning in the testicles, with or without much swelling; orchitis form suppressed gonorhœa, orchitis worse in left testicle (right Bry., Medorr., Rhus., Ars., and Cycl.) Orchitis from suppressed gonorrhœa (Bry.); from getting wet (Rhus); by medicated injections in the early stage of gonorrhœa. (Nux. Medorrh.) Discharge thick, yellowish or yellowish-green. (Similar to Hepar, or Nat. sulp.) with burning and tenesmus on urinating and severe morning chordee. Gleet has also a yellowish discharge. A good remedy for rheumatism, gonorrhœal arthritis, acute or subacute following supression of gonorrhœa in the acute stage; sub-acute forms of inflammatory rheumatism, affecting the knees or ankles, after the suppression of the discharge by medicated injections or douches.

We are apt to find this remedy indicated in mild, gentle, bashful, timid, yielding disposition, who are forever craving sour things and desiring fresh air. They want open windows and out-door exercise and are worse afternoons and evenings, worse lying on left side or back with head low, in a warm close room, before and during menstruation, from eating fats or rich foods. Better in open air, walking slowly about, or gentle exercise; (violent exercise, Sepia); similar to Tuber, in the desire for fresh air.

Case 1. Emma B., age 22, suppressed gonorrhœa in the first stage, followed by gonorrhœal rheumatism, of left ankle joint of a sub-acute form. The leucorrhœa in the beginning was thick, milky in color, bland. There was no thirst at any time, although the fever rose as high as 102. Pain worse in the afternoon and evening; pain relieved by gentle motion and by cool bathing. Tongue coated white. The patient weeps easily and craves cool air.

Case 2. Alice M., colored; suppressed gonorrhœa followed by salpingitis; a tumor the size of a small orange found in the tube, accompanied with fever, pain and much suffering. She had previously had a yellowish leucorrhœa with sharp cutting in the neck of the bladder and frequent urging to urinate, becoming worse when lying on the back or left side. Puls. 50m relieved all her symptoms up to that time. I lost sight of the case after that.

Case 3. Geo. F., age 22. Gonorrhœa for three weeks; treatment by regular school. Symptoms—pain in left testicle which is very much swollen, small bubo of left side also. Discharge very scanty, milky mucus, much burning and cutting in neck of bladder on urinating; symptoms otherwise quite negative; no thirst; no appetite; works every day, but feels very tired and exhausted every afternoon after three o'clock. Tongue coated white; bad taste and no desire for water. Cured with Pulsatilla 1m.

RHUS TOX

This is a valuable remedy in the rheumatic expressions of gonorrhœa or from diseases brought on by getting wet, in patients wih a sycotic constitution, whether the disease was acquired or not. Sycotic patients (men especially) suffer at every change of the weather, and at every falling barometer with stiffness of the joints, pain in the tendons or sheaths of muscles. Such patients become stiff, sore, lame and scarcely able to move, because of a severe muscular prostration that accompanies the disease. Lumbago from the least exposure, from sweating or from getting too warm while at work, or from sitting in a draft. Notice how frequently these imperfectly cured patients have lumbago. Rhus has a broad field of usefulness in rheumatism caused by suppressed or hereditary Sycosis. The symptoms are aching, restlessness, uneasiness, desire to move constantly; pains relieved by motion or change of position; the relief is momentary, however, yet the patient is compelled to move.

Urinary Organs. Urging to urinate with great tenesmus and pain in the region of the prostate; this is like Nux; in severe cases there is also a desire to stool; symptoms are all better by motion; urine hot, scanty, often bloody; either complete retention or it flows very slowly.

In women we have frequent desire to urinate, which ceases not day nor night and occasionally it dribbles away. This is worse in cold air or when cold, better by getting warm or from motion. Rheumatic or uric acid patients needing this remedy frequent, urgent desire, the urine is dark, scanty, becoming turbid on standing and depositing a white sediment. Urine passes in drops with straining and great suffering, Apis, Canth., Mer., or Nux) ; urinary difficulties with much aching, stiffness and soreness about back or kidneys.

Male Sexual Organs. Chordee with desire to urinate. Red spots size of a pin head or larger on the surface of the glans penis. (Medorrh., Thuja, Sulp.)

Orchitis from suppressed gonorrhœa with much œdema and accompanied with rheumatic symptoms; erysipelas of the sexual organs, scrotum in particular, after acute suppression, or during the gleety stage of the disease; erysipelas following gleet or the suppression of the discharge.

Female Sexual Organs. Soreness of the uterus with rheumatic pains in back or limbs; aggravation before storms, in all pelvic difficulties. Leucorrhœa worse after menses, in women with a rheumatic element present. Leucorrhœa, thin, dark, scanty, like dirty water, biting the pudenda. It may be thick, creamy, and acrid, accompanied with backache in the small of the back, and much burning and pruritis of the vulva, causing soreness, redness and swelling of the parts passed over (Ars).

Case 1. Erysipelas of scrotum following suppression of Sycosis in the first stage; began on left side and spread down over perineum and towards the right; temperature 103; much aching and restlessness with shooting pains in lower extremities. Burning, itching, biting, smarting in the skin. Rhus 1m cured in one week.

Case 2. Mrs. R., age 53, contracted Sycosis in the second stage from her husband who was a traveling man. Symptoms, burning, biting, smarting on urinating; urine scanty with urging; desire quick, frequent ; discharge from vagina, thin, scanty, excoriating the pudendum; erythema produced wherever the discharge touches, this smarts and burns like erysipelas. Backache continuous, can scarcely rise from a sitting position, but better when she moves about; better by hot douches and from hot baths, worse during wet or stormy weather ; cured with Rhus tox, given in the 1m then in the c. m. potency, followed by Sulphur c. m.

RATANHIA

Acute or chronic gonorrhœa with burning at the root of penis when urinating. Frequent urging to urinate.

SARSAPARILA

This remedy is syco-syphilitic and is indicated in old men at the close of the secondary and at the beginning of the tertiary stage. It is one of the remedies for old debauchees enfeebled by intoxicants and venereal diseases.

It may follow Nux and may be compared with thuja in gonorrhœa. Symptoms—spasm of the sphincter when sitting down to urinate; relieved by standing; he tries to grasp the neck of bladder with his fingers at the close of urination. There is a severe pain or spasm at the close, which causes him to cry out. Children scream when urinating, but it is usually caused by the passage of sand or a lithic deposit from the bladder. Offensive odor from the genitals (Psor., Thuja); rheumatism following the suppression of the discharge (Ars., Bry., Rhus, Dulc). Gonorrhœa checked from getting cold or wet and is followed by rheumatism. Indicated in the tertiary stage when warts, gouty nodules, and gouty pains follow a suppression in the first or second stage of gonorrhœa; moist eruptions on the genitals; headache, with pain in the back of the head the pain settles at root of nose. Adapted to dark-haired, nervo-bilious temperaments.

SEPIA

Suitable to tall thin women with lax, muscular fiber. She is without natural affection or sexual appetite, especially after child bearing. She is excitable, nervous and fidgety, worse when alone. The face is often freckled or has many moth patches and pigmentary spots. Gonorrhœal discharge milky or thick greenish-yellow; discharge painless; indicated frequently at the close of the secondary stage. It has a drop of discharge of a milky or yellowish color which appears only on the morning and is generally painless. With stricture it has the same symptoms ; discharges stain the linen yellow or yellowish-brown. Frequent desire to urinate ; urine milky and burns like fire (female) ; cutting like knives on urinating it passes involuntarily while sneezing or coughing (Bry. Caust.) Gonorrhœal discharge at night only in men, staining the linen yellow ; painless drop ; no burning on urinating ; urine loaded with urates. Chronic gonorrhœa with loss of sexual power. Great weakness after coition. Urinary organs ; feeling as if a drop was coming out of the bladder, constant pressure on the bladder with inclination to urinate, urine deposits a brick dust sediment, sensation as of enlargement of the bladder. Gleet, no pain, no soreness, subacute or chronic stage of the disease, with only a single drop in the morning, yellowish staining the linen. Meatus glued together in the morning ; sexual organs feel weak.

STAPHISAGRIA

A syco-syphilitic remedy useful after mercurialization ; the patient is easily excited and aroused to anger. Hardness, induration and chronic enlargement of the glands. Prostate gland greatly enlarged causing frequent urging to urinate, passing it in drops with burning before and after. Impotence and complete loss of sexual power ; legs and back weak with loss of mental and vital energy. Sensitive warts about the genitals ; testicles atrophied, very small ; periosteal pains in the long bones ; worse at night.

SYPHILINUM

Urinary Organs. A stopped up, clogged sensation in the male urethra ; urine scalds ; itching at orifice, (Sulph.) ; urinates very slowly, therefore has to strain, (secondary Syphilis) ; color, golden-yellow, (Kali c.) ; infrequent, scanty, slow. After chills, urine quite profuse. Urinary troubles increase at night, (Syphilis).

Male Sexual Organs. Chancres about the glans penis, quite small ; lardaceous floor, everted edges ; glans of a purplish color. Suppressed chancre, where the disease attacks the organism in other places. Pricking or sticking in the chancre is quite a common symptom. (Nit. ac.) Bubo, left inguinal, small, fluctuating, purple, painful ; increased by standing and at night, or from midnight until morning. Inflammation and induration of the spermatic cord.

STRAMONIUM

Urinary Organs. Kidneys secrete very little urine, often none in acute febrile diseases of children. Great desire to urinate, often in acute diseases or after labor or miscarriage. Bladder—retention of urine, after great staining a few drops pass. Not painful like Cantharis, flow increased by drinking vinegar ; urine discharged in drops, after straining and urging. (Canth. Mer. cor. Nux. Apis.) Urinates profusely at night, while during the day it is scanty and only passed with great difficulty. Urinary suppression due to reflex spinal irritation, brain or spinal diseases. Urine very profuse after the delirium of this remedy. Urine often involuntary or dribbling in severe fevers or brain troubles. Temporary paralysis of the bladder sphincter; bladder empty, no urine secreted. Copious passages of pale, watery urine following acute delirium or nervous attacks.

Gonorrhœa. Great irritation of urinary passages; unusual straining and urging in order to empty bladder; flow ceases often, then starts again; shuddering when urinating; urethra feels narrow, as if a band were about it; streams start freely after drinking vinegar; no power in bladder to expel urine.

Male Sexual Organs. Constantly uncovering the genitals (Hyos.), a mental symptom. Temporary loss of sexual power; extreme sexual excitement. Lascivious, exalted sexual passions; onanism following or causing epilepsy; young boys are constantly handling sexual organs; cannot keep hands off them. (Coffea). Intense chordee with unendurable sexual desire. In gonorrhœa it often serves as a palliative.

SULPHUR

Anti-psoric. Sulphur is purely an anti-psoric remedy and it is known as the king of anti-psorics. It stands at the head of remedies for Psora. It often cures chronic disease when Syphilis and Sycosis are blended or banded with Psora, by virtue of its removing the psoric taint or separating the bond of Psora from the other miasms. The symptoms are menstruation too profuse, too early, and too long lasting. Not infrequently the menses will stop completely the fourth or fifth day and then return, and the patient will flow two or three days longer. This to me has been a very reliable symptom of Sulphur. Other remedies have it, but Sulphur has it very markedly. Chronic uterine hemorrhage, with oppression of the chest; distention of the abdomen; constipation; often a dry evening cough; burning of the hands and feet, especially while lying down on first going to bed; great restlessness and tossing about at night, with desire to uncover the feet and limbs, or to find a cool place in the bed. Hot flashes followed by a slight perspiration during menses, about, or at the beginning of the climactric period. She cannot endure a warm room, wants the room about 60 or 65 degrees during menstruation. Severe colic during menses; pains in sides; flashes of heat and feels faint.

Congestion of the blood to the head or chest, heat on the vertex; burning on the vertex during flow. Faint gone feeling in stomach about 10 or 11 A. M., $<$ by eating a few mouthfuls. Bleeding hemorrhoids during menses; flow profuse in the morning with severe colicky pain in the bowels. Standing increases all her sufferings, and at the close of the flow the discharge produces much itching of the pudenda and vulva. Often it excoriates the vulva and perineum ; gnawing hunger ; fainting spells ; hands and feet cold ; flashes of heat to the face, restless and sleepless nights ; wakens often in the night ; peevish ; in great haste in doing anything ; anxious and in doubt about her salvation ; great dryness of the skin ; itching of the eye lids, and of the whole body when in bed and covered up warm ; lips very red ; skin of face and body has a dirty, unwashed look. The lower extremities feel heavy ; she is easily fatigued ; worse ascending a height ; < when standing ; < from heat, bathing when at rest, at night and from changeable weather. > lying on right side, from cool air, and dry warm weather.

Sulphur is well adapted to thin, stoop-shouldered women who are deeply impregnated with Psora or pseudo-Psora. It arouses to action and gives new vigor to every cell in the body, curing a multitude of chronic miasmatic states of the system.

THUJA

The face in this remedy is very characteristic, indeed there is often a typical sycotic cachexia present. We find it greyish, even waxy, again it may have that peculiar greasy, shiny appearance similar to that found in Syphilis at the beginning of the second stage ; I have frequently met with it in the public clinics. Thuja is also a great remedy to antidote animal poisons, such as gonorrhœa, mixed Syphilis, or the bad effects of vaccination. We have the copious perspiration of Mercury, but it is of a sweetish odor, like honey, or again it may be pungent, musty, or like fish brine. Especially is this true of the perspiration about the genitals of both sexes. We notice this symptom in most cases of chronic gonorrhœa as marked perhaps as we do the odor of the feet in Silicea, or Baryta-carb, patients.

Urinary Organs. Burning in the urethra during urination and for a considerable time after ; it is quite a constant symptom of this remedy (after Sarsa) ; cutting, drawing and burning in urethra, with frequent urging (Can, sat. Cann, ind.)

Bladder. Loss of power at times ; unable to fully void the urine ; has to make a number of attempts to do so ; incontinence increases during night ; comes on while coughing (Bry. Caust.) ; urine foamy, often dark with strong odor.

Male Sexual Organs. Nightly painful chordee in gonorrhœa ; discharge greenish, watery, or a thin yellowish-green fluid, stream forked or twisted ; burning or cutting when urinating (Cann. sat. Medorrh.) ; pain < by walking ; urine scalds when he urinates, and urethra very much swollen. Jerking, cutting, burning, with an interrupted stream. Glans penis very red, covered with red sores or spots, elevated red sore points, often exuding a yellowish-green mucus. When gonorrhœal discharge stops, rheumatism begins ; sensation as of moisture running from the urethra (Kali b.) ; dribbling of the urine in chronic cases.

Severe burning in the glans penis; suppressed gonorrhœa with sub-acute or chronic rheumatism. Small tubercles (Sycotic) about the glans penis; warts and warty growths on the sexual organs, or about the anus and perineum, in both sexes. Condylomatous growths after gonorrhœa, usually dry (moist Nit. ac. Cinnabar.); deep, red spots on the glans and inner surface of the foreskin, with slight burning. Gland covered with a thin yellowish-green, badly smelling secretion. Glands red, much swollen in the first and second stage (Medorrhinum.) Symptoms very similar to medorrhinum especially the mental symptoms. Erections violent, long continued, in the morning with increased desire for coition. Voluptous itching in the foreskin. Urine yellow, copious, with frequent desire to urinate night and day. The absence of painful or spasmodic symptoms does not contra-indicate this remedy, indicated in the second and third stage more frequently, however.

General Symptoms. Thuja is a true anti-sycotic, deep and of long action, indicated more frequently in blond or the lymphatic temperament, but it cures in dark as well as light individuals. Skin looks dirty, brownish; sweats on uncovered parts (reverse Sil.), copious and sour smelling, ceases when awake. Sweat about the genitals, sweetish smelling.

TABACUM

Urinary Organs. Renal colic; terrific pains along the ureter (Berb, Coloc. Ver. alb.) with nausea, vomiting, retching (Tart. emet.) and cold sweat. The prolonged use of tobacco sometimes produces a sort of paresis of the bladder with dribbling of the urine, habitual constipation, sticky and pasty stools; tremor of the hands and tongue.

Male Sexual Organs. Nocturnal emissions without awaking. Organs flabby with no erections. Impotence in smokers.

Gonorrhœal discharge renewed or re-established after using tobacco in people sensitive to narcotics (coffee or any of the alcoholics). Many physicians prohibit the use of tobacco during the treatment of gonorrhœa as it prevents their suppressing it, or hinders a cure where homeopathic remedies are used.

DYSMENORRHOEA

Few diseases of women cause so much pain and suffering as this disease. Skene in his splendid work "Diseases of Women," classifies dysmenorrhea in five special forms, "the inflammatory, membranous, neurotic, obstructive and ovarian." All of these are more or less painful and some of them exceedingly so. Each form has been accurately described by many authors in the numerous works on the "Diseases of Women." Each writer has painted his word picture of misery and suffering with all his power of pen, yet none, I believe, has overdrawn this picture of suffering too strongly.

We have no space to devote to a descrpttion of the different forms above mentioned, with their manifold array of symptoms, for such is not the object of this treatise. In the end, all the literature that has been written upon the subject, has not satisfied the majority of practitioners. We feel that the true etiology of the disease has not yet been reached; the true cause is yet unrevealed. Why should the disease manifest itself in so many forms, with hardly two cases of the same form resembling each other? We must look elsewhere for causes, other than the causes specified in the works under which this disease is classified. One form is attributed to congestion, another to neuralgia, another to obstructions, another to the membranes, and still others to malformations of the organs, or to the various pathological states and conditions of the system.

It is true in some forms we do have pathological conditions present that cause great suffering at times, but the majority of cases are functional or neurotic, behind which lies some constitutional dyscrasia. Speaking of the cause of membranous dysmenorrhœa, the same author (Skene) says, "Discarding the current views regarding membranous dysmenorrhœa—that is, that it is due to inflammation, or else to the result of gestation—one is left without any very rational view to offer regarding its cause. While it is not, perhaps, the part of wisdom to discredit the views on any question in medicine until one has something more to offer, still, if the causes assigned can be readily shown to be incorrect, it is infinitely better and safer to be entirely in ignorance of the cause of things than to attribute them to wrong causes." How true this is, but it is only occasionally that some one rises up as a doubter, and throwing to the winds the doctrines of the day begins to investigate for himself, choosing rather to be numbered with the minority and find the truth, than to be numbered with the majority and follow the traditions of men. The world today *would materialize* all *cause*, for *nothing else, seems to satisfy the mind of the materialist*. How happy and satisfied the pathologist is when he can locate the *cause* in some one particular corner or part of the body, in a muscle, in an organ, in a nerve center, in some ganglion, or even in a nerve ending.

When Hahnemann says, "Disease is a disturbance of the life force," it means nothing to many of us, because we know so little about this *life force* that vivifies and animates the human body. It is necessary to understand the Hahnemannian life force theory, and the laws that govern it before we can understand anything clearly and distinctly about disease. We must also know something about the *chronic miasms*, before we can understand the *true cause and the multiple changes in the phenomena of disease*. One will attribute the cause of dysmenorrhoea to a rheumatic diathesis and another to Syphilis; still another to the strumous diathesis; this later is the tubercular, of course. Others have attributed it to external causes, and in a sense they are right, but when we come to study disease carefully from the standpoint of the chronic miasms, a different light is thrown upon cause and effect. We see disease in its true light, we can understand a dysmenorrhea that is due to Psora, pseudo-Psora, Sycosis, or to Syphilis, or to any of the combinations of these great central disturbers of life. We are soon able to classify and to place each form of dysmenorrhea, each individual case where it belongs, calling it, as the case may be, Psoric, pseudo-Psoric, Sycotic, of syphilitic. The writer has given the subject much study and thought, and in practice has seen wonderful results from prescribing the Homeopathic remedy in dysmenorrhea, both from the palliative methods and from the anti-miasmatics. It is of the latter that we wish to speak further.

We notice the tubercular forms of dysmenorrhea more prominently than any of the others. The reason is that we meet it so frequently in practice, and having considerable knowledge of the tubercular diathesis we readily associate the two together. We see the rise and fall of the latent tubercular expression in the organism. No greater field exists for miasmatic action than in the reproductive organs and sexual functions of women.

Today we meet in a great number of women some form of dysmenorrhea. The whole organism is more or less disturbed during menstruation. Often from the crown of the head to the sole of the foot they are disturbed and manifest some form of suffering, all due to the presence of the tubercular element. "No function is ever perverted in a normal healthy organism," and should not be accompanied with pain and suffering. Pain is always a signal of disease ; its meaning denotes a penalty, a fine, or a punishment. A woman should have no suffering at the menstrual period; there should be but a simple consciousness of its presence, a little lagging of the forces of life, a pause, as it were, for the preparation. Indeed, we should have no more than a simple consciousness of the presence and action of any organ, yet we find in the menstrual function of women, who are affected with a sycotic or tubercular taint, every degree of suffering, even to the anguish of death, as the organs attempt to perform their periodical work. The sexual organs of the women of today are the great centers of disease, and especially is this true of the sycotic miasm, whose destructive and disturbing action has become an alarming factor to our best pathologists and ablest therapeutists. Often when therapeutic measures have failed, the surgeon has to be called in to remove a part or even all of the reproductive organs of women. Many times the surgeon's knife is resorted to, simply because, as a therapeutist, he was not familiar with the effect of the sycotic poison (miasm) upon the reproductive tract. His therapeutic knowledge did not reach that far, thus in the end, he demonstrated his ignorance of the disease by removing the organ.

Thus did Pasteur say, when the silk worms of France became diseased, "Kill the silk worm." So they say, "kill everything that is diseased; remove every organ that is diseased." We had better become acquainted with these diseases, and recognize their destructive death-dealing principles, so that we may be able to analyze them

18 F.B.

and meet them on a therapeutic plane, and cure them with therapeutic measures.

The menstrual anomalies of tubercular patients are often pictures of dreadful sufferings from that dreaded miasm pseudo-psora. The flow is always accompanied with exhaustion and weariness. It comes too soon, is too copious and too prolonged, often assuming the form of hemorrhage. The patient feels badly a week before the menses appear and a week afterwards. The menstrual period is accompanied with severe backache, gastric disturbances, neuralgia, headaches, ovarian neuralgia, even diarrhœa and febrile states. Such is the picture of a tubercular case of dysmenorrhea, with all its exaggerated conditions of function, and all its sufferings and phenomena of that exhausting and death-dealing principle, the tubercular element.

The menstruation of the sycotic patient is not prolonged like the pseudo-psoric one, and is seldom as copious. If it is profuse it is not so exhausting, nor so heavy a drain upon the sufferer. It may be very profuse for twenty-four hours or even a little longer, but it does not continue as in the case of pseudo-psoric for a whole week. (The flow of the sycotic patient has more of a spasmodic nature about it.) The tubercular have dark circles about the eyes, are hollow-eyed, pale, a worn-out, exhausted look ; loss of appetite, nausea, vomiting, and diarrhœa are not infrequently present. Hysterical symptoms may arise in these cases in any degree of severity, indeed they are the most difficult cases of the kind we have to treat. The flow is at times pale, watery, and long lasting, as is seen in Calcarea carb. Kali carb and that class of remedies. Again it is profuse even to exhaustion, and of a bright-red color, inducing anæmia in young women whose ages range from seventeen to twenty-four. Occasionally the complexion becomes pale or assumes an ashen or yellowish hue. The menses are not infrequently followed with leucorrhœas, palpitation of the heart, and loss of vitality generally; later on great weakness, flushing of the face, dry tickling cough, vertigo, hoarseness, and finally you have a well developed case of tuberculosis that might have been arrested earlier in life through a careful analysis of the case and a remedy selected on the pseudo-psoric symptoms.

The mental symptoms alone of these patients often furnish us with data enough upon which to base our pseudo-psoric remedy. These patients are sad, gloomy, full of fanciful notions, forboding, are fearful, extremely sensitive, nervous and irritable. Sometimes they may pass through the menstrual period with but little suffering, but it is followed with prosopalgia of a prolonged and distressing nature. I have said little of the neuralgias, the many reflex symptoms, and untold sufferings of these patients. Usually in a marked case where the tubercular element is present, we have retroflexions and all sorts of malpositions of the uterus. Their sufferings date from an early period following puberty, within a year or two at least. In Sycosis, the neuralgias are dis-

THE CHRONIC MIASMS. 261

placed by the rheumatic element. In fact about all the pains of Sycosis are rheumatic. We have muscular rheumatism prevailing in many cases. Of course we have many pains that are similar to pseudo-psora, but on close analysis the rheumatic element can be traced back to the cause. Often they have muscular rheumatism at intermenstrual periods, lumbago or stiffness of the muscles of the neck and aching in the limbs. We have aching of the limbs in the tubercular, but it is accompanied with great weariness, with pelvic congestion so severe that they are unable to stand on their feet any length of time. In Sycosis the uterine pains are spasmodic, colicky, often extending over the whole abdomen, and generally felt in the membranes of the ovaries and tubes.

The remedies called for in sycotic dysmenorrhea are Colocynthis, Chamomilla, Colchicum, Cyclamen, Rhus tox, Bovista, Actea racemosa, Phytolacca, Sepia, Lachesis, Medorrhinum, Nat. sulph, Caulophyllum, Gelsemium, Dulcamara and occasionally Pulsatilla, Arsenicum alb, Lycopodium, Nux vomica, Croton tiglium, Asarum, Viburnum opulus. These are a few of the sycotic remedies, but there are many others that we will call your attention to in giving the indication for the remedies. The miasmatic element will be mentioned under each remedy. The flow frequently comes in gushes with much pain, and is, as a rule, dark and clotted, as we have already mentioned. The menses of a tuberular patient seldom clot, they are more apt to be thin and watery or bright red and copious. The odor of the tubercular menses is like blood, while the sycotic is musty, or it has a fish-brine or stale fish odor. It is often irritating, corrosive, excoriating, producing pruritis at some period of the flow, generally at the close. The pruritis is a biting, smarting, itching sensation, and the discharge quite often excoriates, and produces an erythema of the parts with which it comes in contact. Often we find some form of salpingitis even to complete destruction of the ovarian tubes, or we may find any of the lesions mentioned in the beginning of th' work.

When we have the tubercular element combined wit the sycotic we have the worst form of dysmenorrhea to deal with. There is no worse combination outside of a malignancy than where dysmenorrhoea is based upon a tubercular basis with a sycotic addition to magnify all its phases. Usually in a typical sycotic patient, whether acquired or hereditary, there is some form of irritation of the bladder about the time of the appearance of or during the menses. The urine either passes frequently or in small quantities, or it is copious and frequent with more or less pain or irritation of the neck of the bladder. The menses are almost always dark, clotted, and difficult to wash out. Menstrual colic is frequent with ovarian pains and there is tenderness of the breasts during the flow.

Enough has been said to give the reader some idea of a case of sycotic dysmenorrhea, and a fuller expression of it will be brought out as the indications for the remedies are given. The treatment should be continued until the patient menstruates normally or nearly so, which may take from three months to a year, and in some cases even two years. Prescriptions made during the inter-menstrual period are the most efficacious, as the acute expression has quieted down and the latent expression is shown more clearly, and upon this symptomatology it is better to base your prescription.

THERAPEUTICS OF DYSMENORRHOEA
ACONITE

Aconite will be indicated only when the psoric element is prominent in the case, as it is not a sycotic remedy. The menses are profuse, bright red, and protracted, or are suppressed from cold, cold baths, fright, over-joy, bad news, etc. There is fever with anxiety and apprehension; the pulse is full and quick; there is fear of death, much alarm and excitement; painful menstruation, and a febrile and congested condition. The pains are sharp, cutting, doubling the patient up; hands are cold, even in the febrile state; there is chilliness with flushes of heat intermingled; over-sensitiveness to noise or touch; restlessness with tossing in sleep (like Rhus tox or Arsenicum album). It is adapted chiefly to the sanguine temperament, to young girls of a sedentary habit. Other symptoms are palpitation of the heart, quick hard pulse, anxiety, fear, and hot flushed face.

AURUM METALLICUM

Syphilo-psoric. In this remedy we have a somewhat profuse menstruation with labor-like pains in the abdomen. The flow is acrid, producing great soreness of the parts. There is swelling in the axillary glands and often periostial or bone pains. It is adapted to sanguine, ruddy people with black hair and eyes; in chronic Syphilis and for the bad effects of the over use of mercury. Menstruation with great melancholy, depression of spirits, suicidal tendency, and mental dejection; imagines she is unfit to live; mind turns toward self-destruction, longs for death, < in the evening, at night and at the menstrual period; the least contradiction excites her wrath, and mental labor fatigues her. Indicated more at puberty.

Case: Mrs. A. B., age 27, after birth of second child, suffered with inflammation of right ovary; ovary very much enlarged, sensitive to touch; pain dull, heavy, always < at night, feels well during the day; is cross and irritable at the menstrual period, no living with her, her husband says; wants to die, says she is going to jump into the river if this awful depression keeps on; it begins just before the menses. She is under a fearful cloud all during menses. She was cured with 1m. potency; no return in fourteen years.

ACTEA RACEMOSA

Like all the cohosh family, this remedy is anti-sycotic in its curative effects. It shows the strong rheumatic element of that miasm, while it has the hysterical element.

of Psora. Many of its phases are hystero-rheumatic or the combining of the two elements ; or they alternate, when one is < the other is >. The menses are too early copious as a rule, clotted and dark. During menses the mental field is clouded, there is great sadness and gloominess ; fears that she will hear bad news, or that something awful is going to happen, that she is losing her mind. She is full of imaginations, fears, forbodings, and all sorts of uneasiness. Like Lachesis she is suspicious of everything. The appearance of the flow gives relief to many of her symptoms, especially to the mental. "Rheumatism following the disappearance of mental states." (Kent).

Vertex headaches during the menses ; sore feelings all over the head, and pain in the back extending to the thighs ; much weight and bearing down in the uterus ; a feeling of weight in the extremities ; pain increases until the flow reaches its maximum, then suddenly ceases. Rheumatic dysmenorrhoea in brunettes. There is much weight and heaviness on the vertex (Sepia) ; a sensation as if the head would fly off. Besides, there is much pain in the back of the neck which is rheumatic in character. Pains in uterus darting from side to side ; often the severity of the pain increases or decreases with the flow ; soreness in the uterus or all about that region, and like Arnica, there is a bruised feeling all over. It has also in its lameness, some resemblance to Rhus tox. Her symptoms are changeable like Pulsatilla, yet she is the opposite of Pulsatilla in temperament, irritable, quick tempered, snappish and very emotional. She may be subject to hysterical spasms, even to convulsions; during the menses she has spasms of the uterus, with pains shooting across the abdomen, or from the left ovary to the heart. It acts upon the cerebro-spinal system and is useful in delicate rheumatic, hysterical women with uterine irritation.

ANACARDIUM

This remedy partakes of both the psoric and sycotic element. Its pains and its mental symptoms are characteristically sycotic, especially the mental symptoms. Menses scanty but too frequent. Dysmenorrhœa with pressing pain in the abdomen and uterus. The menses are often accompanied with a severe headache, pressure as of a plug in the left side of vertex. Mental symptoms: Great irritability; desire to curse and swear; great contradiction between understanding and will; a veritable Dr. Jekyl and Mr. Hyde; she has two wills, one hindering her from doing that which the other impels her to do. Dreadfully irritable, always in a controversy with self, lives if in a dream, nothing real. Compare the mental sphere with Hyos., Stram., Bell. She is morose, sulky, sullen, irritable, easily angered, often cruel and malicious, yet feeble. The headache is relieved by eating and by sleep. This remedy follows well after Lyc., and Puls. Plat. may follow it.

AMYLENUM NITROSUM

Indicated in nervous, sensitive, plethoric women during and after change of life. (Lach.) It rapidly dilates the arteries and accelerates the pulse, but later weakens and retards the pulse; intense surging of blood to the face during menses or after menopause. (Bell., Glon.) Craves fresh air, opens clothing, throws off the clothes, and opens windows in the coldest weather. (Arg. nit., Lach., Sul.) Flashes of heat start from the stomach, followed by hot profuse sweating; parts below stomach are cold; flashes of heat from the slightest emotion, much yawning and stretching; angina with tumultous heart action, must loosen clothing and collar when flashes come on (Lach.) It is said to have cured puerperal convulsions after delivery. (Similar to Lach., Bell., Coca, Glon.) It acts better in the c. m. potency.

ALETRIS FARINOSA

Suitable to chlorotic girls and pregnant women. Menses prolonged and accompanied with labor-like pains. Amenorrhœa from uterine or ovarian atony or from a congested state of the uterus or ovaries. Flow copius, black, clotted with fullness in the region of the uterus. During pregnancy, obstinate vomiting with constant spitting of a cottony, frothy mucus. False pains during gestation. General debility with prolapsis of uterus. Similar to Bell., Sab., Hydr., Senega and Puls.

ANTIMONIUM CRUDUM

This is a sycotic remedy, and is helpful in gouty conditions and gouty states of the system. Its symptoms center about the stomach and digestive tract. Menstruation premature and profuse, with a peculiar presssure in the uterus, menses too early in young girls, before the time of puberty ; flow dark, fluid, with coagula ; great tenderness in the ovarian region after menses or after suppression from cold, from cold bathing or from being overheated ; gouty dysmenorrhea ; gouty gastritis ; dysmenorrhea in young girls who are disappointed in their love affairs, this is one of the remedies for the bad results of unrequited affection. Mentally peevish, sentimental ; ecstacy with exalted love ; suicidal tendency with great anxiety about self. Tongue thickly coated white ; eructations after eating, tasting of food ; desire for coffee, pickles, sour things ; subject to warts and gouty pains.

Aggravations from eating and from extreme cold or heat.

ANTIMONIUM TARTARICUM

Syco-psoric. Adapted to pale, sickly, torpid, phlegmatic persons ; menses premature and profuse, or scanty and of short duration. Menses begin with great nausea, pains in the groins, cold creepings all over the body ; dysmenorrhea with nausea and vomiting, and cold sweat on the forehead. Face is pale, sunken, dark circles about the eyes ; lips dry, cracked ; great desire for acids, with much thirst, nausea and vomiting of mucus, or rattling of mucus in chest. (Ipec.)

Aggravations. Dampness, cold weather, also < in spring (Kali sul., Nat. mur., Sul.).

Ameliorations. Cool and open air.

ALUMINA

This remedy is an anti-psoric, but partakes largely of the pseudo-psoric nature also. In it we have one of those rare remedies in which the menses are retarded, scanty and of too short duration; occasionally they are premature, but they are always too brief. The color is pale and watery. Before the menses, headache and disturbed sleep, with a copious discharge of mucus from the vagina. Before the menses, great exhaustion, both mental and physical debility between the periods. The inter menstrual discharge is transparent mucus, very copious, and is relieved by cold bathing. Unnatural appetite in young girls; they desire to eat chalk, starch, slate pencils, charcoal, plaster, coffee, or tea grounds. They have a faint feeling at the stomach, better by eating (Sulphur); sense of constriction in the throat, can swallow but a small piece at a time; rectum feels paralyzed, no desire for stool; a nightly, dry, hacking cough with oppression in the chest. The remedy is adapted to dry, thin, dark women of a mild and cheerful nature, who suffer from constipation and dry itching eruptions. The itching is worse upon getting warm, and in winter.

Aggravations. Cold air, winter, eating potatoes, soups and on alternate days.

ARALIA RACEMOSA

"Menstruation, sudden suppression from cold. There is a feeble state of the nervous system, and much general debility. Chronic catarrh of the uterus, leucorrhœa foul smelling, with pressing down pains in the uterus." (Minton).

ARSENICUM IODIDE

Pseudo-psoric, leucorrhœa bloody, yellow, with hard swelling of the labia, followed by induration in axillae and mammae, with retracted nipples; night sweats, tubercular cachexia and rapidly developing malignancies.

ARSENICUM ALBUM

Menses profuse in pale, anæmic, feeble individuals, who are low in vital energy. Flow is pale red, profuse or scanty, exhausting, producing great prostration; extremely restless with great thirst, worse in the afternoon or after midnight, all her symptoms are relieved by warmth. Flow often thin, pale, watery, acrid, excoriating the parts passed over; much fear, anxiety, restless and uneasiness with thirst for frequent sips of cold water.

Case 1. Mrs. B., 32 years old, thin, tall, with pale face; tubercular diathesis marked, vitality low, reaction poor, heart action weak, pulse small and weak; awakens much fatigued and unrefreshed; flow like thin, dirty water, scarcely any color in it.

Case 2. Mrs. L., age 21, fairly well nourished, but has no vitality, nor reserve strength; menses prostrate her so. Has no life left in her after flow; lips dry, thin, pale, desires to wet them often; cold water disagrees with her stomach, feels better when warm.

Case 3. Mrs. B., age 40, skin pale and white, dark hair and eyebrows, complexion sallow about and during menses; menses begin with an acrid leucorrhœa, corrodes the part with which it comes in contact, very weak and prostrated during flow; fear of dying and of being alone; easily fatigued, always chilly; warmth relieves her pains, suffers much with neuralgia of the head and face at each menstrual nisus. The least pain or suffering prostrates her.

Case 4. Miss A., age 20, nausea and vomiting with cholera like symptoms during menses; thin, watery dysenteric stools, vomiting and purging with great thirst, a sip of water satisfies but it is soon vomited. Severe darting pains in uterus and ovaries; desire for sour things and pieces of ice and ice water; does not care for water unless it is very cold; is very anxious and restless, worse at 1 P.M. or from 1 to 3 P.M. Arsenicum is adapted to poorly nourished, weak, cachetic individuals who have no reserve force; the least exertion or mental worry prostrates them. They represent pseudo-psora, when it has produced anæmia, the red blood cells being deficient in number.

ACETIC ACID

This is a pseudo-psoric remedy, adapted to people who are suffering with diseases in advanced stages, as chest diseases, bowel troubles, prolonged fevers, and after severe injuries. It follows well after Cinchona in hemorrhages, in night sweats, in exhausting discharges, dropsies, extensive ulcerations, etc. Menses profuse, passive; hemorrhages from the uterus, or from the nose, lungs, and bowels in chlorotic or anæmic women. Hemorrhages with rapid emaciation in exhausting diseases. Most of its troubles are accompanied with profuse night sweats, drenching night sweats. Hectic fevers with night sweats; menses do not appear on account of lung troubles; swelling of the feet with night sweats, hectic fevers with rapid breaking down of the lungs.

Case. Mrs. L., age 32, tall, thin, active brunette; came to me in the April of 1896 suffering with lung trouble; right lung badly infiltrated and the tubercular state well advanced. She had painless, prolonged and copious menses; flow alarmingly profuse and bright red, like arterial blood; cough loose, rattling, much phlegm in bronchia, temperature 101 ; night sweats worse in the upper part of the body. For this I gave Acetic acid after Trillium had given great relief, but no longer helped the case. She is still living yet not cured, but Acetic acid has done wonders for her.

ARNICA MONTANA

Premature, profuse menses, after falls, injuries, concussions, railway or carriage accidents. Flow bright red, mixed with coagula. Menses very difficult and painful. After a fall there is nausea, vomiting, and fever at beginning of flow or after injuries. Sore, bruised feeling all over body after injuries, face hot, extremities cold, blood passes hot from vagina. (Bell).

Case 1. Sore and general bruised feeling in the region of the uterus, blood bright red with clots.

Case 2. General bruised sore feeling all over body, cannot bear to move in bed or to have the clothing touch the body. Head is hot, hands and feet are cold. A sanguine plethoric woman who was suffering from a fall.

ANANTHERUM

Menstruation anticipating, copious, ovary painful, generally speaking the flow is light colored, bright red, but if menses are retarded the blood is dark and thick, stitches in uterus during menses ; pressure in uterus during flow ; tightening stitches in womb ; prolapsis of uterus.

Case. Menses begin with bruised pains in thighs and region of kidneys ; pressing pain in womb ; much itching and burning in vulva ; Vulva inflamed, red, excoriated menses followed by a thick yellowish-green leucorrhœa ; mammae swollen, tender, sensitive during menses.

Aggravation : Morning, open air, cold, damp weather.

ARUNDO MAURITANICA
(Reed)

This is another remedy that has too copious and long lasting menses ; they are also black and clotted. They are accompanied with pain in the uterus and with the passage of gas from the uterine cavity ; nymphomania often accompanies the monthly function, she is full of lascivious ideas ; hysterical laughs easily ; violent desire for sexual embrace.

AGNUS CASTUS

Menses are suppressed or retarded, with drawing pains in the abdomen ; melancholy, sad, self-contempt, disgust with life generally, complete obliteration of sexual desire, or sexual desire greatly increased. Sterility, with suppressed menses and loss of sexual power ; impotence complete ; mind greatly depressed during menses. It is said that the Jewish women used this remedy to destroy sexual desire while attending their passover services. Sterility with suppressed menses; fears she will die, keeps repeating it; absent minded, cannot recollect anything, due often to sexual over-indulgence; sexual desire diminished or completely lost.

ASAFOETIDA

Menses premature, too short and too scanty, often ten days too soon. Labor like pains in the uterus, with much bearing down during menses; empty gone feeling in the epigastrium, with pricking flatulent colic, constantly belching large quantities of gas. Nervous flatulence, *globus hystericus*, gas chokes her, it comes so fast from stomach. Sense of constriction in throat, or sensation of ball in the throat; gas forms so fast that she cannot belch it fast enough; nervous flatulence, no disturbance of digestion; syphilitic or carcinomatous ulceration of the cervix with carrion-like odor from the discharges. Breasts become large with milk in them during menses.

Case 1. Nervous, hysterical, plethoric woman, about forty years of age. Her husband said something to her that made her angry, which was soon followed by great nervousness and a spasm of the œsophagus; belched gas so fast that she lost her breath for a short time. There was much anxiety with great fear that she was going to die; constantly swallowing a ball in the throat (Ignatia, Lachesis); menses came on with pricking colic; Asafoetida 30 relieved all her symptoms in about an hour.

Case 2. Mrs. L., age 27, confined to her bed for three months with nervous prostration ; suffers with globus. The least disturbance causes nervous belching such as a few minutes' talk with a friend or the receiving of a letter ; she has to be kept perfectly quiet, cannot even go to her meals, for the least exertion brings on this awful belching. There is much fear and trembling with twitching of the muscles ; spasms of the throat and constant belching ; no odor whatever, no disturbance of digestion ; cured with a few prescriptions of this remedy. Compare Ignatia ; Lachesis, Argentum nit. The menses are followed by a profuse greenish, thin, offensive leucorrrhœa, causing swelling and inflammation of the parts.

ASARUM EUROPAEUM

Menses too early, too long lasting, accompanied with violent backache ; pain in lumbar region some time before and during menses. The backache is worse than that of Puls., Kali carb, or Rhus tox. Accompanying the flow is great nervous sensibility ; cannot endure the least noise, the whole body seems too light, as if she was hovering in the air ; great nervous irritability and exaltation during menses.

Case. Mrs. B., an undersized, but stout, a woman of about 34 years, came to me for treatment for backache. Continuous backache, very severe during menstrual period ; she was holding her back with both hands as I came into her home. She complained that the pain was awful and she could not endure it a moment longer. She was indeed in agony with it ; could scarcely take a full breath. The flow was dark, clotted, with colicky pains ; she was so nervous that the rattling of a paper or the least noise would set her wild. The backache grew better, she said, as the menses appeared. On examination of the uterus, it was found to be retroverted considerably. Asarum cured this case ; the backache did not return at next menses. It is followed well by Bismuth.

AMBRA GRISEA
(Anti-psoric)

Menstruation too early too profuse ; appears a week before the time. Between the periods, discharge of blood in small quantities. Mental condition : Great restlessness with extreme nervousness ; talks hastily, jumps from one subject to another ; mind weak, forgetful ; spells of mental excitement followed by great depression ; the presence of strangers aggravate all her symptoms ; vicarious menstruation from the nose ; *great weariness on awaking in the morning* ; frequent urination of sour-smelling urine; urine burns, smarts, produces itching and titillation of vulva ; menses produce soreness, itching and swelling of the vulva ; this itching of the pudendum becomes violent during the menses. Aggravations.—Music, touching hair or scalp, lying down in a warm place ; adapted to thin people or people who are prematurely old and of a nervous, bilious temperament. Many of her symptoms are better by open air or by walking (Puls).

AMMONIUM MURATICUM

This is a pseudo-psoric remedy and adapted to fat and sluggish or fleshy, large women who are indolent. The menses are premature, profuse, dark, black, clotted (Ammonium carb.). She has contractive and compressive pain in the small of the back; flow < at night and on lying down; choleric symptoms at the menses as in Ammonium carb. During menses, great exhaustion with labor-like pains in abdomen and small of back, with frequent urging to urinate, menses accompanied with diarrhœa, nausea, vomiting, pressure and contraction in abdomen, afterwards with pain in the feet, and much languor and weakness in the lower extremities. The mind is apprehensive, gloomy, not inclined to talk; stools hard, crumbling; menses flow freely during stool.

Aggravations. Night, 2 p. m., and during menses. (Puls, Phos.).

AMMONIUM CARBONICUM

This is a true pseudo-psoric remedy, it has the hemorrhage of that miasm, and is indicated in fleshy women who lead a sedentary life. About the time of the menstrual period there is an inclination to weep, as in pulsatilla; she has a tendency to faint, often feels faint; all her discharges are acrid—the saliva, tears, urine, leucorrhea, menses, etc. Her tendency to faint is due to enfeeblement of the heart.

The menses are premature, abundant, dark, clotted, blackish clots, (Magnesium carbonate, Crocus sativus, Sabina), acrid, excoriating; flow < at night, when standing, or after riding in the cold air. Before menses the face is pale with a tendency to faint; griping, pains, like colic, violent pains in small of back between scapula; choleraic symptoms at beginning of menses (Veratrum alb., Arsenicum alb., Capsicum, Viburnum Bovista). Great fatigue in whole body, especially in thighs, with yawning and chilliness, and pains in small of back; violent cutting pains in abdomen. The sleep is full of dreams, dreams of dead people, of the dying, danger, ghosts, and all sorts of offensive things (Lachesis). Great swelling of external genitals due to acrid discharges; sensation of soreness and rawness in whole pelvis, worse at 3 A. M.; it has weakness of chest like Stannum. It is inimical to Lachesis.

Aggravation: Cold air, wet weather and washing.

Amelioration: Dry weather, and lying on abdomen (Pulsatilla).

ABSINTHIUM
(Wormwood)

This remedy when first taken has a very pleasant and soothing effect. It contains a volatile oil (Absinthol) upon which its activity largely depends. It effects especially the central nervous system and produces symptoms closely resembling epilepsy, twitching of the muscles, especially of the face, clonic and tetanic spasms of muscles; cries out; grinds the teeth, urine passes involuntarily; salivation; convulsions followed by a period of unconsciousness. After epileptic attacks no recollection of them. It is one of the remedies that will bring on the menses, its dysmenorrhea begins with darting pains in uterus and ovaries, followed by trembling all over the body, and with epileptic spasms and stupor (similar to alcohol, Belladonna, Hyoscyamus, Stramonium).

AESCULUS HIPPOCASTANUM

This remedy is indicated in the pseudo-psoric as well as the sycotic miasms. The hemorrhoids of the remedy are found in the tubercular diathesis, and are often worse at the menstrual period; especially in those patients with abdominal plethora and portal congestion. It is very markedly a venous remedy. Great weakness across the sacro-iliac region, with a constant backache across the hips, a sacral backache, with a throbbing behind the symphysis pubis. The backache is aggravated by walking or stooping. The pain is often a severe aching, a sensation as if the back would give out when walking. Hemorrhoids large, purple, painful, with cervical headache; another sensation is that of a fullness of the hands and feet during menses. This venous plethora is worse in warmth, or after a hot bath. Its congestions are all venous. The lower part of abdomen feels full and heavy before and during her menses. Varicose veins are common in this remedy. The bowels are sluggish, constipated with hemorrhoids; sensation of sticks or splinters in rectum; this latter has always been considered a leading symptom, but I have found the same under Sulphur. A dry, full, aching, uncomfortable feeling in the rectum is more like Aesculus. The mind is gloomy, despondent, irritable. It has many gouty pains, showing the sycotic element.

Aggravations: Walking, stooping, hot bathing, warmth in general.

Ameliorations: Quiet, rest, and cool air.

AGARICUS

Agaricus is a syco-psoric remedy, it is adapted to light-haired women with lax skin and muscles. This is one of the strange and peculiar acting remedies; many of its symptoms are spinal or reflex in their character. Its reflexes are manifested by twitchings, jerkings and tremblings of the body even to chorea. All sorts of abnormal sensations are present during the menses; strange feelings and sensations, as of a cold, of heat, of insects crawling over the body, a sensation as of hot needles entering the flesh, as of stinging, burning, itching, pricking, and tingling, especially on the extremities. Menstruation is profuse with titillation in the genital organs and strong desire for sexual embrace. The flow is sometimes attended with very severe pains in the back and abdomen, which are pressing and tearing; itching and burning of the ears or of the feet, like frost-bite; palpitation of the heart during menses; twitching of the facial muscles; great sensitiveness of the spinal column; at every turn of the body, pain in the spine ; nervous symptoms worse while awake and better when asleep. Spinal irritation often due to sexual excesses; whole mind is sluggish, stupid at times; cannot remember; co-ordination of muscles bad; drops things, and is clumsy, similar to Pulsatilla and Sepia in its menstrual symptoms. The heart, spinal and chest symptoms are worse during the menses.

Aggravations : Eating, motion, cold air, mental work, coition, and before a thunder-storm. (Phosphorus).

APIS MELLIFICA

Menses diminished or suppressed with congestion of the head, or of the ovaries. Flow intermittent, scanty, dark, mixed with mucus. Before menses, congestion of blood to head and stinging pain in right ovary; eruptions like bee stings (urticaria) ; sharp, cutting pain in uterus and right ovary; often œdema with the urticaria or œdema of the lower limbs and feet, incidental anasarca; much tenderness over region of uterus. Menorrhagia attended with bearing down pains, heaviness in abdomen, yawning and faintness, red blotches or maculae like bee stings. Stinging in region of ovaries, restlessness, irritability, constantly changing position. (Rhus tox., Arsenicum, Aconitum.) Irritable, jealous, constantly changing occupation; awkward, breaks things, drops things from her hand and then laughs about it.

Case 1. Swelling of lower extremities; bag-like swellings under eyes; stinging, cutting pain in right ovary. Eye-lids much swollen; œdematous, skin pale, clear, transparent, no thirst, better in cool air or by bathing the eruption in cool water. Eruption itches and stings; urine dark, smoky, and scanty.

Case 2. Severe stinging pain in right ovary; very sensitive to touch; œdema about the face and eyes, red spots upon the skin which come at every menstrual period (Dulcamara). She is very awkward and let things fall, often breaking them. Tips of ears red and swollen; skin dry and hot for a short time, then perspires freely; urine scanty, dark, like beer; mucous menses; much tenderness of left ovary; labia swollen and sensitive.

ALOE SOCOTRINA

This remedy is adapted to phlegmatic women. The menses are too early, too profuse, long lasting and exhausting. Uterine hemorrhages occurring in women who are nervous. Flow is dark red, clotted and there is fullness and heaviness in the uterus or in the rectum, with a feeling as if she must go to stool, choleraic form of dysmenorrhea; muscus stools with much straining; stool often involuntary with escape of much flatus, rumbling and gurgling in abdomen before stool; dysentery during menses with fullness and weight, and dragging in pelvis, worse when standing; pain in small of back, and pressing down in rectum with hemorrhoids which protrude during menses.

Aggravations. Morning, hot weather, or cool nights and hot days, eating, drinking, standing, walking, and during the autumn.

Ameliorations. Cold bathing of parts affected; passing of stool or flatus.

APOCYNUM CANNABINUM

Dysmenorrhea with general dropsy; flows begins with drowsiness and headache; great irritability of the stomach with vomiting; flow expelled with large clots, with bloating of the abdomen and general anasarca; general or local dropsy with profuse urination; œdema of the feet.

ARGENTUM NITRICUM

Menses too profuse and usually too long lasting; mental symptoms predominate; all mental symptoms aggravated during menses. Patient complains of palpitation of the heart; pulsation all over the body (Actea). Desire for open air (Puls.); trembling all over the body; great fear when alone, with nervous trembling and palpitation of the heart; patient feels anxious; sensation of trembling internally; wants to eat or drink or do all things in a hurry, tremulous weakness with great general debility; much flatulence with rumbling of gas in the abdomen; great fear at night when she awakes; labor-like pains in abdomen at beginning of flow. Metrorrhagia at change of life or in young widows and those who have not borne children. She is always in a hurry, for time passes too slowly for her; great desire for sweets (Sulp.); stomach feels full of gas as if it would burst; great debility and weariness of the lower extremities.

Case. Profuse flow of menses, with cutting pains in small of back and groins; great nervous excitement and trembling all over the body; fears she will lose her mind; is afraid to be alone; time passes too slowly; is in a hurry to do everything; can't wait for the nurse to bring her anything; retroversion of the uterus; dizzy, confused; head feels enlarged; much nervous sneezing and belching of gas; gas forms faster than she can belch it. (Asafoetida).

ANGUSTURA

Menses delayed, menses appeared with pressure in the right ovary and a sensation of swelling in the uterus; complains of lame feeling in sacrum; difficult to stoop down; all symptoms better when the flow appears, yellowish or milky-white leucorrhœa before menses appear (Kali carb.). Large pustules on labia; itching and tickling sensation on labia before menses, itching and swelling of the genitals, compelling her to scratch, better by cold bathing. This remedy was proven by Hahnemann, yet it is seldom used in practice.

Case. Weariness in lower limbs before the appearance of the flow; lame feeling in the sacrum; stiffness after sitting, like rhus tox. Milky leucorrhœa before menses, better by cold bathing; uterus feels swollen.

Aggravations. Before menses, and at 3 P. M. Leucorrhœa relieved by cold bathing (Alum.). Given some times after Puls.

BARYTA CARBONICA

Menses scanty, too short, lasts but a day; preceded often by a toothache, and a pinching colic. Flow often resembles bloody mucus; the principle pain is described as a bruised pain in the back; sensation of weight over the pubic arch; heaviness in feet and lower extremities.

Case. Ella W., age 17, stout, thick-set, scrofulous; cervical glands enlarged and hard; always chilly; never warm enough; weak physically, although she appears very strong; very offensive foot sweat, only palliated by Psorinum; profuse leucorrhœa before menses, bloody mucus; great weariness of mind and body during the flow, with constant desire to lie down; toothache before and during menses; suitable to thick set dwarfish women.

BELLADONNA

Most Belladonna patients are pseudo-psoric or have a tubercular taint; menses are too soon and copious, or tardy and scanty; often indicated in congestive dysmenorrhea in what appears to be typical Calcarea carb. patients. Flow is bright red, hot, with congestion to head; menses with acute febrile attacks and congestion; rush of blood to face and head. Menses begin often with high fever, congestive headaches, bearing down pains, pressing down in abdomen; very suitable to young, plethoric subjects. Pains are cutting, colicky, bearing and pressing downward in pelvis; pains paroxysmal, spasmodic, and severely acute. Pressing in genitals as if everything would be pressed out (Sepia); worse sitting, and better standing or walking; pains come and go quickly; back aches as if it would break, pains go straight through from front to back, reverse to Sabina (Sepia, Plat., Berb., pains go around).

Concomitants, mental symptoms; nervous, anxious; tries to escape, laughs, cries, sings, tears clothing, bites, strikes; over-excitability of all her senses; starting as if frightened; face red, flushed, hot, glowing; just as she drops off to sleep starts up with a jerk (Ign.), frightened, delirious, sings, shouts, talks incessantly in delirium of fever; drowsy, sleepy stupid in fever with twitchings of muscles and startings in sleep; pupils dilated, eyes glassy, sparkling bright; face red, hot; great dryness of mouth, desire for frequent sips of water during fever, often a dry spasmodic cough.

Case 1. Jessie L., age 15, inclined to be fleshy, had a severe chill followed by high fever and a severe congestive headache; face flushed, red, glowing, carotid throbbing, pulse very rapid, skin is dry and hot.

Case 2. Mary B., age 20, took cold from sitting in a cold schoolroom during menstrual period. She had a severe chill, accompanied with severe backache and suppression of flow followed with high fever and active delirium.

BORAX

This is a pseudo-psoric and anti-psoric remedy; menstruation premature and profuse; suppression with great nervousness. Patient is very anxious and nervous about trifling things; indescribable feeling within that is greatly aggravated by a downward motion, as descending an elevation, a stair or in an elevator; will walk down many flights of stairs rather than go in an elevator; even rocking produces a nervous excitable state (Nat. carb.). It has cured membranous dysmenorrhea; sometimes it has violent labor-like pains during the flow. Pain extends sometimes from stomach to small of back or it has stitching pains in thighs. Pains keep up until membrane is expelled, which is often long after flow begins.

Concomitants: During menses, lassitude; throbbing in head and rushing in ears; very nervous, starts at least noise; dreads downward motion; menses followed by leucorrhœa like white of egg, or albuminous, starchy leucorrhœa. Leucorrhœa often midway between the menstrual periods, or about the time of ovulation. Sterility from leucorrhœa. Borax has as profound an action upon the female genital organs as Pulsatilla. It is a much neglected remedy, however, and is indicated in lax constitutions and sensitive nervous women.

Aggravations : Downward motion, rocking, sudden noises, cold damp weather, at menstruation.

Ameliorations : Pressure, holding the painful part.

Case : Mary L., age 30, has suffered with painful menstruation all during her menstrual nisus; passes shreds of membrane every other menstrual period; suffers great pain; always has a sore mouth during and before flow begins; extremely nervous during that time. I had given this patient a number of remedies with but little relief; finally, during one of her visits at my office, she spoke of dreading to go down the elevator unless someone held her steady, an indescribable feeling that came over her so that she could not enter the elevator car alone. Borax 1m cured in a few months.

BOVISTA

Syco-psoric as well as pseudo-psoric. Menstruation too often; every two weeks in some cases; too scanty; flow is generally clotted, dark, (small clots), like Crocus; in a few cases the flow is delayed and profuse, but it is usually too frequent, dark and clotted, and accompanied with much pain. It is one of those remedies that has a choleraic form of dysmenorrhœa (Verat. alb., Cup., ars.). The flow often begins with diarrhœa, bearing down towards the genitals; hemorrhages or menstrual flow$<$ at night or in the early morning.

Concomitants: Lassitude during flow; soreness in the mons veneris; diarrhœa, headache, sad, despondent, gloomy, sensitive, moody, and easily vexed. *Nausea, vomiting with urging towards the genitals, much urging and tenesmus while moving; diarrhœa when flow begins; relieved when flow is well established.* "Heart feels enormously enlarged with oppression of chest and palpitation after a meal or during menstruation." (Farrington) (Croc., Verat, Trill, Secale, Ustil, all of which have uterine engorgement).

Case: Lila B., age 19, brunette, vivacious, lively, active, pleasant and agreeable disposition; unmarried; is perfectly well during the month, but suffers much during the menstrual flow; flow is dark, clotted, worse in the early morning; diarrhœa before the flow or as long as the uterine pains continue. Bovista c. m. a few doses given during the flow for four or five months produced a complete cure.

BERBERIS VULGARIS

Syco-psoric; menses scanty, intermittent, of too short duration, accompanied with labor-like pains beginning in lower uterine region; much chilliness; pain in the limbs and in region of the kidneys; severe pains in the sacrum and loins; menstrual flow often of a greyish color, bloody or slimy mucus. After the flow, great weariness; vagina hot, sensitive, dry; soreness of the labia, vagina often sore and painful. Leucorrhœa albuminous.

19 F.B.

Concomitants: Sleepy, tired, desire to lie down during the day; stools hard like sheep's dung; burning in anus; sharp pains in the region of the kidneys; shooting, darting pains in renal region; pains run around towards the bladder; urine dark with a mealy sediment; feeling of stiffness in back so that it is difficult for her to rise from a sitting position; adapted to women with renal troubles; backache worse when lying in bed; pains persistent, continuous; complexion pale, dark circles about the eyes; rheumatic and gouty complaints; tertiary Sycosis; gouty state of the bladder (Benzoic acid); acts well I find after Bryonia. Its general aggravation is motion, or jolting in car or carriage. It comes in between Kali, carb and Bryonia.

BURSA PASTORIS
Proving by Fincke

Menses protracted and profuse with violent cramps; uterine colic and pain in brests. This is one of the few remedies in which the flow is slow in starting; the second day we usually have a severe hemorrhage; flow dark, clotted, and accompanied with colic and sometimes vomiting; lots large and dark (Sabina). Constipation, stool hard and dry; sometimes the pains in uterus have bearing down character in which it resembles Sepia. It seems to me to be a remedy which comes in between Sepia and Pulsatilla, yet it has features of other remedies. Occasionally in the proving, the menses were of a bright red color when they began and when they ended were dark and clotted. Pains drawing; aching in small of back; worse sitting down; pain low down in the uterus; worse in the morning before rising and on rising. Weakness in the uterus; pain in lower back; consciousness of uterus all the time; tired faint feeling all day; bitter taste in mouth and hunger after eating. Better from cold bathing and open air.

BRYONIA

Menses dark red; too early and profuse; nose bleed during menses or in place or menses in pseudo-psoric individuals; severe headache, with nose bleed during menses; congestion of blood to head and chest, (like Bell) during the flow. Nausea on sittng up or moving about; better lying quiet; hemorrhage greatly increased on motion. Bleeding from the nose or spitting of blood in place of the menses. Constipation; stools dry, hard as if burnt. Great thirst for large drinks of cold water; dryness of lips and mouth with great thirst. Extremely irritable, gets angry at the slightest cause. Tongue dry, thickly coated white with a bitter taste. Rheumatic dysmenorrhœa with general Bryonia symptoms; pains sharp, shooting and stitching. Great congestion of the ovaries at menstrual period; flow suppressed from drinking cold water, from over-heating or over-exertion. Threatened peritonitis after suppression of the menses or metastases to internal organs, as ovarian congestion, headaches, gastritis, acute rheumatism or arthritis. Aggravations, warm room, motion and in the morning.

BROMIUM

Pseudo-psoric; flow premature and copious of the bright red blood; hemorrhage with much exhaustion; membranous dysmenorrhea; contraction or constrictive like spasms in the abdomen; great soreness of the abdomen following the attacks. The contractions are at the beginning or commencement of flow ; pain in the abdomen and small of back, with discharge of pure, red blood and membranous shreds; gas passes from the vagina during flow; passes with a loud noise like Lycopodium. She has vertigo from looking at running water like Ferrum; sensation of spiders web on face (Mag. carb.) ; ovary hard and swollen; much hoarseness and rawness in the throat. Adapted to fair, light haired women with blue eyes.

BUFO

Dysmenorrhea with burning in the ovaries, or in both uterus and ovaries; occasionally extending to the external genital organs. The malignant conditions and carcinomatous pains (like Arsenicum) burn like fire. All its discharges are very offensive, horribly so; spasms or epileptic attacks during menses. All these symptoms are worse just before or during menses. In Bufo we have a wonderful remedy for the malignancies arising from the mixed miasms Pseudo-psora and Sycosis; all of its diseases are of a low form. Aggravations, warm room, putting feet in warm water; better in cool air.

CINNABARIS

This is a syco-syphilitic remedy, indicated in mixed Syphilis, or where both venereal diseases are present, (Thuja, Nit. acid, Medorrh.) especially where condylomata are present. At menstruation she suffers with an intense frontal headache; during and before menses increased flow of saliva or copious flow of urine; aching in small of back, and bruised feeling in the spine; cramps in the bowels; diarrhœa and much prostration; fullness in the throat with desire to swallow; great lassitude and prostration with a feeling of lameness all over the body. Indicated in syco-syphilitic or syco-tubercular patients, where there are bleeding warts or discharging condylomata. She has a sanguine temperament, and is aggravated at night, and by touch. Her headache is better from pressure.

COLOCYNTHIS

Syco-psoric. Suppression of menstruation from chagrin or anger. All its pains are crampy or colicky. Severe crampy pains during menses, causing her to draw her limbs up to abdomen; pain in left ovary as if squeezed in a vice; colicky pains in abdomen coming on in paroxysms, doubling her up and increasing in severity. Severe cutting in abdomen, better by hard pressure with the hand and worse by gentle pressure; better from heat, such as hot applications, hot plates or fomentations. When the uterine pains are at their height, nausea and vomiting come on. Pains are clutching as if the parts were grasped by a hand (Cactus).

Case 1. Miss B., aged 20, weight about 140; found her lying in bed with her limbs drawn up, with a hot plate over abdomen, and was pressing down upon the plate with all her strength. She was moaning and groaning with pain; every now and then she would raise up, lean forward, and press with her hands upon the abdomen. Menses had just made their appearance. Colocynthis 30th potency relieved her in a few minutes, and she resumed her housework in a few hours.

Case 2. Alice H., age 40, widow. Found her suffering with severe colicky pains in lower abdomen while menstruating. These pains were cutting colicky, came in paroxysms, increasing in severity, and when pains were at their height she had nausea; was better from heat and pressing over the affected parts. She had diarrhœa with yellowish, watery stools, and bowels began to move when pains became severe.

CUPRUM METALLICUM

Anti-psoric and pseudo-psoric. Menses too late and too protracted. Suppression of foot sweat or sweat in general. Before the menses, violent palpitation of the heart; dyspnœa, rush of blood to the head, nausea, vomiting, purging, and convulsive motion of the limbs, with spasms of the muscles, cramps in limbs and abdomen. Menses with nausea and vomiting. Vomiting is relieved by a drink of cold water; reverse of Arsenicum, taste in mouth metallic; face pale or bluish; lips blue or earthy color. Choleraic dysmenrrhœa; spasms, contractions and convulsions of the muscles. Tonic contractions of hands and feet; limbs drawn up violently, cries out when spasms come on; dysentery with rice-water discharges; face a picture of fear; fear of death (Ars.); spasms often begin in fingers and toes. Hysterical and nervous symptoms often a marked feature. Indicated in young girls just beginning to menstruate (Aconite, Bell., Puls., Nux. Verat Album, Gel., Bovis), or those who have menses suppressed getting wet in rain, or from going in bathing and remaining in too long; anæmic and chlorotic states.

CINNAMONUM

Menses regular, or too early and profuse. "This," says Dr. Minton, "is one of the best general remedies that I know of for postpartum hemorrhages, especially if the flow is sudden, profuse and of a bright red color." (Ipec., Bell., Mill., and Sabina). It stands high as a remedy when the hemorrhage is due to lifting, or when there is a threatened miscarriage, caused by a strain in the loins, or from a sudden jar to the body, from a false step.

The flow is bright red, arterial blood. It has nausea while riding in a carriage (Coccu). It is one of the best remedies for the vomiting of pregnancy, after lifting or straining. She vomits mucus (Hydr.), has much nervousness and hysteria, and is better by eructation of gas. (Asaf.).

CANTHARIS

This is an anti-sycotic remedy and its whole sphere of action portrays that miasm. The menses are dark, even black, retarded, and often copious. The pains are of a burning nature and are almost always accompanied with irritation of the neck of the bladder and vesical tenesmus. Uterine hemorrhages with straining and vesical tenesmus, or in other words membranous dysmenorrhœa with severe dysuria, burning in the vulva and vagina, and pain in the region of the kidneys, with painful urination.

Concomitants : Anxious, restless, head hot, with much mental sufferings (Ars.) often ending in rage ; in the sexual sphere there is amorous frenzy with shameless gesticulations ; complexion sallow or pale, sickly looking. Constant desire to urinate, passing but a few drops at a time ; urine bloody, turbid and scanty, with burning and smarting in neck of bladder after urination.

Case 1. A violent itching and burning in vagina ; extremely painful urination, screams when urine passes, says it is as hot as fire, menses dark and clotted; she was a recently married woman who had contracted gonorrhœa from her husband. Cantharis 1m cured.

Case 2. Mrs. A. B., age 30, dark complexion, severe burning in neck of bladder; much bearing down in uterus with a burning pain in the left ovary; pruritus vulva; strong sexual desire; severe pains in the region of the kidneys with frequent desire to urinate; desire comes on with the pains in the back. The urine was not examined in this case. Relief in a few hours after taking the c. m. potency in water. This potency I made myself with a gravity potentizer.

Aggravation: Touching the larynx (Lach.), bright light (Stram., Bell.,), drinking water; dysmenorrhea brought on by cold; indicated in disease of the bowels, bladder, lungs, brain, puerperal states, and gonorrhœa.

CUBEBA

Anti-sycotic. Menses scanty and retarded or suppressed; menses too soon; preceded by leucorrhœa, or flow consists largely of leucorrhœa, yellowish, greenish, very acrid and offensive, producing very severe erythema on inner surface of thighs; pruritus volva, or a severe urethro-vaginitis during flow; womb painful; intense desire for coition during menses; urine often albuminous and bloody. Desire for oranges, acid fruits, onions, nuts, brandy, and stimulating things. During flow dragging pains in ovaries, worse in the right ovary. This remedy acts better in bilious temperaments, in gonorrhœa of the first and second stages. It is sometimes indicated in dysmenorrhœa due to gonorrhœal poison; it affects the whole genito-urinary tract. It is worse at night, and better from motion.

CROTON TIGLIUM

Anti-sycotic. Menstruation scanty, often comes on with an exhausting diarrhœa; choleraic form of menstruation, with nausea and vomiting (Verat. alb., Cup.,). Stools watery, yellow, gushing; worse from drinking and eating. Intense itching of the genitals during menses; vesicular eruption on external, genital organs during menses (Rhus); eruptions, burning, itching. Drawing pain in the nipple of the breast, as if something were pulling on it (Kent). Drawing pain in umbilicus or in uterus during menses. The eruption and diarrhœa often alternate, when one is better the other is worse. Intense itching of the genital organs, better by gentle rubbing and scratching. Pain from nipple through to shoulder blade when child nurses.

CROTALUS HORRIDUS

This is a sycotic remedy. It is indicated in malignant or specific cases, with anæmia, face yellow, jaundiced, pale, waxy; menses suppressed for a long time due to anæmia (Ferrum, Mang.); vicarious menstruation in a severe form; bleeding or oozing of dark fluid blood from ears, eyes, nose, gums, and teeth. Menstrual flow continuous, either dark and clotted or thin, and fluid with no tendency toclot. (Naja., Lach., Elaps., Carbo veg.). Malignancies (Conium, Ars.) and puerperal States (Secale). She bleeds from every orifice of the body as well as the uterus. Indicated in sycotic diseases, in menstrual troubles, in typhoid or low septic fevers, abortions, septic poisoning, and puerperal states.

Concomitants: Fearful dreams, of murder, dead people, grave-yards, etc. (Lach., Lac. Can.).

Face besotted looking, cadaverous; craves intoxicants; aggravation after sleep (Lach.); she sleeps into an aggravation; all discharges offensive, fluid, black, continuous, character of disease rapid and malignant.

COCCULUS INDICUS

Many of the symptoms of this remedy will be found in the pseudo-psoric patient. The menstruation is too early and too copious. There is hemorrhage when rising to the feet, the blood comes in gushes. In this remedy the menses are also very scanty, often but a few drops of black or very dark blood, and usually coagulated. There is often a leucorrhœa instead of menses. Great weakness in the back with crampy colic; spasms of the chest, and marked hysterical symptoms (Minton); menses with great nausea; extreme vertigo and spinal irritation. There is a painful pressure, with crampy pain in the chest and great nausea. Violent cramps deep in the abdomen during menses; so weak she is scarcely able to walk; *occipital headaches during menses, with vertigo nausea when rising from a recumbent position, or riding in a train or carriage*; vomits a sour substance. She has a dry, fatiguing, laryngeal cough during menses, and much dryness of the larynx. It is adapted to light haired women of a lively disposition, who are subject to uterine and nervous complaints; always full of trouble and imaginary fear. Another symptom is uterine colic, with sensation as if sharp stones were rubbing together in abdomen (Coloc.). Distention of the abdomen with sharp, cutting, contractive, colicky pains and a scanty flow; severe spasmodic pain in the neck of the uterus, with cramp like pains in the chest; fainting and nausea.

CROCUS SATIVUS

This is a syco-psoric remedy, but very markedly sycotic in its menstrual phenomena. Menses too early, too profuse, black, clotted; clots small (large, China and Sabina); sensation as if menses would make their appearance in a few hours. She has colic and dragging down in region of sexual organs. Pressing in the pudendum with great sexual excitement. Flow comes away in fibrous clots or in long strings. Flow passes dark, clotted or stringy; much commotion in abdomen during menses, not infrequently a sensation as if something alive were in abdomen (Thuja, Lyc.); abortion at third month. Mental symptoms: disagreeable mood; she sings, laughs, dances, whistles, wants to kiss everybody (Hyos.). Ill tempered, sad and anxious or full of hilarity; great debility, with palpitation of the heart; hemorrhage from any orifice of body, with or without pain; sensation when moving the head as if the brain was loose.

CINCHONA

Anti-psoric. "Indicated in stout, plethoric, robust people who have suffered from loss of blood or exhausting discharges." (H. C. Allen). Menstruation too early, very copious, dark and coagulated, or pale and watery with coagula, suppression from chagrin (Anacard.); great fullness in the uterus during menses, with pressing towards the genital organs. Severe, painless hemorrhages with prolonged vertigo; fainting often during the hemorrhages with desire to be fanned violently (gently, Carbo veg.); sight suddenly disappears, and everything becomes dark about her during severe hemorrhages. Sometimes the extremities become cold and the whole body is covered with a cold clammy perspiration; there is ringing in the ears, together with vanishing of vision, a very marked set of symptoms for china. Everything tastes bitter or sour. The veins are distended and are very blue; under the nails it is blue (Carbo veg.); blue rings around the eyes, face pale or sickly looking often of a sunken appearance with pointed nose; red lips, much thirst for cold water. She is aggravated by the slightest draft of air or touch; worse every other day, and better from hard pressure.

COLCHICUM AUTUMNALE

Anti-sycotic. Indicated in the gouty and rheumatic expressions of Sycosis, especially when the digestive process is so disturbed that the uric acid diathesis develops. Menses too early and scanty, or there may be suppression of menses during rheumatic or gouty attacks ; metastasis to the internal organs ; often suppression of the menses. It acts upon the periosteum and synovial membranes. The urine is dark, scanty, looks like beer, and has a white sediment. All the symptoms are aggravated in cold, damp weather, and are often worse on such days in summer (Dul.). She is super-sensitive to odors, especially to that of cooking foods. There is nausea from the smell of cooking food, not alone in pregnancy. Great distention of the abdomen during the menses ; colic with tenderness and soreness ; worse from cold, eating and motion. She has autumnal diarrhœa and dysentery, coming on when the nights get cool ; stools are bloody, jelly-like or white mucus with much tenesmus ; often when the stool becomes cool, it assumes a jelly-like consistency ; burning in the stomach or icy coldness with much flatulent distention ; great heaviness of the body and especially of the feet ; tired feeling in lower limbs and feet.

CICUTA VIROSA

Syco-psoric. The menses are apt to be delayed and when they do begin, they are accompanied with cataleptic attacks or spasmodic nervous affections. During menses there is a constant pain under the right shoulder blade at the inner border (Chelidon); sensation of coldness in the occiput ascending from the nape of the neck; complexion sallow or jaundiced; taste bitter, tongue coated yellow; choking in the throat as from hasty swallowing; dry, hollow, spasmodic cough; sensation as if something were about the throat, or as if a fish-bone were in the throat (Hepar). Epileptic or choreic convulsions during menses, violent, with fearful distortion of the limbs, loss of consciousness with opisthotonus, renewed by the slightest touch or jar. Quite often the spasmodic symptoms calling for this remedy arise from injuries to the head or from suppressed eruptions. Aggravated by touch. (See mental symptoms and desires in Dr. Kent's Materia Medica, pages 410 and 411.)

COCCUS CACTI

Syco-psoric. Menstruation too early, and too profuse. This is another hemorrhagic remedy. This patient passes large clots, has sudden suppression of menses about the second day, with some form of vicarious menstruation; profuse spitting of dark blood when menses cease; urging to urinate during menses, with passage of large black clots. There is a brick-dust-like sediment in urine (Sepia, Phos., Lithium carb.). Burning, throbbing, or shooting pains in the pudenda during menses. Pudenda extremely sensitive and tender. She cannot bear pressure of napkin over the parts (Lach, Plat.).

great hunger with empty eructation ; great lassitude and weakness with tendency to perspire from least exertion. General action upon mucous membranes, larynx, urinary tract, and nervous system.

CYCLAMEN

Menses too frequent and too copious ; they may also be suppressed or scanty and painful. The discharge is black, clotted and occasionally membranous. The pains are labor-like and attended with distention of the bowels ; patient feels better during the flow (Puls., Actea, Sep., Lach., and Sulp.). She is worse in the cold air ; weeps during menses but it does not afford her any relief (reverse of Puls.). Menses suppressed, with vertigo, headache, melancholia, palpitation of the heart, loss of appetite and desire to be alone. After menstruation the mammae swell and secrete milk; membranous dysmenorrhœa in blonds. Leuco-phlegmatic patients who are subject to fainting spells and great chilliness during the menses. Dull vertical or occipital headache which is better by bathing with cold water. Tongue is coated white ; taste putrid or flat ; sensation as if air streamed from nipples. She is aggravated in the evening and from rest, cold, sitting down, open air, exercise, and fatigue. Is better when walking and from warmth.

CONIUM MACULATUM

Conium is a deep acting remedy. It cures even where all the miasms are present, but it fits especially into those cases where the presence of the acquired sycotic element induces a malignancy. For instance a wife contracts Sycosis from her husband ; the uterus becomes envolved and she is treated locally by medicated lotions, or what is more probable she has been curetted for a subinvolution due to Sycosis, and from this, cancer develops. Conium comes in early when the hemorrhages begin to show themselves, or a continuous bloody discharge which is extremely offensive. Menstruation too early and feeble, or too late and scanty. The discharge is dirty, offensive, brownish colored blood. The menses and most of the complaints of this remedy are painless. The glands become involved, early in most diseases. Symptoms, trembling, weakness with vertigo, vertigo worse on turning over in bed ; mentally she is sad, gloomy, depressed, unhappy, takes very little interest in things. She is slow in her movements, passive, often her symptoms border on the paralytic. During the menses the breasts swell, become sore and tender, hard, often painful. The flow excoriates the external genitals producing severe pruritus. She dreads to be alone, avoids society, very easily excited, has loss of memory early in the disease (Natrum mur.). Face earthy, sallow, pale, or sickly looking. This remedy is adapted to women of rigid fiber, nervous and easily excited, to old maids' troubles during the menopause, in indurations, and malignancies.

COCA

Pseudo-psoric. Menses flows in gushes, < at night ;

it awakes her at night. She has loud ringing and buzzing in the ears during the menses (China); nervous prostration, voice weak, palpitation of the heart from flatulence; trembles with weakness following nervous depression from over-work; mental anxiety; sexual excesses. Great lassitude and weariness during the menses. Indicated in very nervous, plethoric women; great nervous erethism, with timidity, melancholy, and nervous exhaustion. "It implants buoyancy; cheers the heart, brightens the mind, and renews the bodily strength for the vigorous tasks of life." (Hering Guiding Symptoms).

CHIMAPHILA UMBELLATA

From a careful study of the pathogenesis of this remedy we find it is well adapted to sycotic troubles; indeed its pains and aches call our attention at once to the sycotic taint. The mammary symptoms show that even if all the chronic miasms be present, it would still prove the curative remedy. Menses suppressed, followed by cancer of the mammae or uterus. Flow copious, offensive and accompanied with large lumps in breast, enlarged glands. Great dysuria during menses, suppressed menses with atrophy of the breasts. Ulcers in mouth during menses; urine bloody, ropy, dark, and clotted. On sitting down, sensation as if a ball pressed against perineum. This remedy is indicated in lymphatic women with a tubercular or strumous diathesis, who are affected with acquired Sycosis in the tertiary stage. Toothache during menses relieved by cold water (Coff. Sepia.). May follow Cistus canadensis.

CHAMOMILLA

This is a true anti-sycotic remedy ; it follows all the expressions and actions of that miasm, whether physical or mental ; from infancy to old age, we see the sycotic element present. A typical sycotic patient will have symptoms resembling those of this remedy very much, especially in women and children. They are cross, irritable, extremely sensitive to pain, to impressions, to persons, and to their surroundings in general. We see this clearly in its colicky stool, mental states, dentition, and sufferings of every description. Menstruation early, profuse, clotted, dark, often offensive. There are clutching, cramping pains in the uterus, sometimes these pains are violent, or they seem so to the patient, who is one who cannot endure pain (Coffea). She is irritable and quarrelsome. The pains are followed by the passage of large clots and the pains make her angry, hot, thirsty, and fretful. Toothache during the menses is a common symptom ; eructations and diarrhœa with green, watery stools with much colic, are present. This remedy is indicated in very nervous excitable women with brown or light hair. Pains < at night or before midnight.

CARBO VEGETABILIS

This remedy may either have profuse or scanty menses, pale or dark in color, or they may be thick, corrosive, and of a pungent odor. During the menses there is a drawing pain from abdomen to small of back, swelling of the pudenda with much itching and burning in vulva. The menses, like those of Carbo animalis, are accompanied with an excoriating, thick, milky or yellowish-green leucorrhœa. This remedy is indicated often in prematurely old women, and at or about the menopause, or when menstruation is prolonged beyond the regular period ; odor from menstrual discharge, carrion like and very offensive ; knees cold all the time ; desire to be fanned when the pains are severe. (China).

CARBO ANIMALIS

This remedy is one of the most profound and deep acting of the carbon group. It is more frequently indicated than we think for. It should be carefully studied ; in exhausting diseases, it spends its force largely upon the venous system, and almost all of the diseases for which it will be called, will present venous congestion. All its diseases are sluggish, and most of its inflammations show dark purplish venous involvement. Menses too copious, and prolonged, premature ; sometimes the flow is pale, but generally it is a thin, dark, fluid, acrid, ichorous, and excoriating ; exceedingly protracted menstrual period ; she seems to sink down to almost death's door at each monthly flow.

Concomitants : Aphtha often appear upon the external organs during the flow ; itching, soreness, burning, smarting in vulva and anus. Burning in the hands and feet (Sulphur, Phosphorus); desire to be fanned during all its hemorrhages (Carbo veg., China); knees and extremities often cold, with heat or rush of blood to head and face. The face is often greyish-yellow or greenish, or there is great pallor, eructations frequent and violent (Lyc., Carbo veg., Argent, nit.); morning and evening aphonia; flow very offensive, often carrion-like. Indicated in low physical states of the system at the climacteric period; cancerous and malignant affections, old age, advancing senility, enfeebled circulation, with lack of vital heat.

COFFEA CRUDA

Coffea is an anti-psoric remedy. Menses too profuse, long-lasting, dark in color, and attended with great nervous excitement, excessive sensitiveness of the sexual organs with voluptuous itching; great exaltation of the senses; with nervous excitement there are mental symptoms only. Great hyperesthesia of all the senses, hearing, sight, smell, touch; they are all extremely acute. She is full of fanciful ideas and has an excited and exalted imagination. Her pains and all her symptoms are mentally magnified; a mole-hill becomes a great mountain. Her troubles come on from over-joy, excessive laughter, anger, disappointed affections, fright, or from coffee drinking. During menses she whines, moans; is afraid she will die; weeps with her complaining (Puls.,

Ignatia), her pains are unbearable, with great mental excitability. She has severe paroxysms of colic, great insomnia during menses. lies awake all night, can give no cause for it, simply an inability to close the eyes and go to sleep. This remedy is adapted to nervous sanguine women. She is aggravated by touch, contact, motion, and open air.

CAUSTICUM

The menstrual flow is bright red, hot, delayed, flows feebly and in the daytime only. Flow ceases when lying down. Before the menses there is great weakness; cramp-like pains in the sides and back; great melancholy and sadness during the menses (Nat. mur.). Complexion very sallow. She has a sensation as if the scalp were too tight; eyes feel weak, can scarcely hold the lids open; great aversion to sweet things and to fresh and smoked meats. Urine passes involuntarily when coughing and laughing. There is often aphonia during the menses. She is extremely sensitive to noise and touch and is easily startled. Generally she is ameliorated by heat and aggravated by dry weather. Great mental and physical fatigue; must lie down during menses; severe cramp-like pains in the back just before the flow begins.

CALCAREA PHOSPHORICA

Calcarea phosphorica is a true pseudo-psoric remedy, it has all the weakness of its sister Calcarea carb. and has added to it, the nervous and the hemorrhagic element of Phosphorus. It is especially indicated in youth, while Calcarea carb. is indicated at any period of life. The menses as you would expect, are too frequent in yong girls, every two weeks; flow bright red; in adults the flow is apt to be dark and delayed in coming. Before menses the patient is often annoyed with rheumatic pains, or a stitching pain in the left side of the heart; drawing pains and a sore feeling in the pubic region.

Concomitants: Mental anxiety—always finding fault with others; desire to go from place to place; love-sick girls, or young women disappointed in love; headache of school girls, frontal or on the vertex, accompanied with rheumatic pains; uterine displacements with rheumatic pains, a feeling of great weakness in the sexual organs during menses; great weariness in all complaints, especially while walking or ascending stairs or a height, (Cal. carb.)

During menses great sexual desire; parts feel full of blood; pulsation in all the parts, (nymphomania); all the parts erect with insatiable desire.

Case 1. Miss B, age 18, tall, slim, weak in body, no muscular strength, face pale but flushes easily, cheeks become hot and flushed at least excitement, palms of hands sweaty, menses every two weeks, which are copious and bright red. After Cal. phos. cm. was given the menses became normal in two months and my patient has greatly improved in general health.

Case 2. Alice M, age 20, has been running down in

health all winter ; thinks her school work is too much for her. She suffers with rheumatic pains in her shoulders and arms, which are < during the menstrual period. Her muscles are soft, flabby, and have grown more so of late ; feet damp, cold and clammy, easily affected by change of weather, < at the approach of a storm ; tires very easily ; wishes to sit or lie down all the time ; leucorrhœa after menses, albuminous ; feeling of great weakness in sexual organs. 45m cured her.

Case 3. Age 16, dark hair and eyes, suffers with frequent menses, blood bright red, accompanied with drawing pains over the pubic region ; during menses weary and tired all the time. 45m. cured her.

EUPIONUM

Menses too soon, copious, thin, and fluid. During menses great irritability and disinclination to talk (Nux. Cham.); full pressive feeling in the head ; stitches in the chest ; vertigo; things suddenly become black before her. (China). Backache very severe, relieved by pressing hard against something hard, the pain extends from the back to pelvis, < stooping (Rhus.). Backache always < when leucorrhœa begins, which is acrid and exceedingly copious.

ERIGERON CANADENSES

Menses premature and profuse, accompanied with violent irritation of rectum and bladder ; often diarrhœa and dysuria at the commencement of the flow; pains spasmodic, colicky; flow profuse, bright red, and < with every movement of the body. Post-partum hemorrhage or severe hemorrhages after abortion; constant, painless flow during pregnancy. Pallor and weakness when flow is severe, bleeding from nose, gums and mouth, bright red. Severe pain in lower dorsal region during menses; low spirited and very languid. She is aggravated by motion and rainy weather.

FERRUM METALLICUM

The menses in this remedy may be either scanty and late, or profuse and too early, but we usually look to Ferrum for a copious and prolonged, pale, watery fluid. Often it is intermittent, pale, and watery, or it may be suppressed or delayed. It may come on as a flood with colicky pains and with excited circulation, flushing of the face, alternating with pallor. The patient often has the appearance of plethora in the face, but it is a false plethora. Again the face looks flushed as if she had taken stimulants. Hemorrhages followed by prolonged oozing, palpitation of the heart, more or less shortness of breath, general debility and weakness. It is a typical tubercular or pseudo-psoric remedy; all its expressions are tubercular. Menses suppressed or delayed in young girls about seventeen or eighteen who have a tubercular taint. Hectic conditions and a rapid development of pulmonary tuberculosis. The flow is often long in establishing itself. Rush of blood to the head with congestive headaches during menses. Flow ceases then returns; weariness with desire to sit or lie down. After hemorrhages, things grow dark or black before her on rising from a recumbent position; (China), vertigo on descending or on crossing a stream; hands, feet and face oedematous. She is < standing, (Sulph.); < in cold, wet weather; > from warmth, sitting or lying down, gentle motion, and is adapted to delicate chlorotic women where there is a tendency to anæmic conditions with frequent flushing of the face.

GLONOINUM

Instead of the menses, great congestion of blood to the head with throbbing and surging sensations. Tearing pains in the head; surging of blood to the heart; great disturbance of circulation during the menses; fullness in the head; sensation as if too large; face red, dark; pulse full, quick; arteries raised like cords, with throbbing in arteries; vomiting with cold extremities; face and head hot, flushed, often purple; < from heat, and after taking stimulants; > from cold applications, quiet, pressure. Adapted to florid, plethoric, sanguine, nervous temperaments, about the period of the menopause, and to disturbances and congestions of the brain with the above symptoms.

GOSSYPIUM HERBACEUM

Menses delayed, scanty, watery, accompanied with stinging pains in the ovaries and drawing pains in the uterus. Flow only lasts a day, and is watery, pale, scanty ; there is soreness in vulva and thighs when the flow is thin and watery. Pains jump from place to place ; (Cal. phos.), great uneasiness, with much sighing during the menses, sometimes nausea and vomiting. It is a remedy to be thought of in the early morning sickness of pregnancy.

GRAPHITES

Pseudo-psoric, very decidedly in all its actions. It has like all pseudo-psorics, a great tendency to hemorrhages ; often vicarious and apt to be venous. Menses delayed, retarded, scanty, thick, black and occasionally watery. Menstruation suppressed, with flow of blood from the anus. Great weariness and lassitude with heaviness of the limbs during the menses ; violent colicky pains in the epigastrium, as if torn to pieces ; heaviness and weight in the anus. Itching blotches here and there on various parts of the body ; soreness of the parts between the thighs, with blotches and pimples. Nails grow thick and crooked ; fingers cracked and fissured, bleeding or oozing a thick, honey-like, sticky serum. Skin of hands very hard, thick, dry, rough and fissured. Vicarious hemorrhages from the nose or spitting of blood in place of menses, or bleeding piles, very copious at times ; sometimes there is a burning sensation on the vertex or on soles of the feet during menses (Sulphur) ; stools large, hard, knotty, covered with a white slimy mucus (**Alum.**).

Mentally, the graphites patient is sad, despondent; thinks of death or that something dreadful is going to happen. (Actea). Anxious about her spiritual welfare. Skin cracks behind ears, lips, corners of mouth, nose, fingers, toes, etc. Taste salty, sour or bitter. All her symptoms are aggravated during menstruation or from cold, except the skin symptoms. Adapted to tubercular women when there is a tendency to obesity, skin eruptions and venous stagnation.

GELSEMIUM

Anti-sycotic. This remedy is the Aconite of the prairie country; we seldom find aconite indicated in fevers in and about Chicago. Rhus tox, Ferrum phos., or Gel., and Bell. are more often indicated in febrile conditions. Almost all its diseases have a sycotic taint and a febrile state. Menses are often greatly delayed or suppressed in this remedy. Menses with convulsions or suppressed with great aching all over the body; pain at the base of the brain; fever; muscular prostration; and a general muscular soreness, aching and lameness. Menses with congestion to the head; face red; fever high; pulse soft, slow, with sharp labor-like pains in uterine region. Menses suppressed from embarrassment, shock, fear, sudden surprises; great anticipation or excessive joy brings on menses too soon. Menses come on too soon in LaGrippe. Menses with fever, diarrhœa, red face, painful aching of the whole body; with great heaviness of the limbs, delirium; with a drowsy and sleepy condition of the senses (Bell., Opium). She is often very irritable. Menses accompanied with a wild crazy feeling in the head alternating with uterine pains; pain lingers at the back of the head or spreads over it; relieved by passing large quantities of urine (Ign.). Pain in uterus as if squeezed by the hand; complete relaxation of the whole muscular system, with trembling of the body. Adapted to nervous, rheumatic, excitable women; often indicated in people who have a tubercular taint blended with the sycotic element, whether the Sycosis be transmitted or acquired.

GRATIOLA OFFICINALIS

The menses are usually too early and too profuse, accompanied with darting pains in the chest, more especially in the right breast (Conium). There is pressure in the forehead, or a full feeling in the head; burning heat in the face, yet feet and hands are cold. Hunger yet without appetite. Cold feeling in abdomen; diarrhœa of a yellowish-green color.

HYOSCYAMUS NIGER

Anti-psoric. Menses profuse, bright, red, too late; often suppressed with muscular excitement; mental aberration and spasmodic symptoms; convulsions, and contractions of the muscles; menses begin with convulsions; jerking and twitching of the muscles. Sometimes there is fever, delirium, and great mental excitement ; she talks all the time ; is full of illusions and hallucinations ; imagines all sorts of things ; suspicious, jealous, talks or calls to imaginative people ; prays ; scolds one minute, the next laughs boisterously ; picks at the bed-clothes ; mutters to herself ; tears her clothing off ; wants to go naked ; exposes the sexual organs. In Hyoscyamus niger we have a severe maniacal form of dysmenorrhœa or amenorrhœa. The patient is violent, kicks, strikes, bites, and talks incessantly ; is lascivious or erotic. There is mania during the menses or when they are suppressed, as in exanthematous diseases. There is violent sexual desire during the flow or when brain troubles threaten. She has a short, dry, tickling cough (Rhus) ; coughs until she is exhausted, profuse discharges of pale urine during an attack ; there is great mental and nervous excitement at each menstrual period. She falls suddenly with a shriek ; is afraid of being left alone, or of being poisoned. Her eyes sparkle, twitch ; are constantly in motion ; stares as if in fear ; has constriction of the throat with inability to swallow (Lach.). This remedy is adapted to nervous, irritable, excitable subjects of a sanguine temperament ; hysterical people ; young girls soon after puberty, whose mental balance is easily disturbed. It is indicated principally in the tubercular or psoric subject.

HELONIAS DIOICA

Pseudo-psoric ands yco-psoric. Menses usually dark, flow passive, offensive, coagulated, profuse and exhausting. The pains are sharp, cutting, and extend from the uterus backward. Severe flooding at the climactric period, attended with severe uterine and ovarian pains. Indicated after excessive child bearing, and in atonic conditions of the uterus ; marked cases of subinvolution and displacements, retroversions, etc., women who are worn out with hard work ; also women who are enervated by indolence and luxury ; who suffer from prolapsus and uterine atony. Great soreness in the uterus with sensation of great weight (Sepia). Consciousness of a uterus ; a dragging weight in it ; feels it move as she moves her body. In the proving of this remedy there was great uterine hemorrhage with severe backache. Flow passive, coagulated, offensive ; complexion sallow and earthy. During menses great weariness, lassitude weakness, heaviness, languor and drowsiness. Dysmenorrhœa in delicate women of lax fiber, or who are chlorotic. She is aggravated by motion, standing during the climactric period, and by pressure of clothing, and is > when mind is engaged.

HAMAMELIS VIRGINICA

Pseudo-psoric in its action. This is a prominent venous remedy ; venous plethora ; venous stagnation ; clogging of the portal and great venous centres of the body. Menses profuse ; dark venous blood ; active in the daytime ; while the patient is moving and exciting and pushing ahead the circulation, but ceases at night when the patient is still. Passive, non-coagulable uterine hemorrhage, or a profuse steady flow of black blood. Vicarious menstruation ; varicose veins in lower extremities enlarged and very marked. Active hemorrhage ; flow bright red ; seldom any pain during hemorrhages. During menses the small of the back feels as if it would break ; tired, weary feeling in the lower extremities, due to the venous stagnation. Great lassitude and a feeling of weariness. A sore, bruised feeling in abdomen. In hemorrhages from the nose there is a tight feeling in the bridge. Taste metallic or brassy.

IODINE

Iodine meets all the miasms, and especially the tubercular and syphilitic. The menses are premature, copious, and the patient suffers much during the flow. It may, also, be too late, or retarded. When delayed the patient suffers from severe vertigo and palpitation of the heart. The flow is unusually acrid, it excoriates the thighs, and is followed by an acrid, slimy leucorrhœa. She is very hungry during the menses. There is great weariness that is aggravated by going up stairs or ascending a height (Cal. c.). She has hemorrhages with cutting pains in abdomen, and aching in the back and loins ; pains extending from right ovary to uterus ; ovary very painful and sensitive during menses. During the menses the breasts are much smaller than usual (reverse Con.) Leucorrhœa always < at menstrual period Mentally she is sad, and of a melancholy mood ; feels as if she had forgotten something ; very irritable ; constantly moving about. Face dark, brownish, spotted like Sepia. Indicated in tubercular diathesis more especially. There is great irritability of the whole nervous system ; rapid failing of strength, a chronic slow form of emaciation, and a low cachetic state of the system. She is > after eating and when in motion, always hungry, and < when quiet, or when the weather is hot.

IGNATIA

Anti-psoric. Menses too early ; discharge offensive, dark, coagulated ; this is more especially true after great mental sorrow, grief, or fright. Suppression from grief, great joy, or unexpected bad or good news. It is one of the heart-breaking remedies. It often meets the nervous state that comes as a reaction from overjoy or sorrow. It is indicated in those highly sensitive women who readily take on hysterical manifestations ; they seem all right until they are stirred up mentally, and have any unusual mental strain, then they go all to pieces. They have, in other words, the hysterical diathesis ; overmental efforts bring about in them an ignatia state. During menses they have a uterine spasm or a crampy pain which is > by pressure. The patient is constantly sighing, often weeping ; the slightest contradiction irritates her ; she has difficulty in swallowing as if there was a lump in her throat ; has nervous sore throat ; is peevish, fretful, irritable, yet weeps easily. Her symptoms are constantly changing from mental to physical and from physical to mental. She has all sorts of vivid fancies ; < when crossed or contradicted ; < often at menstrual period after having company, or from least excitement. She often has hysterical insanity (Hyos. true insanity) ; she trembles ; has twitching of the muscles ; complains of empty feeling in stomach ; is constantly sighing and complaining ; is full of dread, fear, anxiety, apprehension, and all sorts of imaginary troubles. She is > from quiet, rest and warmth ; and when this remedy ceases to act we think of Natrum mur.

KALI BICHROMICUM

Great anxiety and timidity before the menses ; easily frightened and apprehensive. Flow ropy, with tenacious mucus in it ; swelling and itching of the vulva. Sometime the flow is accompanied with nausea and vomiting of sour food, giddiness and rush of blood to the head. The menses come occasionally with severe headaches, that begin with blindness ; adapted to fleshy, light-haired, blue-eyed women.

KALI IODATUM

Syphilo-psoric. Menses late ; begin with chilliness ; icy coldness of hands and face ; severe shuddering ; colic, diarrhœa, cramps and severe squeezing pain running down the thighs. Aching pains as if bruised in groins and small of back; constant urging to urinate, which ceases when flow begins. Saliva copious, often bloody, viscid and smells like onions. Severe pains in the bones, which are $<$ at night and $>$ from heat; $>$ from motion and $<$ from rest.

IPECACUANHA

Anti-psoric and pseudo-psoric. Often indicated in the gastric irritation of tubercular patients and in their hemorrhages. Menses profuse, premature; comes in a flood of bright red blood with nausea. Before the menses, nausea, often vomiting with pain and heat in head. Pain about the umbilicus with great nausea and vomiting. Flow profuse, bright red; with this there is some cutting pain in the umbilicus with nausea. Face pale, heat in the head; constant nausea, restlessness, general coldness; very weak, must lie down, as the nausea increases. Pain and pressure towards the uterus and rectum with great nausea and vomiting. Hemorrhage after accouchment, bright red, profuse, continuous, with nausea and vomiting.

KALI CARBONICUM

Anti-psoric and strongly pseudo-psoric. The menses are either too early, copious and long-lasting, or they are too late o suppressed with anasarca and ascites. The menses are usually pale, but may be bright or dark red; they have a pungent odor and are apt to be acrid and excoriate the parts, producing eruptions of papules or vesicles. *She feels badly a week before menses; awakes tired*, (Cal. c.) weary, with worn out feeling and constant backache. The pains are in the back and abdomen. The pain in the back as if it would break, with a tired, worn-out feeling; in the abdomen the pains are colicky or shooting. During menses awakens about 3 a. m. and does not go to sleep again. She often awakes with a severe headache, and a backache as if it would break; feels as if she had not slept. She is peevish, irritable; has sac-like swellings over the eyes; foul taste in the mouth, with bitter eructations; often nausea, rumbling in the bowels and a griping colic. Menses pale, acrid, excoriating the thighs. She is full of apprehension, sadness, timidity, and has great aversion to being alone; constipation during menses, dry, large, difficult stool (Graph.); she may have night sweats, dry, hacking or gagging cough, with scanty, viscid expectoration; stitches in the lungs with palpitation of the heart. The pale menses show the anæmic condition of the blood; the skin is usually pale looking; the blood is deficient in red corpuscles; there is a tendency to anasarca. She wishes to lie down or sit all the time; the back and limbs give out, and she seems to have no strength left in her body. Indicated in pseudo-psoric young people, who are threatened with incipient phthisis or to broken down women in advanced life.

KREOSOTUM

Menses too early, too long-lasting and copious. Before the flow begins, there is an acrid-smelling, bloody discharge which produces itching and burning of the parts passed over. The flow is usually dark, coagulated, acrid and offensive; flow intermittent, stops and starts again (Sulph.); always chilly; swelling, heat, and hardness of the labia with voluptuous itching deep in the vagina and external sexual organs. Indicated in old ladies, blond and delicate young girls who grow rapidly, and are very tall, and who have despondent and irritable dispositions.

LAC CANINUM

Anti-sycotic. Menses too frequent, profuse, bright red; when put into water forms itself into long strings; smells like ammonia; when it dries on the napkin it becomes a dark or olive green color; it washes out easily, however. A flow of bright red blood relieves a severe pain in the right ovary (Lach., Zinc.). Menstruation seems to relieve all her symptoms; she is very hysterical at other times. Bearing down or dragging sensation in abdomen with a sensation as if the contents of the pelvis would burst out above the pubes. She cannot bear any weight over the abdomen (Lach., Bell.); she is extremely despondent and hopeless during the menses; thinks she is incurable; has fearful dreams of dark water, dead people, snakes, as if surrounded by them, or as if they were running over her body. Abdomen swollen, hard, sensitive; breasts sore and sensitive, often with hard lumps in them ; flow of milk from breasts during menses (Ver. vir.). Great heat in the ovarian region during the menses ; < in the right ovary, extreme soreness and tenderness in the uterus during menses, pains as if knives or needles were darting upward from the uterus ; menses too soon, bright red, comes in gushes ; of a sticky consistency; breasts enlarged and sensitive to touch. Indicated in tertiary Sycosis and in individuals of a highly sensitive organism who are extremely nervous. The pains are erratic and the symptoms have a great tendency to shift from one side of the body to the other. She is very forgetful and absent-minded ; < from a jar or moving.

LOBELIA INFLATA

Anti-psoric. Menses too early and too profuse. It is sometimes indicated where the menses are suppressed in prolonged fevers like typhoid. During menstruation, severe pains in the sacrum with fever ; great weight and heaviness in the genital organs ; severe pains in the right side of the face and temples with retarded menses ; in consumptive patients, with neuralgia of the face. Profuse saliva with pungent taste ; dryness in the throat with frequent expectoration of frothy mucus. She gulps up a sour fluid from the stomach with incessant nausea ; nausea with a copious flow of water from the mouth. Hysterical asthma with a slight respiration or a desire to take a deep breath ; great soreness, pain and tenderness in the sacrum, with weight and pressing toward the genitals; nausea with great weakness toward the pit of the stomach, a sensation as of a lump in the throat or pit of the stomach with nervous dyspnea. All symptoms > in the evening.

LACHESIS

Menses delayed, scanty, dark, even black, lumpy, acrid; pains and general complaints > during the menses. Pains and all complaints < on the left side of the body and after sleep. Great desire for open air during the menses (Puls.); has to loosen neck bands and to have her clothing loose on her body. Hot flashes; hot spell before the menses and sometimes during; mental symptoms > during flow. The patient is apt to be suspicious and jealous. She thinks people are talking about her. The face is often flushed, hot, or mottled, spotted, purplish and puffy looking or bloated; very sensitive to pressure over uterine region or over abdomen generally.

LYCOPODIUM

This is a powerful anti-sycotic, so deep in its action that it will, when indicated, cure in almost any miasmatic state of the system even to a mixed miasm or malignancy. Menses profuse, usually late and of long duration; the flow may appear a part of the time dark and clotted, and a part of the time bright red blood mixed with serum. Great sadness and melancholia often accompany the menstrual nisus. In Lycopodium there is always much distension of the abdomen, great flatulence and accumulation of gases ; a true uric acid state of the system is presented in this remedy which usually has Sycosis as a miasmatic basis. Great fullness in abdomen from partaking of any food ; much fermentation and rumbling in abdomen ; < in the left side ; frequent eructations with rumbling of gas in abdomen ; there is a constant sense of satiety ; the least quantity of food partaken causes an uneasiness, fullness, gas, rumbling, distension, and belching. The pains are generally due to gases and distension of the colon, although we have also pains in both ovaries. Before the menses appear, there is a bearing down pain as if they would appear ; this same pain often comes on after the menses have ceased and the leucorrhœa makes its appearance. The flow as well as the leucorrhœa produces swelling, itching and burning of the pudenda. The flow is < in the afternoon after 4 p. m. Concomitants ; great dryness of the vagina ; frequent spells of shivering during the menses ; escape of air from the vagina. The patient is low-spirited, sad, desires to be alone ; she has great doubts about her salvation ; has a sallow, earthy complexion, dark rings and circles around the eyes, frequent flushes of heat to the face ; always hungry, but the least food produces discomfort in the stomach and intestines ; red sand in urine ; shortness of breath, and palpitation of the heart from the accumulation of gases in stomach and abdomen ; desire for open air (Puls.). Aggravation : 4 p. m., eating oysters, tight clothing, strong odors, cold food ; > from warm food, drinks, walking, uncovering and loose garments.

LAC DEFLORATUM

Tubercular. Menses delayed, dark, scanty, or suppressed from putting hands in cold water ; drinking a glass of milk has suppressed the flow until the next period. A drawing pain across the ovaries with a downward pressure in the uterus is said to be often present in the proving of this remedy ; menses delayed with dragging weight in the ovarian region ; great lassitude and even extreme prostration during the menses. Hemicrania every month during or after the menstrual period in pale, thin, anæmic, tubercular women, between the ages of 36 and 40. I have cured a number of such cases with this remedy. It has one of the most profound headaches in the materia medica, often lasting a week at a time. The headache begins in the forehead and extends to the occiput ; the pain is a bursting or a hard ache, sometimes throbbing ; begins early in the morning and is usually accompanied with nausea, blindness, sometimes vomiting, and is greatly aggravated by light, by sitting up and by movement ; > from quiet, lying down in the dark, and fasting. The face becomes pale, the lips white, and the breathing is prolonged and slow. She has no desire to eat or drink or to be annoyed in any way. It is relieved by profuse urination, (Gels) and by quiet, rest, pressure or bandaging tightly, and sometimes by heat. This remedy is adapted to thin, tall, tubercular women who are very anæmic and highly sensitive and nervous.

LILIUM TIGRINUM

Anti-psoric and pseudo-psoric. Menses normal as to time ; flow usually thick, dark, offensive, and < when the patient is moving about, ceases when she lies down (Kreos., Mag. carb.). During the menses great bearing down in the uterine region with a sensation when on the feet as though the whole pelvic contents would issue from the pelvis (similar to Murex, Bell, Sepia), relieved by pressure of the hand against the vulva or by sitting down ; heaviness in the region of the heart, or as if the heart were squeezed in a vice ; fluttering of the heart awakens her ; severe palpitations when lying on the left side. During menses sensation of pushing or bearing down of the uterus with a sharp pain in the left ovary extending down the anterior surface of the thigh. The bearing down in the uterus is often extended to the rectum and bladder (Nux vom., Aloe., Sepia, Bovista). Mentally she has a wild crazy feeling on vertex (Actea rac.) ; weeps easily like Puls., is tired and fearful ; again she is disposed to strike, or to curse, to do things in a hurried aimless manner ; fears to be alone ; fears that her disease is organic, and that it is incurable ; she < is after eating, standing, lying on left side ; often the crazy feeling spoken of comes up from the back of the head and finally settles on the vertex. Like Pulsatilla she wants a cool room, and likes to walk in the open air ; also aggravated by consolation (Igna., Nat. mur.), adapted to nervous, hysterical blondes who suffer from atony of the uterus, uterine displacements especially retroflection ; heart troubles due to uterine displacements, or uterine irritation. Remedies to compare with Lilium are Sepia, Belladonna, Podophyllum Platina, Helonias, Murex, Nat. Phos., Cactus and Actæ.

MAGNESIA CARBONICA

Syco-psoric. Menses too late, thick and dark ; flow < at night, or while walking or standing ; again we have the flow scanty, even suppressed; flows more in the afternoon, menses retarded ; flows in large clots. This is one of the few remedies with a flow that is < at night with absence of pain. In a typical Mag. carb. dysmenorrhœa the flow is dark, thick, acrid, often pitch-like, viscid, and is washed from the napkin with difficulty. There is a cutting pain in the uterine region or a colicky bearing-down pain with pressing towards the pelvis or a cutting in abdomen ; menses often preceded by sore-throat (Lach., Bell.) ; toothache during menses (Sepia) ; stool soft, like clay or putty, and crumbling. If diarrhœa accompanies the menses the stool is typically sycotic. Greenish, sour smelling, frothy, accompanied with a cutting colicky pain ; great restlessness and weariness during the menses ; she feels so tired (Cal. carb., Kali carb.) ; many of her symptoms are relieved when the flow is established (Lach). Face pale, sickly ; sensation of white of eggs on face, bitter, sour taste ; thirst for acid drinks, such as lemonade. She is aggravated every three weeks, by rest, during menses, and by cold air.

MAGNESIA PHOSPHORICA

Menses eight days too soon ; menstrual colic precedes the flow ; pains, cutting, drawing, pressing, cramping and intermittent. Another form of pain occurring in membranous dysmenorrhœa is shooting, like lightning flashes, comes and goes suddenly (Bell.) yet does not entirely disappear. Pains decidedly intermittent and < on the right side, also from lying down ; pains < in the lower part of the abdomen and frequent, coming in shocks, darting and paroxysmal until flow starts.

Rheumatic, membranous dysmenorrhœa. Much rheumatism or neuralgia and aching in the limbs ; tingling in different parts of the body like electric shocks ; pains often so severe as to cause fainting ; colic relieved by bending double (Colyc.), by heat or external warmth, rubbing ; a drink of cold water often starts the colic. Dull aching in the occiput extending to the brain, > by eating and from eructations of gas. Dull drawing pain in the lumbar region ; pains > by gentle and continual motion (Puls.).

MILLEFOLIUM

Millefolium is pseudo-psoric ; menstruation profuse,

of long duration, of a bright red color, and with no pain. Although the books speak of colicky pains, I have never heard these patients complain of pain. I have given it frequently to women who were markedly tubercular; some of them had a cough, but at each menstrual period they almost flooded to death; complete atony of the uterus, no pain, no contraction; flow increased by motion and exertion. The flow is always < after exertion and may be confined to the uterus, but as this is one of the hemorrhagic remedies, it has also hemorrhages from the lungs, nose and bowels all of a bright red color. There is no anxiety or alarm in this remedy, as found in many others during a severe hemorrhage. There is some oppression of the chest, and often severe palpitation of the heart. A confused, dull feeling in the head if often present and a cough with spitting of blood. It resembles Trillium, I think, more than any other in uterine hemorrhages, in other ways it resembles Cinchona. The blood is bright red, and there is very little, if any, clotting. This remedy follows Arnica in hemorrhages after falls, mechanical injuries or over-exertion. The patient is a tubercular one and naturally hemorrhagic.

MERCURIUS

Anti-syphilitic and pseudo-psoric. Menses always too copious and quite often dark and clotted; menstrual flow often between the periods; flow makes its appearance two or three days before it really becomes established. During the menses, great heaviness and weight in the limbs, with anxiety. Breath very offensive ; teeth sore, feel long and loose ; gums bleed easily ; tongue thickly coated and flabby ; taste bloody or metallic. Breasts enlarge during menses and feel tender ; sore and swollen, with milk in them. Much rawness and soreness in the vagina and about the labia. Face often pale, earthy and sickly-looking ; general anxiety and apprehension < in the evening ; fears she will lose her mind ; is peevish and suspicious. Much vertigo when lying on the back ; head feels as if in a vice and the whole scalp is sore and painful to touch. Dragging in the loins and in the lower abdomen. Occasionally we have trembling of the whole body, with general weakness and copious perspiration, which is < at night.

Aggravations : At night, by heat, warmth of bed on perspiring, and during wet or stormy weather.

MERCURIUS CORROSIVUS

Menses too early, too profuse, with burning and heat in genitals ; useful in syphilitic diseases in general. Taste is bitter, salty or metallic. Intense vesical tenesmus with burning in the urethra ; violent tenesmus of the rectum and bladder, passes only a few drops of urine at a time ; bloody mucus with violent tenesmus ; screams with pain as a few bloody drops pass ; terrible cutting, colicky pains during menses.

MUREX PURPUREA

Syco-psoric. Menstruation too early and profuse,

with soreness in the uterus. During menses, pains in the uterus extending to chest (Actea), especially in the direction of the right breast; sharp cutting pains in the uterus; sensation of constriction of the uterus; feeling of great heaviness in the vagina; weak, gone, empty feeling in the stomach during menses (like Sepia); violent sexual desire during menses. Throbbing in uterus; heaviness in the labia majora; severe sexual excitement, which is greatly increased by touching the external genitals (Plat.) Her pains are < when lying down, so also is the weariness in the lower limbs. Pains in the back with great weakness and a downward pressure in the uterus (Sepia, Lil., Bell.). This pressure extends to the rectum (Aloe), like Plat. it has great sexual desire; it is the reverse of Sepia in this respect. She is not hysterical, but very irritable during the menses. Cancer of the uterus, with menses every two weeks or with severe hemorrhages and sharp cutting pains in uterus; after the flow ceases, a severe watery or bloody, greenish or yellowish-green leucorrhœa appears (Kreosotum); < during the daytime; sanguine, lymphatic temperament, indicated at all ages of the menstrual period of women, and at the climacteric age.

MOSCHUS

Anti-psoric, menstruation very irregular, profuse, too early, with violent drawing and downward pressing pains in the genitals; pressing and pulling in the parts like labor-pains at the beginning of the menses. "Intolerable titillation in genitals." (Minton.) Great anxiety with palpitation of the heart, and *great dryness of the mouth*; sexual desire greatly increased during the menses; very hysterical; hysterical spasms of the chest, suffocation in chest, and sensation of great constriction, palpitation, prostration, fainting; fears she will die in her nervous attacks; hysteria at every menstrual period. Complains that have their origin in the sexual sphere o women often call for Moschus. She does everything in a great hurry, so that things fall out of her hands. There is a great tendency to be frightened; she is thoughtless, foolish in her gestures, peevish, tearful, quarrelsome; breaks out into fits of laughter or rage, trembles when frightened; has fear of death during the menses, with intense sexual excitement and titillation of the sexual organs. She is > in the open air, < when moving about, < in her room; her nights are restless, and full of dreams and strife, with tossings about the bed, and with a desire to uncover. This remedy is suitable to spoiled, humored, sensitive, nervous and hysterical women.

MEZEREUM

Mezereum, anti-syphilitic, and pseudo-psoric. **Menses** too soon, profuse, long lasting, accompanied with **severe** prosopalgia. Mentally low-spirited and weeps **much**; dread to be alone. Leucorrhœa like white of egg **after** menses. See General Symptoms of Remedy.

MURIATIC ACID

Anti-psoric and pseudo-psoric. Menses too early, too profuse; usually there are more or less pressing and bearing down pains during the flow, or a pressing as if the menses would appear long before they do appear. During the menses the genitals are exceedingly sensitive to touch, and even to pressure of clothing (Plat.). There is an aching pain in the small of the back, heaviness of the anus, and great weakness of the thighs, interfering with walking. Headache from 9 a. m. to 1 p. m. every day; menses dark, thin, liquid blood. Hemorrhoids very sore, swollen, dark-blue in color, sensitive to touch; urine passes slowly because of the weakness of the bladder; suitable to women with dark complexion and black eyes. Aggravated at 9 a. m. by walking, and lying on right side (touching genital organs).

NUX VOMICA

Anti-psoric. Menses too early, profuse and long lasting. The peculiar thing about Nux vomica is its antidotal power; its power not only to antidote the poisonous effects of drugs, but its power to cure diseased conditions of the organism produced by drugs. It also antidotes or counteracts the bad effects of over-eating and over-stimulating the organism. The prolonged, copious and painful menses of this remedy are induced very often by irregular eating, by over-eating, by rich foods such as fats, meats, pastries, wines and stimulants. The menstrual discharge is dark, thick and coagulated attended with griping pains in the uterus and spasmodic pains in the abdomen, resembling indigestion. Menses cease and then reappear again; very irregular, indeed never on time. Before menses she is very sensitive to external impressions; noises, loud talking, strong odors are intolerable. She is cross and irritable. Nausea in the morning with chilliness; constipation with urging to stool accompanied with uterine pains; urging to stool and urination with menstrual pains. During the menses she wishes to be alone and to lie down where it is quite and warm. She is self-willed, headstrong and irritable, with much debility and lassitude; wants to be let alone and to be quiet in a dark room; head aches as if she had not slept well, < on arising in the morning. Griping, dragging pains in the uterus with nausea and discharge of dark clots; pains in the small of the back as if broken; longs for stimulants such as beer and spiced foods; severe pains in the uterus extending to the rectum causing a desire to stool, with nausea and bitter bilious vomiting. Suitable to thin, irritable, choleric, women, with dark hair and motive-bilious temperament, who are addicted to stimulants, spices and condiments.

Aggravations: Eating rich foods and stimulants; cold in general; morning, touch, noise and mental exertion. > from rest, quiet, heat, lying down, being alone and in the evening.

NATRUM CARBONICUM

Pseudo-psoric. Menses too late and scanty or too

soon and profuse, almost to flooding; during menses great pressure in the hypogastrium as if everything would come out. This pressure is toward the genitals; there are sensations of movements in the uterus as of a fœtus. Menses sometimes preceded by drawing pain in the neck with headache; sensation as if head were too large, as if it would be drawn back. (Gel.)

Concomitants: Sad and despondent during menses; is made < by music, especially piano music (reverse Tarantula), and by a thunderstorm; great aversion to men (Puls.); she experiences great debility from the least mental effort; < from heat of summer; pale looking skin; dark rings about the eyes; inability to think; wholly taken up with sad thoughts; no sunshine in her life whatever. Flashes of light before the eyes on awakening; over-sensitive to noises; thick, yellow or yellowish-green discharge from the nose, especially from the posterior nares.

Aggravations: Music; during thunderstorm; exercise; heat of sun; mental or physical exertion; during full moon; headache from mental efforts. This remedy follows well after Sepia in bearing down pains; compare also with Lilium, Murex, Nat. sulph., Phos., Sil. and Nat. mur.; ameliorated by gentle pressure, and rubbing of the affected parts. It is adapted to leuco-phlegmatic women with weak ankles and inability to do mental work.

NATRUM MURIATICUM

Pseudo-psoric. The menses are either too early and

profuse or too late and scanty. Suppressed menses in young women; first menses are slow in appearing, and difficult; Jahr says "the primary effect of the salt is to shorten the menses and its secondary action is to prolong the flow." The flow is usually dark, and continues day and night, accompanied with great sadness; low spirited, and despondent, < in the morning. Gloomy, anxious, very sad; severe headache on awakening in the morning or beginning about 10 a. m. and lasting until sun-down. Headache, frontal, with sensation of little hammers beating in the brain, or headache beginning with blindness accompanied with zigzag flashes of light before the eyes. Dysmenorrhœa with bearing down and pressing towards the genitals, which is only relieved by sitting down. Fluttering of the heart with a weak feeling about it. Menses a week too soon; thin, watery, scanty; more at night; chilliness, with goose flesh during the flow or at the beginning of the menses. Herpes simplex, usually appear about the mouth or chin at the beginning of the monthly period; constipation with depression of spirits; fluttering and palpitation of the heart, with weeping; weeps easily (Puls., Ign., Tuber., Cycl.). Bitter or salty taste with craving for salt; wants food highly seasoned with salt or eats it raw. She has numbness of the fingers, toes, lips, tongue; very absent-minded, forgetful; heaviness of the hands, legs, or feet; feet or hands go to sleep; loses flesh while living well (Iod.)

Indicated in pale anæmic, tubercular individuals, where the tubercular taint produces despondency; also in hysterical conditions peculiar to the tubercular taint. It is complementary to Ignatia and is the chronic of Ignatia; we often have to differentiate it from Cal. carb., or Silicea.

Aggravations : At 10 a. m. in the morning ; sea air ; lying down ; sitting still ; lying on the left side ; > lying on something hard ; evening ; lying on the back, and walking. There is frequently a great desire for much salt in the food, or the saliva tastes salty.

NICCOLUM

Menses are late, scanty, and of short duration. They are accompanied with much pain in the small of the back, great debility, and much bloating of the abdomen with severe colic. There is much thirst day and night, with burning flatulence ; nausea ; much distension of the abdomen, and sour eructations. Mentally the patient is apprehensive, low-spirited and despondent, is easily vexed and made angry ; at night she is much < ; being very restless (like Rhus. tox.) ; changes position frequently ; often her restlessness is accompanied with colic and vomiting when menses are suppressed. In the morning vertigo and pressure in the vertex.

ORIGANUM

Psoric miasms very marked. During menses and long after, great sexual irritation, erotomania ; nymphomania, with suicidal tendencies ; intense sexual excitment as if she would lose her mind, driving her to onanism; practices it often; rapid failing of memory and loss of mind from it. Lascivious impulses; dreams of sexual intercourse, and thinks of sexual subjects continually during the day; voluptuous tingling in sexual organs; sexual inclinations so strong she cannot overcome them; she is dull, listless, morose. This remedy is to women what Staphisagria is to men; it has the intense sexual irritation of Cantharis, but not the physical symptoms. Unlike Lachesis, the symptoms are largely confined to the sexual organs. It is a much neglected remedy and a little known one. Tuberculinum is another remedy often indicated the sexual irritation of women. When the tubercular and sycotic or psoric elements combine and spend their forces upon the sexual organs, we can expect severe sexual irritation in sensitive nervous women.

OLEUM ANIMALE

Menstruation too early and scanty, with great languor in hands and feet; discharge usually dark and very scanty (Sepia). Before the flow appears, cutting, colicky pains in abdomen, also sticking pains in small of back which is < while sitting.

Concomitants: Sad, peevish; ill-humored; filled with grief; a sensation of giddiness when in the open air; blood rushes to the base of brain in a warm room (reverse Puls.); morning vertigo with pressure over the eyes and quivering of the eyelids; complexion earthy.

Her thoughts vanish suddenly; dry prickly heat in different parts of the body; burning, biting itching on the skin like flea bites.

OLEUM CAJEPUTI

Menses suppressed or greatly diminished in quantity; they may be suppressed by a sudden check of perspiration, with constant choking sensation in throat; nervous distension of the bowels from nervous uterine reflex; tongue feels as if swollen, and when speaking she lisps. Spasmodic coughing; nervous hiccough; nervous vomiting, nervous dyspnœa, and nervous dysmenorrhœa.

OLEUM JECORIS ASELLI

Pseudo-psoric and syco-psoric. Menses premature and very copious; rheumatic dysmenorrhœa; pains in sacrum and back; great soreness of the ovaries; menses cease suddenly from taking cold; dysmenorrhœa in advanced stages of tuberculosis; chronic sore throat or diarrhœa due to tuberculosis; expectoration yellowish-green; great weakness in chest and back; burning heat in chest with cough; rheumatic pains in all the large joints and back; constant loss of strength with emaciation. The patient is $>$ in the summer, $<$ in winter; cough and rheumatic difficulties, also $>$ from heat; adapted to pale cachectic tubercular women who have engrafted upon that diathesis, a tertiary sycotic taint. Often the tuberculosis has been stirred up by receiving the sycotic infection; after a few years the mixed miasm presents itself in a malignant form. It is more frequently indicated in thin nervous blonds, with a white transparent skin in which the blood vessels show through of a bluish tint. Great hunger is almost always present, like Psorinum, Iodine, Sulphur and Tuberculinum.

OPIUM

Menses profuse or suppressed with rush of blood to the head. During the menses, violent colic, compelling her to bend double; labor-like pains with drowsiness and desire to sleep; restless all night from heat of bed; tosses about, searching for a cool place; unconscious, often in a comatose state; face red; congestion of blood to the head; climactric states, very imaginative; full of illusions and fancies; very sensitive to sounds, odors and noises. Her sleep is heavy and accompanied with snoring. Indicated in corpulent and good natured women, who suffer with stubborn constipation and a prolapsed or an atonic relaxed condition of the uterus. She has spasms or convulsions from fright, anger, shame, overjoy, or any great emotions; sometimes attacks of epilepsy at night followed by stertorous breathing, red face, and a semi-comatose condition following. Quite often there are no symptoms whatever, excepting the stupor of this remedy. Suitable to elderly women who are fond of stimulants, and narcotics (Bell.), also adapted to school children in certain mental states. Delirium, staring, wide-open eyes, constantly talking, flushed or pale, hot, and bloated face following suppression of the menses. Skin covered with cold sweat; threatening collapse; aggravation during and after sleep, perspiring warmth of bed, > from cold or walking.

PULSATILLA

Indicated more frequently in the pseudo-psoric; it being the acute of Silicea, you can readily see the dyscrasia behind it; sometimes the remedy that meets fully a pseudo-psoric state will cure almost any disease. Menses retarded, delayed, especially in young girls, at or about puberty. Pains, cramp-like, colicky, accompanied with chilliness; menses scanty, dark, thick, even black, coagulated. It may, however, be normal in color or pale and watery. Menses suppressed from cold, from becoming chilled; the pains as well as the mental symptoms are changeable; menses accompanied with chilliness; she weeps with her pains. Before menses, *weeping, sadness, moody, melancholy; goose flesh during menses*, (Nat. mur.); *nausea, often vomiting, with heaviness and pains in abdomen*; colic with vomiting; *she is pale; feels faint; shivers as if cold; weeps often and easily; tongue coated white, no thirst.* Breathing difficult, *cannot get a full breath when in her room, must throw windows and doors open, which relieves her at once.* Menses with pains in back, sides and abdomen, with pressure in abdomen and small of back as of a stone, with ineffectual desire for stool (Nux); *adapted to mild, cheerful, gentle blondes, of a yielding disposition, whose symptoms are constantly changing; to lymphatic constitutions; pale-faced, light-haired, blue-eyed women who have a great tendency to catarrhal troubles and leucorrhœa.* She craves ice cream, butter, fat things which aggravate her very much; milk in breast during menstruation (Mer. sol.); breast sore and tender during flow (Mer. sol. Con.); milky leucorrhœa during menses. Sleeps with hands over head (Plat.), and cannot sleep on left side as it aggravates her heart symptoms; chilly; thirstless; veins distended; puffy about the face and eyes during menses. She is aggravated in warmth; evening; on beginning to move; lying on left side; by fats; rich pastries; warm applications; > from gently moving about; cool air; eating cold things, and cold applications.

PRUNUS SPINOSA

Menses too early too profuse, with severe pains in the small of the back and sides; flow light colored; small of the back feels stiff as from over-straining (Rhus); severe cramps in abdomen during menses that are relieved by walking about ((Puls.). Fullness and distension in stomach, a little satisfies (Lyc.). Hard, dry, scanty stool, with burning in rectum (Nux); anxious, short respiration which is < when climbing a hill or even walking; spasm of the bladder, with much tenesmus and burning in sphincter and continuous urging ; pain relieved by urination ; severe itching in ovaries ; > by rubbing.

PHOSPHORUS

Flow too long lasting, and usually profuse ; bright red blood. Indicated in tall, thin, narrow-chested women who are strongly tubercular. Face often pale, sickly, with dark circles around the eyes. Chlorotic girls who grow too rapidly ; small wounds bleed much, and there are hemorrhages from the nose or lungs during menses. She is very sensitive to light, noise, odors and touch. The least exertion causes exhaustion (Tuber.), she is anxious and apprehensive in the evening about twilight or when alone during a thunderstorm. The nervous symptoms of Phosphorus induce hunger (similar to Sulph.). Sometimes we have a cough with spitting of blood and aphonia with weakness and heaviness in the chest, or a tight heavy feeling in the chest.

PODOPHYLLUM

Anti-psoric and pseudo-psoric. Menses often suppressed in young women, with bearing down in the hypogastric and sacral regions, relieved by lying down. Painful pressing down in abdomen and back, with a numb sensation running down the thighs. Podophyllum is adapted to blonde women who are subject to bilious attacks who have a sallow, sickly complexion, foul breath, thickly coated tongue (Mer.); congestion and torpor of portal system with diarrhœa; severe colic and rumbling in the transverse colon; dark yellow stools; stools very offensive coming on in gushes with much flatulence and sputtering of gases. Gagging as if she would vomit when at stool; prolapsus of uterus with severe aching pains in lumber region, with much aching pain in ovary; hemorrhoids with prolapsus ani. Aggravated, in the morning, by hot weather, or by hot days with cool nights.

PALLADIUM

Said to be a good remedy for dysmenorrhœa while nursing. Jelly-like discharge before and after menses; heaviness and weight in the pelvis as if it were sinking down; during menses pain in left hypogastrium shooting from umbilicus to pelvis; bearing down and drawing in the region of right ovary with a full feeling in the bladder; frequent urination; bladder feels full to bursting; urine scanty although it feels as if she could pass a great quantity at any time; > when lying on left side (reverse Puls.); < standing or moving; aversion to work or exercise and during the flow she must lie down. Sharp knife-like pain in the uterus, > after stool (Minton).

Aggravation: Standing; motion; wounded pride; mental excitement; lying on right side during menses. > when lying on left side, from quiet, and after sleep.

PLATINUM

Platinum has many symptoms of an anti-psoric and

pseudo-psoric nature. I have not studied it close enough to give its true miasmatic setting. The flow is too early, too profuse, and lasting but a short time. The flow is dark, even black, thick, clotted, it may be viscid or ropy. The menstrual flow is preceded by great mental depression, backache, spasms, labor-like or bearing-down pains, and pressing towards the genitals with desire for stool. It is one of those hemorrhagic remedies in which the flow is usually dark and fluid. Dysmenorrhœa usually develops the third day of flow; pains drawing, pressing down and crampy. During the menses there is much sadness and disposition to cry; she is suspicious and jealous (Lach.). She has great self-exaltation; fears she will die or that she will lose her senses; she is full of anguish; her limbs tremble; her heart palpitates; very changeable, weeps, and laughs alternately. She has a sensation as if her body were growing larger, as if other people were very small, or as if they were inferior to her. Nymphomania during menses, with voluptuous tingling in external and internal genitals. Sexual excitement will often bring on all her symptoms; great sexual erethism in young women. Sexual excitement is unendurable; great sensitiveness of the vagina; an examination is impossible, cannot bear the pressure of a napkin she is so sensitive; ovaries very sensitive, especially the left one; uterine hemorrhage with prolapse and bearing down or pressing down pains. Pains increase and decrease gradually (Zinc); stools constipated, soft, clay-like, adhesive; after movement weakness in abdomen and chilliness.

Spasmodic yawning like Ignatia; while asleep lies on her back with her hands over her head (Puls). The pains in the ovaries are spasmodic and of a burning character. Platinum is suited to neurotic women with dark hair and rigid fibre; she is $<$ when at rest, $>$ when in motion; mental and physical symptoms often alternate.

RHUS TOX

Menses too early, too profuse and of too long duration in rheumatic individuals. Flow is light colored, or like dirty water or the washings of meat; it is also acrid, causing biting and itching of the external genitals. Menses suppressed from getting wet, especially getting the feet wet. Rheumatic dysmenorrhœa with labor-like pains, and with much lameness and stiffness in the back and limbs; very restless; especially at night during menses. Prolapsus uteri from over-lifting or straining; aching in back and limbs with a bruised feeling all over the body; better by walking and motion. Occasionally the flow is very much clotted with labor-like pains; backache is relieved by lying on something hard. The symptoms are usually $<$ at night while at rest and $>$ in the daytime and by heat and motion.

SYPHILINUM

Anti-syphilitic. Menses too soon and profuse, often two weeks before the regular time; flow bright red, or occasionally of a pinkish color. During flow, the uterus is very sensitive; shooting pains in uterus, and darting pains in ovaries; worse in left ovary; mammae sensitive and sore both during the menses and between; profuse, yellow leucorrhœa; it soaks through the napkin, running down the limbs (Alumn.). The menstrual pains increase and decrease gradually and are worse from dark until near morning. She dreads the night, on account of periosteal and bone pains. She has great loss of memory (Medorr., Nat. mur.); she begins to grow worse at 4 a. m. (Lyc., Bell., Kali iod.). She feels much worse after sleeping (Lach.).

Hereditary or acquired syphilis; round or irregular shaped ulcers in the mouth at every menstrual period; <at night (Nit acid, Merc. sol.); ulcers with salivation; lardaceous bottoms; firey-red edges; walls straight cut; tongue shows imprint of teeth; taste putrid or metallic; herpetic eruptions about the mouth; desire for alcohol, and aversion to meat. (Desire for meat, Tuberculinum, Cal. c.). Heavy aching in the back, or neuralgic pains that begin at 4 p. m. and last all night. Sleepy at the beginning of the menstrual period (Bufo.); epileptic convulsions after each menstrual period. < at night, dreads to be alone. Asthma or cough in summer only; aching in pelvis and extremities, tibia especially, which is sensitive to touch. Syphilitic eruptions break out during the menses or in the summer time. Aggravation: Night; change of weather; heat of bed. All pains and sufferings < at night (Mer. sol., Kali iod, Aurum, Asafoe. (reverse Medorrhinum).

STANNUM

Pseudo-psoric. Menstruation too early and profuse, often accompanied with pain in the malar bone, or facial neuralgia of some form. Great mental distress and anxiety, which is relieved as soon as the flow begins; the menstrual pain comes in paroxysms, increasing gradually until very severe, then decreasing gradually to disappearance. Mental symptoms quite significant; anxiety, restlessness, great anguish, irritability, sadness, despondency, aversion to men, very hysterical, weeps, sings, prays. Great heaviness with trembling; her weariness comes on suddenly and is < in the morning; has to sit down to rest a number of times before she completes her toilet (tubercular people); anus and limbs feel heavy; great weakness in the chest, which extends to the throat.

Her condition is aggravated by talking, reading, and singing (Phos.). Dry cough, < in the evening (Phos.) until midnight; expectoration is of greenish-yellow mucus with a sweet or salty taste, musty odor from perspiration and from expectoration, smell like old hay. The colicky pains are better from hard pressure or lying on the stomach (Puls., Colocy.).

STAPHISAGRIA

This remedy is anti-sycotic, but meets also those cases of mixed Syphilis or a syco-syphilitic condition which are often as baffling. This will be seen by a careful study of the remedy. A syco-spyhlitic taint in a pseudo-psoric patient is the true field for the use of this peculiar remedy. Menstruation too soon, or absent; discharge pale at first but grows darker; the flow is often irregular, late, profuse, and affected by anger or chagrin, which often delays or suppresses it. Sharp, shooting pain in the ovaries with extreme sensitiveness to weight or pressure; nymphomania during menses, mind cannot be drawn from sexual subjects; during and before menses anger easily aroused; Staphisagria wrath if pent up brings about the physical state peculiar to this remedy "The whole mind and nervous system is in a fret." (Kent)

The menstrual pains are griping and colicky (Colyc.) The cervical glands enlarge and become hard; the patient suffers from gouty nodosities, especially on the fingers; condylomata, warts about the sexual organs (Thuja); pruritus vulvæ with great sensitiveness to touch or pressure. It is indicated often in the first menstruation after marriage or after surgical operations upon the abdomen; a menstruation following mental or surgical shocks, or from extreme, pent-up anger. Touching the sexual organs in making an examination will often throw a Staphisagria patient into spasms (Plat). Another symptom is extreme nervousness and mental symptoms developed from sexual excesses; styes on the lower lid, very painful, or toothache during the menses. "Aggravation:" Mental affections; grief; indignation; mortification ; sexual excesses ; tabacco ; touching affected parts" (H. C. Allen).

SILICEA

Silicea is a pseudo-psoric remedy in every sense of the word. It vies with Natrum mur., Sulphur, Arsenicum, and Psorinum in its depth of action. It searches into every cell and changes every fiber of the organism. The menses may be too early and profuse or too late and profuse. When menses are suppressed, they are followed by an acrid, excoriative milky or watery leucorrhœa (Puls). Discharge of water from the uterus instead of the menses. Milky, watery, or brownish leucorrhœa in place of the menses. Menses smell strong and are acrid.

TABACUM

This wonderful remedy is more frequently indicated than we think for in dysmenorrhœa, especially about the climactric period. The menses begin with vertigo, heaviness in the head when moving ; there is qualmishness of the stomach ; sinking sensation at the pit of the stomach ; palpitation of the heart ; coldness of the lower extremities from the knees down, deadly pallor of the face with an indescribable sickness at the pit of the stomach ; terrible nausea, with vomiting, cold sweat on face and forehead (Ipec., Lob., Verat. alb.). Menstrual headache coming on early in the morning (Nat. mur. Nux, Bry., Lac def.) growing much worse towards noon. It lasts often two or three days and is brought on by fatigue or excitement; pain as if the head would burst or was bored into; vomits mucus and bile, with great nausea, faintness and weakness as pit of stomach; painful retching; straining and gagging. Face pale, anxious, sunken; skin pale, covered with cold clammy sweat (Verat. alb.).

Case 1. Sickness at stomach, violent efforts to vomit, deadly nausea, pallor, coldness; vomits sour mucus (Nux), worse from the least motion (Bry.); dreadful faint feeling at pit of stomach. Lymphatic temperament. Sickness while on the sea.

TEREBINTHINA

Resembles Berberis in its pains in back and kidneys and its bladder symptoms although they are usually more severe. To it we may add great hemorrhages and its great power to suppress diseases. It vies with Camphor in that respect. Camphor and Turpentine are two drugs much abused; they do great harm in domestic practice; both are powerful suppressers of discharges and secretions. Menses too late, scanty, accompanied with much meteorism; great tympanitis and burning in uterus and bearing-down pain.

Concomitants: Burning in uterus and on urination; urine a violet odor, albuminous, dark, scanty, smoky, bloody, like coffee or coffee grounds; drawing pains in the kidneys; worse from motion like Berberis. Fever with red, dry tongue ; mucous surfaces feel dry ; much thirst ; pulse hard and frequent ; profuse sweat ; great prostration. Passive hemorrhages, with general anasarca, etc.

USTILAGO MAYDIS

Menses too frequent, profuse and long lasting ; flow dark, fluid ; blood intermixed with small, black clots ; flow with profuse gushes of bright red blood (Ipec.) or a persistent long continued oozing of mahogany-colored blood, blotted or in strings (Crocus) ; !menses every three weeks of either dark or bright red blood ; active or passive uterine hemorrhages ; climactric flooding ; heavy, dragging backache during the menses and for some time after. Indicated in slim, tall, light complexioned, tubercular women. Similar to Secale.

XANTHOXYLUM

We have a very imperfect proving of this remedy. Generally speaking the symptoms of the urinary and genital organs are both very meager. In the urinary organs nothing of importance is noted ; but in the sexual sphere, especially in that of women, we have a more extended proving.

Female Sexual Organs. Menses too soon ; scanty ; the pain extending down the genito-crural nerves. The earlier the menses appear, the more severe the pain is apt to be. Neuralgic dysmenorrhœa, with profuse flow, in tall, lean women of sedentary habits ; excruciating pains in the loins and low down in the uterine region. These pains are very severe and unbearable in nervous patients ; who are apt to be tubercular. They begin twenty-four hours or so before the menses appear. She fears she is going to die ; is extremely nervous, and sensitive to noise ; pale face with dark rings around the eyes ; she has dreadful headaches with sensation as if the top of the head would fly off. In this respect it is similar to Actea. Membranous dysmenorrhœa, with severe, uterine pains low down in abdomen ; pains agonizing, running to the knees ; she screams with pain. The flow is dark, black, clotted, prolonged to ten days or two weeks. Sometimes the face or other parts of the body become œdematous.

Concomitants—Great despondency with anguish about the chest ; a terrible nervous, frightened feeling, heaviness, fulness of the head, with pressure and throbbing at root of nose, and a sensation as if the top of the head would fly off. Oppression in the chest is here a nervous symptom

LEUCORRHOEA

The word leucorrhœa, like many of the old pathological terms, does not express its meaning in fullness. The word really means a white flow from the vagina, yet it is only occasionally found to be white ; almost any color or shade of color presents itself in this disease process, if I may be allowed to use that term. The ancient physicians did not understand it, and not much has been added to that meager store even in this day of great learing and research. Any discharge that is not blood is called leucorrhœa, yet there are discharges from the genital canal that are as far from being a leucorrhœa as anything can be. It is not a disease, but the product of a diseased state or condition of the system. The genital canal is one of the waste gates of the body. Through these discharges it becomes an eliminative exit, and when these discharges are suppressed (dried up locally), the organism becomes affected unfavorably. The patient who is comparatively well with a leucorrhœal discharge, is in some way made sick when the flow is suspended by local treatment. All sorts of morbid phenomena have ensued from bad treatment at the hands of physicians, who do not understand the nature and cause of the disease that lies behind them. Clinically we have four divisions of leucorrhœa, the vulvular, the vaginal, the cervical, and the uterine. The first form we find oftener in children, and in aged women, but the other forms we find all during the child-bearing period. The vulvular discharge is sero-purulent, viscid, unctious, having an odor of old cheese or at least an offensive smell. It comes largely from a rapidly developing sebaceous fluid. The vaginal occurs in young women and is creamy or white, purulent; it may be either bland, or excoriating. The cervical discharges are thick, tenaceous, ropy, or stringy, showing the albuminous elements. The uterine is similar to the cervical but is more watery. It may be tinged with blood or mixed with pus. After the menopause it is thin watery, and often excoriating. Histologically the cell structures of the canal will often show the origin of the leucorrhœa, if you wish to go that far into the investigation. Some women suffer all their lives with such discharges, while others suffer only occasionally as the result of temporary congestion due to fatigue, cold, exhaustion febrile states or acute disease processes which pass away in a few days, leaving them once more normal. It is the permanent conditions with which we have to deal, and it is those sufferers who call upon us for treatment, and if we do not understand something about the nature of miasmatics, we will soon lose ourselves in the labyrinth of pathological names and conditions to which leucorrhœa is attributed. I will mention a few of them, so as to give you some idea of the confusion which puzzles medical men, who believe in those doctrines, menstruation, foreign growths, laceration, congestion, parturition abortion, sexual over-indulgence, uterine displacements, efforts to prevent conception infections of all kinds, specific diseases, such as Syphilis and gonorrhœa, gouty states of the blood, tuberculosis, struma, and a thousand other causes. These make an interesting study to the lover of etiology and pathology, but Homeopathy searches deeper than this; although pathological states are not to be despised or overlooked, as they always have some bearing on the case. We have eyes and glasses to look through, which the rest of the medical world know not; they were bequeathed to us by Samuel Hahnemann. All men may wear them if they will, and to put them on, is to put on the habiliments of truth, and to use the telescope of law, that searches the labyrinth of disease to its fountain head and reveals its hidden mystery. Then we see leucorrhœa to be only a symptom, a cleansing and sanitary process to eliminate that which taints the stream of life. A few of you have seen these truths, and many have passed through this life without knowing them, and there are many, however, living to substantiate the truth and leave their seal of approval, that it may be known to all men that homeopathy, the law of cure, is truth.

The symptoms of leucorrhœa like those of all other chronic disease processes are changeable and numberless; our voluminous Materia Medica testifies fully to that fact. Some of the more prominent and constant symptoms are pain in the back, head, and loins, languor, often loss of strength, and general debility, which is made worse by standing or by working, and is worse about the menstrual period. In the treatment of leucorrhœa, I always study my case from the standpoint of the Chronic Miasms and from the light thrown upon disease by Hahnemann's teachings in his Organon and Chronic Disease. Then I am never disappointed; Hahnemann's etiology of disease becomes mine, and from what I have learned of disease by experience and from what he has taught me, I get the best results obtainable. Through his revelations in the Organon, I have seen a great light and am not in darkness any longer ; I have come into that light, and with every case I study the phenomena of some chronic miasm, active or latent in the organism, slumbering by virtue of the presence of the leucorrhœal discharge or awakened by its suppression. "The constitutional or symptomatic treatment of leucorrhœa is of the greatest importance," says Dr. A. C. Cowperthwaite. He further says : "It must be continually borne in mind that leucorrhœa is, in itself, but a symptom, either of some constitutional dyscrasia or of some local existing cause." The question arises what is a dyscrasia ? Here are some of the many definitions given : "A sin process or something that makes the body healthier," (Jeremy Taylor) ; a disease of an undefined character ; a general impairment of health ; a degeneration, a faulty condition of the body ; a morbid diathesis, and a predisposed condition of the state of the organism. In all these we see nothing fixed or definite, but when we say a syphilitic, gonorrhœal or a psoric diathesis, we begin to see cause and definite cause at that. When we speak of a tubercular diathesis, we all know just what we are talking about. We may say the same thing of a leucorrhœal discharge. Let us first learn whether it be tubercular ; if so, it will have the characteristics of the pus, of the anæmia, of the mental and physical phenomena of this diathesis. And the same thing may be said of every form of disease. (See Vol. I, Chronic Miasms, under Sexual Organs.) The leucorrhœa of the tubercular patient is thick, and yellowish, creamy, or greenish-yellow; it often has a sweetish odor, at other times there is no discernable odor. The leucorrhœa of Psora is whitish, albuminous, odorless, and usually bland; that of Sycosis is thin, watery, greenish-yellow or dark, like dirty water and usually acrid, and excoriating, producing pruritus of the parts passed over. The odor is pungent, musty, like fish-brine or stale fish. Often every symptom that presents itself in the organism, will correspond with the whole leucorrhœal discharge. A careful study and acquaintance of the miasms will soon reveal this to be true. It will not require much study, if the observation is at all acute, for you to prescribe from a miasmatic basis. There is no disease that requires a more careful study and analysis of the constitutional symptoms than does this disease. The tubercular forms must be treated as you would a tubercular patient suffering from any other process. They should have a nourishing diet, plenty of fresh air and sunshine, exercise, appropriate bathing, and anything that will restore the vigor and tone to the system. A tubercular leucorrhœa is the one that produces a great drain on the system, due of course, to the blood changes and the death of the red blood cell. In the true sycotic we see no such blood changes, no such anæmia or loss of strength; in the sycotic the body is usually well nourished, although when we find a mixed miasm as in Syco-psora of Pseudo-psora, combined with a sycotic element, then a cachexia and diathesis may develop, that approaches malignancy with its blood changes greater even than the simple tubercular. Each case must be carefully studied and a remedy based usually upon the totality of the active miasm ; only in the sycotic form do I prescribe douches or injections and then not oftener than once a day, using sterile water at about the temperature of the body ; too much douching is bad practice as it balloons the vaginal canal, producing reaction of the tissues and in the end becomes a local irritant. Besides this the organism soon demands the stimulant effect produced by the hot water, and it is not long until the patient cannot do without it. I have found better results come from the non-use of them ; at best you can only cleanse the vagina and the real trouble is entirely confined to the uterus. I often prescribe raw eggs, milk, cream, olive oil, cereals, vegetables, fresh air, sleeping with windows wide open and so on so as to get the best results from the environment. The raw eggs replace the loss of albumin that is more or less a factor in the case ; raw foods and fresh air are also splendid in renovating the system. The olive oil increases the amount of fats in body, so necessary to assist in overcoming the work of the tubercular element. The loss of adipose tissue being about the first change we see taking place in these patients, together with blood-cell changes. We see the same changes taking place in children suffering from worms. The urine will soon be found to be covered with fat globules. Take away potatoes and meats for a short time or give them sparingly and increase the fats. The best fat is olive oil ; two desertspoonfuls a day are sufficient, it being about all the system will take care of. Eggs, pure butter and cream follow in their order as fat producers, fresh air and plenty of walking together with the indicated remedy will soon restore these patients' health.

THERAPEUTICS OF LEUCORRHOEA

ACONITE

Acute, simple vaginitis; vagina hot, dry, sensitive; urine scanty and scalding; fever with restlessness; discharge is white or yellowish, even bloody, coming on after taking cold or getting wet. Tendency of blood to head and chest, with fear of death; sanguine, plethoric women of sedentary habits, after acute febrile conditions. Aconite is one of the best remedies for retarded or suppressed menses.

ACTEA RACEMOSA

Vaginal or cervical leucorrhœa in rheumatic women; sensation of weight and bearing down in pelvis; prolapse of the uterus in nervous, sterile women. Sensation as if top of head would fly off. Constantly full of forebodings and fear of future happenings. Leucorrhœa watery, with weight, and torpor in uterus and lower extremities.

AESCULUS HIPPOCASTANUM

Dark yellow, sticky discharge which is worse after menses and after walking. Constant backache across the hips and sacrum ; worse from walking or stooping ; stiffness in lumbar region (Rhus) or sore, lame feeling in small of back, as if back would give out when walking. Leucorrhœa corroding labia and surrounding parts ; very uncomfortable feeling in the rectum. Prolapsed feeling in rectum with dry, hard stool ; hemorrhoids purple, like grapes that burn and have a full and aching feeling.

AGARICUS MUSCARIUS

Profuse, dark colored leucorrhœa ; accompanied with aching and sensitiveness along the entire spine ; great sensitiveness of spine. Titillation in sexual organs with strong sexual desire. Trembling of hands ; itching, burning, and redness of fingers and toes. Leucorrhœa from inordinate coition; spinal irritation ; women of light hair, lax skin and muscles. Dribbling of urine, dragging down sensation in uterus (Fluoric acid).

AGNUS CASTUS

Transparent leucorrhœa, yet it stains the linen yellow ; complete obliteration of sexual desire. Indicated often in women who prostitute themselves ; in premature old age, mental apathy, impotence after attacks of gonorrhœa ; sexual organs relaxed with coldness.

ALETRIS FARINOSA

Leucorrhœa following general debility from loss of fluids ; defective nutrition ; profuse between the menses ;

prolapse from muscular atrophy; weakness of mind and body; sterility from uterine atony. General debility with weight and heaviness in the uterine region. Suitable to chlorotic girls (Helon., Senega).

ALLIUM SATIVUM

Leucorrhœa excoriating, producing soreness of the thighs and pustules, with bright red spots on the labia majora and vulva, which sting and bite. Herpes with itching and burning.

ALOE

Leucorrhœa bloody, mucous, slimy, preceded by colic. Bearing down sensation when standing; heaviness and fullness in the groins; sensation as if a plug were wedged in between the symphysis pubis and coccyx. Hemorrhoids that protrude like small bunches of grapes and are relieved by cold bathing. Fear as if a stool would escape with flatus, heat and burning in rectum.

ALUMINA

After menses great exhaustion both mental and physical with copious discharge of mucus from vagina during menses. Leucorrhœa profuse, yellow, corroding or acrid, creamy or transparent, and worse after menses. Leucorrhœa like cream, causing itching in the pudenda, copious only in the daytime ; sensation as if everything would fall from the vagina, with much weakness. Leucorrhœa chronic, painless, from the cervix ; copious, running down the limbs (Medorrh.). Leucorrhœa relieved by cold douches, worse when walking. Pain in back as if iron was thrust through lower vertebrae. Burning in the spine ; sensation as if a tight cord were around the body. Numbness of the head, trembling in limbs, and great exhaustion. Gonorrhœa and leucorrhœa of long standing ; a whole week passes before she gets over the effects of menstruation which is prolonged by leucorrhœa.

AMBRA GRISEA

Discharge thick, or bluish white mucus, or in lumps ; stitches in the vagina before the discharge ; violent itchings ; soreness and swelling of labia ; discharge of blood in between menstrual periods. Adapted to thin aged people, and those of a nervo-bilious temperament. Aggravation, evening and warm room.

AMMONIUM CARBONICUM

Leucorrhœa watery, profuse, acrid, causing much burning and smarting ; smells like ammonia ; much fatigue of whole body especially of the thighs ; suitable to sickly, weak, delicate women. Leucorrhœa with swelling, itching, and burning of perineum ; sleep in daytime and not at night. Cholera-like menses with exhaustion; hysterical women who faint easily and who always carry a smelling bottle. Sensation as if inner parts were raw, as if soreness were deep in; averse to walking in the open air.

AMMONIUM MURIATICUM

Leucorrhœa like white of eggs, preceded by griping pains around the navel; leucorrhœa constant, painless, brownish, slimy, albuminous, great distension of abdomen and violent backache at night.

ANACARDIUM ORIENTALE

Leucorrhœa with itching and soreness of the perineum; greatly aggravated by scratching or rubbing (Rhus tox). Very irritable and full of strange notions, ideas and impulses. Alternation of moods; skin burns and itches wherever the discharge touches it.

ANANTHERUM

Leucorrhœa fetid, thick, light-colored, or clear and watery, or milky with a bad odor. In gonorrhœa it is thick, purulent, greenish.

ANTIMONIUM CRUDUM

Leucorrhœa acrid, producing a smarting and biting

sensation down the thighs. Profuse discharge of acrid water mixed with lumps of pus. Thick milky coating on the tongue; desire for pickles, eructations tasting of food; tendency to grow fleshy; leucorrhœa due to chronic Sycosis, or to gastric disturbances and gouty states of the system.

APIS MELLIFICA

Leucorrhœa profuse, yellow or green and acrid, attended with stinging sensation in the perineum; frequently painful; urgent desire to urinate; ascites; cutting and stinging pain in the right ovary; eruption like bee stings on the body. Puffiness and swelling of the ankles; absence of thirst; scanty, dark urine; adapted to frivolous and jealous girls, who, though generally cautious and careful, drop things or let them fall while handling them.

ARALIA RACEMOSA

Leucorrhœa is acrid, foul smelling; pressing down pains in the uterus; great debility and feeble states of the nervous system, together with chronic catarrh.

ARGENTUM NITRICUM

Leucorrhœa like pus, ichorous, bloody, offensive, scenting the whole room. Leucorrhœa of a mucous nature with much pain in the back and great debility of the lower extremities. Aggravated by riding in a carriage or car. Often indicated in sterile women and young widows. Pain in uterus as from sticks or slivers; induration of os uteri; cervix bleeds easily; prolapsus uteri; she is always in a hurry, time passes too slowly; desire for sugar; debility of the lower extremities is characteristic; much flatulence in abdomen of a nervous origin.

ARNICA

Leucorrhœa after difficult labor, after injuries, falls, etc. Sore, bruised feeling over the whole body; head hot; extremities cold. Bruised feeling in uterine region and sacrum. Heaviness of the limbs; tendency to boils that are exceedingly sore and sensitive. Bad effects from falls, contusions, and other mechanical injuries.

ARSENICUM

Leucorrhœa acrid, excoriating, thin or thick; producing erythema of the parts it comes in contact with; leucorrhœa worse, while standing. Often under Arsenicum we have leucorrhœa in place of menses in very anæmic women. Indicated in women of a pale waxy complexion, who have the tubercular cachexia well marked, who are always chilly and easily fatigued. The least exertion causes exhaustion; œdematous swelling of eyelids or a puffiness about the face; bloody, offensive, watery discharge, often menses cease and leucorrhœa begins; flow profuse; she is easily exhausted, desire to lie down all the time; lips and mouth dry, always thirsty for small drinks which usually disagree with her stomach. She is nervous, sad, anxious, irritable, fears death, and is worse about 1 a. m. or 1 p. m. Leucorrhœa in scirrhus of the uterus with burning pains, which are worse after midnight.

ASAFOETIDA

. Indicated in syco-syphilitic individuals (Nitric acid, Thuja, Mer. sol., Cinnabaris), leucorrhœa profuse, thin greenish-yellow; urine offensive. Ulceration of the cervix; ulcers have a hard edge and are painful and very sensitive; bleed easily in malignancies and Syphilis. Bearing down in genitals when riding in a carriage. Leucorrhœa producing swelling and inflammation of the genitals; nervous affections follow suppressed discharges; turgidness of the mammae during the menses with milk in breasts. Globus hystericus; spasm of the œsophagus, as if a ball were rising from the stomach; gas forms so rapidly that she cannot belch it fast enough (Arg. nit.).

ASARUM EUROPAEUM

Leucorrhœa, long, yellow strings of mucus, with dreadful backache; backache low down as if it would break; no other remedy has a more severe backache than Asarum; lumbar backache, scarcely can breathe because of it ; leucorrhœa tenacious and yellow, food tastes bitter ; exceedingly nervous, cannot bear the rustle of paper ; much lassitude in lower extremities ; great nervous irritation, the least unpleasant noise thrills every nerve. It is often indicated in women who are addicted to stimulants.

AMMONIUM MURIATICUM

Leuchorrhœa profuse, yellow or white, thick, corrosive, with burning and smarting of the vulva. It often excoriates the whole perinium and inner surface of thighs ; it constantly runs from vagina ; scrofulous and syphilitic leucorrhœa in despondent and melancholy individuals, whose minds are constantly turned towards self destruction ; leucorrhœa from prolapsed uterus ; leucorrhœa with redness and swelling of labia majora ; burning and pricking in the vagina ; large red pimples on labia. Adapted to despondent, suicidal, sanguine temperaments ; muddy complexions ; light haired women or girls at puberty. Aggravated at night, and from getting cold.

BARYTA CARBONICA

Leucorrhœa, thick, white, copious, passive ; worse before menses ; slightly bloody, with a continuous troublesome weight over the pubes ; indicated in scrofulous girls whose development is greatly retarded by the excessive tubercular element present ; young girls of slow development ; mind and body dwarfed by the tubercular element; usually the tubercular element hurries the development too rapidly as seen in Calcarea carb., but under Baryta it retards it. Leucorrhœa in these cases often prevents lung difficulties. We find the glands hard, knotty, and indurated all over the body; abdomen and head large, and limbs usually emaciated; children or young women who look prematurely old; they are bashful and timid, and grow worse by thinking about their case. Dwindling of the glands with sterility or induration and hardening of the glands.

BELLADONNA

Leucorrhœa sanious, mucous, always before menses, followed by more or less congestion; leucorrhœa with colicky pains and bearing down in the uterus. It appears and disappears suddenly, and is more copious in the morning. Leucorrhœa after acute febrile states (Aconite). Great dryness of mucous surfaces and sense of constriction. Discharges feel hot, as they pass from the body. Leucorrhœa after acute inflammations of uterus or sexual organs. Congested feeling in uterus. Better when sitting or lying down, and much worse when standing, parts affected very sensitive to touch. Leucorrhœa white mucous attended with colic. Worse in the morning.

BORAX

Leucorrhœa white, albuminous; feels hot like warm

water while passing over the parts ; appears midway between the menstrual periods ; like starch or white of egg ; bland and without pain ; between the menstrual period it may be corrosive. While she has the leucorrhœa she is very nervous, is easily startled, cannot bear a downward motion, such as descending stairs or going down in an elevator. Even rocking affects her. Adapted to lax, sensitive, nervous women. She is subject to aphtha in the mouth during the menses, or to herpetic eruptions about the mouth (Nat. mur.); urine hot, burns like fire. This remedy has cured some cases of leucorrhœa, especially in children where there was an aphthous condition of the mouth and external genitals.

BOVISTA

Leucorrhœa following the menses, thick, slimy, tenacius acrid and corrosive. It, like Borax, has a leucorrhœa like the white of an egg. It comes out coagulated when walking, or it is of a yellowish-green color and leaves a green stain on linen. It excoriates the labia, perineum, groins and thighs by its acridity. The menstrual flow is only at night.

BERBERIS

Leucorrhœa albuminous and worse before the menses ; region of the vagina sensitive, and hot. Leucorrhœa is accompanied with intense burning on urination with much soreness in the urinary canal. A yellow mealy sediment in the urine. There is much prostration while the leucorrhœa lasts; grayish, mucous leucorrhœa which is very acrid; stitching and shooting pains in kidneys.

BUFO RANA

Leucorrhœa purulent, fetid, or it may be clear and without any odor; sometimes it is thick, yellow, creamlike, or like the washings of meat. Leucorrhœa from polypi of the cervix. It produces pruritus vulva, burning heat and stitches in the ovaries (Cactus grand.). The leucorrhœa of this remedy has nothing characteristic about it, so we have to confine our study to the general symptoms. A sense of constriction seems to be the guiding symptom in this remedy. Constriction about neck, chest, heart, as if uterus or heart were grasped by a hand or in a vice; rush of blood to chest and heart. It is quite decidedly a sycotic remedy as seen in its rheumatic, gouty and cardiac symptoms. Her menstrual pains cause her to scream. This remedy is adapted to young plethoric women who are subject to sudden congestions. The heart symptoms usually call your attention first to the remedy. Aggravation, 11 a.m. (Sulphur, Nat. mur.).

CALCAREA CARBONICA

Leucorrhœa after menses like mucus or milk; worse

after urination ; albuminous leucorrhœa from cervix with lassitude and debility ; leucorrhœa of little girls ; the least excitement brings on the leucorrhœa or menses. The leucorrhœa is thick, yellow, acrid or bland. This remedy is indicated in pale, blond, light-haired anæmic women Tubercular leucorrhœa in pale, fleshy, soft-muscled blonds ; perspiration about the face or head ; hands and feet cold and damp always. Thinks she will lose her mind ; much anxiety with fear of death. Leucorrhœa is thick, yellow, acrid, continuing from one menstrual period to another. Leucorrhœa following copious long lasting menses.

CALCAREA PHOSPHORICA

Leucorrhœa looks like the white of egg, odor sweetish, worse in the morning on arising, also worse after stool or urination (Cal. cab.). Feeling of great weakness in the sexual organs. She takes cold at every change of weather. This remedy is indicated in school girls, who develop too rapidly and who suffer with rheumatic pains in their extremities. Albuminous leucorrhœa comes in gushes, worse from walking, or running sewing machine.

CALENDULA OFFICINALIS

Constant sense of weight and fullness in pelvis ; leucorrhœa profuse, offensive and watery ; cancer of the uterus ; discharge causes much exhaustion.

CALADIUM SEGUINUM

Very forgetful; absent minded; forgetfulness induced by onanism or sexual excesses. It cures a white mucous discharge from the vagina, that is induced by onanism; violent sexual desire with complete loss of sexual power, and gonorrhœal leucorrhœa in old debauchees. The discharge produces intense prutitus; the patient is compelled to scratch or rub the parts; the discharge produces pimply eruptions.

CARBO ANIMALIS

Leucorrhœa watery, causing burning and biting; yellowish leucorrhœa; discharge stains linen; worse when walking or standing; offensive, bloody in cancer; quite often it is thin, watery and dark. Induration of the cervix uteri malignant ulceration with foul discharges; venous plethora in elderly women.

CARBO VEGETABILIS

Leucorrhœa often accompanies the menses and continues after they cease. It produces aphthæ, itching, burning, swelling, soreness and smarting of vulva; sore spots on vulva like little ulcers. Leucorrhœa a milky mucus, or thick, yellow or yellowish green; < in the morning, before menses and after urination. Flatulent distension of abdomen; great debility from least exertion ; low state of vital power ; knees and joints remote from the center of circulation are cold ; all discharges are offensive ; desire for cool air and to be fanned.

CASTOREUM

Leucorrhœa thick or watery, with burning ; great weariness in thighs.

CAULOPHYLLUM THALICTROIDES

Leucorrhœa profuse, mucous, acrid or bland, with congestion of the uterus and bearing down pains, often indicated in little girls. Leucorrhœa with aching and dragging in the small of back, and rheumatism in the small joints ; spasmodic dysmenorrhœa in young girls ; upper eyelids heavy ; moth spots on forehead ; very similar to Pulsatilla. Leucorrhœa with uterine congestion or sensation of congestion ; articular rheumatism of the small joints.

CAUSTICUM

Indicated in women with a yellow, sickly complexion ; leucorrhœa flowing only at night, like the menses and is of a similar odor. Leucorrhœa preceded by colic or abdominal cramps, with emission of flatus ; weariness in thighs, and soreness in the small of back ; great aversion to sweet things. (Reverse to Sulph., and Arg, nit.) A feeling as if the scalp were too tight; much melancholy and sadness and threatening paralysis. < in fine, clear weather : > in damp, warm weather. Appetite vanishes as soon as she begins to eat.

CHAMOMILLA

Leucorrhœa yellowish, corrosive, smarting, burning in vagina as if excoriated; leucorrhœa acrid, watery, gonorrhœal leucorrhœa, crampy, pains in back and abdomen. She is whimsical, snappish, irritable, fretful; flies into a rage in a minute; over sensitive to pain and impressions of every kind; constantly criticising and finding fault. Adapted to cross, irritable, black-haired women. Aggravated by heat, evening, open air, and anger.

CINA

Indicated often in the leucorrhœa of little girls suffering from pin worms; much itching about genitals; hemorrhage from uterus before the age of menstruation; masturbation of little girls due often to the irritation of ascarides; urine turbid, and milky; fat globules on the urine; appetite very ravenous or changeable; breath smells sweetish or like new corn on the ear; spasmodic dry cough, < in the evening; temperature rises about three in the afternoon and lasts all night; the child is peevish, fretful, irritable, impulsive, and cannot bear to be touched ; picks and bores in the nostrils with fingers. Leucorrhœa bloody serum alternating with pus.

CINCHONA OFFICINALIS

Leucorrhœa often bloody and attended with spasmodic, uterine contractions which supercede the menses ; leucorrhœa purulent or bloody ; bloody serum alternating with discharges of pus ; countenance pale, yellow, sickly, pointed, after abortion or childbirth, after hemorrhages ; < at midnight, in least draft of air, and every other day ; debilitating night sweats ; congestion of the uterus with a feeling of fullness ; aversion to exercise ; bitter or sour taste in the mouth, after severe hemorrhages ringing in ears ; black spots before the eyes ; desire to be fanned (Carbo veg.).

COCCULUS INDICUS

Leucorrhœa between the menses or in place of them ; flesh-colored leucorrhœa which gushes out when bending over ; leucorrhœa bloody or like the washings of meat; bloody serum; distension of abdomen with cutting colic ; much vertigo with spinal irritation ; great nervous exhaustion aggravated by riding in a car or carriage ; nausea, vomiting, great vertigo or sick headache caused by riding in a car or carriage. Headache in occiput or at base of brain and cervical region as if tightly bound by a cord ; time passes too slowly (Arg. nit.).

COCCUS CACTI

Leucorrhœa mucous in its character and accompanied with constriction in the abdomen or drawing pain in the inguinal region. Sweet metallic taste in the mouth ; she passes great quantities of ropy mucous during the day from the vagina ; catarrhal leucorrhœa worse in the winter time ; jelly-like mucus (Kali bich.). The mental symptoms are depression, anxiety, and sadness ; inflammation or congestion of the vagina or uterus with copious discharges of thick, white, ropy, jelly-like mucus ; worse from excitement.

CAPSICUM

Adapted to plump, fleshy, flabby, sandy-haired or red-faced people, who are sensitive to cold and have no physical endurance. Leucorrhœa thick, yellow, cream-like ; tenesmus of bladder with strangury.

COFFEA

Leucorrhœa mucus-like, milky, more profuse while urinating ; occasionally it is bloody with great hyperesthesia and sensitiveness of the external genitals ; hyperesthesia of all the senses, hearing, taste, smell, sight and touch ; full of fanciful imaginations and ideas ; all the physical and mental faculties seem exalted and carried far above the normal plain ; great excitement of the genitals and excessive itching of the vulva ; cannot keep hands from genitals (both sexes) ; trembling of hands ; does not know what to do with them ; bad effects on the whole nervous system from the use of coffee ; has no appetite until she partakes of a cup of coffee ; eats nothing to speak of. Diseases brought on by over-joy or excitement ("The nervous system is in a fret." Kent).

COLCHICUM AUTUMNALE

Leucorrhœa jelly-like mucus, bloody and stringy (Crocus, Kali bich., Coccus cacti.). Leucorrhœa during pregnancy with nausea and loathing of food ; dreads the smell of cooking food or odors of the kitchen in general. Soreness and tympanites of whole abdomen ; numbness œdema, and swelling of limbs; gouty joints, finger joints enlarged ; urine like beer, very strong and acid ; sudden suppression of menses followed by dropsy.

COLLINSONIA CANADENSIS

Leucorrhœa with obstinate constipation and pruritus ; stools are dry, hard, light-colored balls ; hemorrhoids ; pruritus vulva ; loss of appetite ; violent itching of the genitals ; parts are badly swollen ; dysmenorrhœa ; stubborn constipation ; hemorrhoids ; pruritus and uterine displacements.

CONIUM MACULATUM

White, acrid leucorrhœa causing a burning sensation ;

mucous leucorrhœa with great weakness and paralyzed sensation in small of back. It sets in a few days after menstruation, ceases, then alternates with a fresh flow of the menses; this is apt to occur in malignancies. Leucorrhœa in old maids; foul, bloody, or brownish discharges from the uterus in fibroid or cancerous growths of the uteus; carrion-like odor from cancer in early stages, no pain, and indeed a lack of any general symptoms, simply the dirty brown offensive discharges from the vagina, vertigo when lying down or when turning over in bed. Face is sallow, earthy; breasts painful, hard, sensitive with shooting pains in them. Nipples sore and tender with a tendency to retraction. I have made many cures of uterine cancer and malignant disease of the breast in women of a tubercular diathesis who had acquired and suppressed Sycosis, appearing as a malignancy at the beginning of the change of life.

CROCUS SATIVUS

Leucorrhœa dark colored, even black or bloody viscid, stringy; smells badly; sometimes it drops out in viscid strings of mucus. It is aggravated by the slightest motion. Sensation as if menses would return, or as if something were moving or were alive in abdomen (Cocculus).

CROTALUS HORRIDUS

Leucorrhœa with ovaritis or ovarian neuralgia; leucorrhœa offensive and bloody ; discharges from malignant growths about cervix or uterus in puerperal states, which are dark and even black, very offensive ; pruritus vulvæ ; large dark vesicles on external genitals that burn severely, very sensitive, cannot rub or scratch the part ; vicarious menstruation from any orifice of body (Lach.).

CROTON TIGLIUM

Leucorrhœa with herpes about genitals ; intense itching of genitals, aggravated by scratching or rubbing ; eruption vesicular, like Rhus tox

CUBEBA

Leucorrhœa profuse, acrid, yellowish, or greenish, and of a very offensive odor ; it produces erythema of inner surface of thighs and vulva, with intense pruritus of vulva. Mensus scanty, preceded by copious leucorrhœa ; much weakness and fatigue in loins ; uterus swollen and painful.

CURARE

Leucorrhœa scanty but thick, clotted, purulent, foul-smelling with heat, itching and burning in vulva ; much burning and contraction in uterus.

CARBOLIC ACID

Leucorrhœa copious, of fetid, greenish-acrid matter
22 F.A.

from vagina ; ulceration of cervix after cauterization, after severe burns. Dragging sensation through the loins and pelvis ; excoriating discharge worse after profuse menses ; frequent urination with burning pain in the urethra.

CYCLAMEN

Membranous leucorrhœa with constant chilliness, indicated in blondes or in leuco-phlegmatic subjects who have scanty and retarded menses ; mental symptoms better when menstruating ; more cheerful, feet do not feel so heavy ; much distension of abdomen ; pains in the heels ; swelling of the mammae with secretion of milk in the breasts ; inclination to weep easily, and yet ill-humored ; aversion to open air (reverse of Pulsatilla). Pork disagrees ; saliva has a salty taste ; better when walking (Cal. carb., Coc.).

COPAIBA

Sycotic leucorrhœa in first and second stages, bright-yellow in color, purulent ; burning and itching in urethra and vagina. Discharge of thick bloody mucus from uterus. Profuse, greenish, gonorrhœal discharge with much distress and burning when urinating ; itching of vulva ; sensation of warmth or heat in the vagina.

DULCAMARA

Leucorrhœa with menstrual suppression from taking cold, from acute catarrh of the sexual organs, from getting wet, from a sudden change to wet weather, wading in water, too much bathing in lake (river, China) (sea, Nat. mur); urticaria before the menses appear. Aggravation from cold, getting wet, suppressed menses and eruptions.

DAPHNE MEZEREUM

Leucorrhœa like albumen; chronic in malignant cases; much discharge of mucus from the vagina.

DICTAMNUS

Leucorrhœa tenacious mucus, first brown then white, lastly streaked with blood; leucorrhœa attended with frequent discharges of urine; itching of the anus and perineum, with erosion of these parts. Uterine leucorrhœa (Minton).

ERIGERON

Chronic leucorrhœa, profuse, uterine or vaginal, attended with spasmodic pains and great irritation of rectum and bladder; epistaxis of bright red blood; bleeding from the jaws or from the cavity of a tooth; menstruation with much suffering in lower dorsal region; itching and distress in bladder; all symptoms < in wet weather.

EUPION

After menses, leucorrhœa yellow, painless with bland discharges; colors the linen yellow, and is attended with emaciation, great lassitude and trembling of the whole body; leucorrhœa with a terrible backache; when the backache ceases, the discharge comes on in gushes; it runs from her in a stream; during urination, burning, itching and swelling of the labia; pressing against something hard relieves the backache of menstruation; sacrum feels as if broken; vertigo with confusion of the head; things turn black before her (China.).

FERRUM

Leucorhœa like water or milky; smarting and corroding the parts; dragging pains, weight and pressure in sacrum and loins. Leucorrhœa in chlorotic patients, like boiled starch, generally during stool; sallow, earthy complexion; palpitation of the heart; flushing of the cheeks; rush of blood to face and chest; occasionally a discharge which is mucus and in shreds; young girls suffering with incipient tuberculosis; great weakness and relaxation of genitals and bladder. Leucorrhœa from masturbation or developing from a tubercular cachexia. Quite often in these chlorotic girls the menses will cease for months and a severe form of leucorrhœa take its place, and the longer it exists the more sallow and chlorotic they become. Great hunger all the time; food tastes bitter. She is ameliorated by walking slowly about (Puls.).

GELSEMIUM

Leucorrhœa after onanism with great weakness and

trembling; lack of muscular co-ordination. Headaches in occiput. Heaviness in uterine region with leucorrhœal discharge; a feeling of fulness across the sacrum; great depression of spirits and excessive languor. Leucorrhœa after febrile states, after LaGrippe, after a rheumatic attack; violent headache in occiput with pulsations, like a pulse beating. Leucorrhœal discharge white, with aching across the lower part of the back or severe aching across the sacrum.

GRAPHITES

Leucorrhœa profuse, white, thin, mucous, with great weakness in the small of the back when sitting or when walking; discharge more profuse in the morning, often in gushes during the day; painful pressing towards the pudenda; soreness of labia with a rash; leucorrhœa sticky, glutinous, copious; flowing down the thighs and producing erythema of the part, even ulceration; smells like herring pickle, or is very offensive. Nails hard, thick, crippled, break or split easily. Stools hard, large, knotty, and are often covered with a viscid white mucus (similar to Pulsatilla in many of its symptoms), but is more apt to be indicated near or at the climactric period. Skin unhealthy, everything suppurates; cracks, and fissures in feet, toes, fingers, lips, face. (Follows Sepia well in leucorrhœa.)

HAMAMELIS

Leucorrhœa very profuse, with relaxation of the vaginal walls; discharge usually bloody, copious, constant, with debility and lassitude; venous congestion generally; bruised feeling in abdomen; varicose veins; hemorrhoids, adapted to passive hemorrhages, venous (complementary to Ferrum); general lassitude and a feeling of weariness, especially in her extremities, after hemorrhages or when suffering with varicose veins.

HELONIAS DIOICA

Leucorrhœa with an atonic state, or due to an atonic state of the uterus; prolaps with ulceration of cervix; discharge copious, continuous, foul-smelling, and profuse, serous, with backache, tenderness in the breasts, and a sore heavy sensation in the uterus. This is a remedy which has a constant consciousness of the uterus; very irritable, cannot bear contradiction, always fault-finding; loss of sexual desire with sterility; uterus either retroverted or low down in pelvis; always conscious of the uterus, dark, fetid discharge from uterus; labia and pudenda hot, red, swollen, covered with apthæ; indicated in women who are worn out with hard work or enervated by overindulgence and luxury; burning-aching in back when sitting; soreness and weight in uterus.

HEPAR SULPHUR

Leucorrhœa thick, creamy, yellow, with a sweetish odor; smells like hydrogen sulphide; cervical glands enlarged; indicated in pseudo-psoric patients, blondes; scrofulous leucorrhœa, yellowish or bloody, smelling like old cheese; slight wound and sore ulcerate and produce much yellow pus. Symptoms and patient very much like Cal. carb., very sensitive to cold, and > from warmth. Glandular enlargements all over the body, also a tendency to the formation of abscesses; sour smell from body; urticaria from every change of weather, aggravated by uncovering, and relieved by warmth and in damp, wet weather; wounds or sores very sensitive to touch, and patient very irritable.

HYDRASTIS

Leucorrhœa viscid, hangs from the os uteri in viscid strings, ropy, yellow, tenacious; cheese-like discharges from vagina or uterus. Leucorrhœa complicated with hepatic difficulties and constipation; superficial ulceration of the cervix uteri with tenacious leucorrhœa, debility and general prostration. Patient cachetic-looking, sallow; leucorrhœa discharges very offensive in the early stages of uterine cancer; fissures about the mucous openings of the body; weakened, debilitated, scrofulous subjects with ropy catarrhal discharges; gastric and hepatic difficulties.

HYPERICUM

Leucorrhœa in children milky; leucorrhœa with violent, lacerating pains in genitals and frequent desire to urinate; with delayed menses and heaviness and pain in small of back; diseases brought on by injuries to nerve trunks or nerve endings; wounds of the coccyx; stitching, tearing pains after injuries to nerves, surgical operations on sphincters, mechanical injuries of spinal cord and concussions, nervous shock and depression following nerve wounds.

IGNATIA

Leucorrhœa purulent and corrosive, preceded by bearing-down labor-like pains; leucorrhœa in low-spirited, hysterical, nervous subjects who are always sighing or complaining; in very hysterical women who suffer from nervous prostration, from grief, joy, and disappointed love.

IODINE

Leucorrhœa thick or thin, yellow, corroding, aggravated at the menstrual period, and attended with great weakness; hunger with emaciation; swelling and induration of cervix; leucorrhœa makes thighs sore. Leucorrhœa with great weakness; dwindling of the breasts; when it becomes corrosive it is usually scanty; very nervous, irritable, melancholic; dull pressure like a wedge between the right ovary and uterus.

KALI BICHROMICUM

Leucorrhœa yellow, ropy (Hydrast), may be drawn

out in strings; stiffens the linen, yellow; much weakness across the back; dull heavy pain in the hypogastrium, suitable to fleshy light haired women; syco-psoric affections or pseudo-psoric; sycotic or sphilitic leucorrhœa; yellowish or greenish, stringy, ropy, comes out in fine strings of a gleety nature; voice often hoarse, metallic; leucorrhœa preceded by membranous dysmenorrhœa, greenish, bloody, ropy, stringy leucorrhœa; gonorrhœal leucorrhœal, white or yellow and tenacious.

KALI CARBONICUM

Pseudo-psoric leucorrhœa with severe constant backache; back aches as if it would break; marked tired feeling; very tired in the morning and unrefreshed when she awakes; discharge yellow mucus, with itching and smarting of the vulva. Leucorrhœa very acrid and excoriating; *mucous leucorrhœa with pain in back as if it would break.* Frequent sour eructations; constipation, stools dry, large, hard, difficult. Dry, hard, tight, spasmodic cough in tubercular patients, < in the morning. Backache with night sweats and dry cough; bag-like swellings above the eyes. People with dark hair, lax fiber, inclined to obesity, very sensitive to touch, especially the feet; wandering, stitching pains. Indicated in the gouty stage of Sycosis.

KALI FERROCYANATUM

Leucorrhœa after menstruation, pus-like or yellowish,

creamy, profuse, non-irritating; "uterus tender and sensitive to touch." Minton.

KALI HYDROITODICUM

Anti-psoric and anti-syphilitic; syphilitic leucorrhœa discharge is greenish, thick, copious and offensive. Leucorrhœa white with lameness and stiffness in small of back or nightly bone pains after mercurialization.

KALMIA LATIFOLIA

Yellowish leucorrhœa which is < in the morning; pain in back and lumber region; weariness of the extremities.

KREOSOTUM

Leucorrhœa, thick mucus with bad odor, excoriating the perineum; menstrual and leucorrhœal flow intermittent; patient always chilly; discharges almost cease then begin again. Leucorrhœa acrid with voluptuous itching of pudenda, and swelling, heat and redness; whitish leucorrhœa, bland, smelling like green corn. It may be bloody in the beginning, then yellowish-white and acrid, causing much irritation and itching of the vulva. It stiffens the linen and turns it yellow; leucorrhœa like washings of meat, acrid, dark and bloody with stitches in the vagina and great debility of the lower extremities. Frequent urging to urinate at night; burning between

23 F.B.

the thighs on urinating. Leucorrhœa flows from her like milk with urinary irritation and burning in the small of the back. Indicated in delicate blondes, who are tall for their age; irritable and despondent, complexion yellow and sallow, even cancerous; gums often spongy and bleed easily; leucorrhœa with burning in abdomen like a ball of fire.

KALI MURIATICUM

Leucorrhœa milky white, thick, mucous, bland with chronic hypertrophy and congestion of uterus.

KALI PHOSPHORICUM

Leucorrhœa often bloody, acrid, scalding the parts passed over; great depression of mind; lassitude and nervous debility.

LAC DEFLORATUM

Leucorrhœa, light-yellow with great lassitude and disinclination to work; sensation as if cold air were blowing over her even when covered up warm. Chronic constipation, stools large, hard, with great straining. Indicated in anæmic patients with a well marked tubercular diathesis; she feels completely tired out and exhausted. I have found it to be called for in thin, tall, anæmic blondes with a quite disposition; subject to cephalalgia, lasting for a number of days after each menstrual period. Supraorbital headache; urine scanty during headache but pale and copious and gushes out with a hot sensation as headache is getting >. Face and lips pale, pulse slow and thread-like; patient < sitting, > lying down when quite, at rest, and in the dark.

LACHESIS

Leucorrhœa greenish, thick, or yellow just before the menses; as menses become scanty leucorrhœa increases; very sensitive over region of uterus, about waist and throat. Cannot bear clothing tight in any place. Leucorrhœa beginning three days before menses, copious, acrid, thick, yellowish, stiffening the linen; leucorrhœa in place of menses at climactric period, with hot flashes, pains, and suffering, all relieved when menstrual flow begins.

LAPIS ALBUS

Leucorrhœa white, mucous, copious, painless with some smarting in perineum; whining mood; frequent desire to urinate with scanty emissions; "bruised pain in small of back." (Minton.)

LAUROCERASUS

Leucorrhœa about the time of the climactric period,

copious, jelly-like mucus, pain in sacral region extending to pubes. Colicky during menses, a feeling of weariness in small of back ; urine pale yellow.

LAC. FELINUM

Leucorrhœa dark yellow with furious itching of the vulva and vagina ; dragging pains in left ovary ; nervous trembling all over as if intoxicated.

LAC CANINUM

Leucorrhœa yellowish, bland, occurring only in the daytime ; general symptoms erratic ; discharges from nose acrid ; intense unbearable backache, > by rest and on first moving ; membranous dysmenorrhœa followed by sore-throat or sore-throat during menses (Lach.); escape of gas from the vagina (Lyc., Sars.); great heat in ovarian region during menses with great sensitiveness and soreness ; sharp pains in left ovary ; gonorrhœal leucorrhœa, acrid, excoriating, causing swelling of labia ; raw, herpetic eruption, much swelling of labia and thighs ; breasts sore and sensitive to pressure ; sleep disturbed ; fearful dreams ; sensation as if there were a ball in throat.

LYSSIN

Leucorrhœa whitish, sometimes slimy, with pain in back ; it makes her very weak, has an offensive, whitish discharge from uterus for several months (proving); vagina and womb very sensitive, painfully so; complaints greatly aggravated by the sound of running water; desires to urinate; dread of dogs; saliva ropy, frothy, (Merc.). Breasts swell at night; a sore lameness in back and lower abdomen; cold sensation in spine. Aggravation: Touch, bright light, riding in a carriage. Adapted to blonde women of white skin, blue eyes, quick temper, and very sensitive to medicine or external impressions.

LEDUM PALUSTRE

Leucorrhœa profuse, with copious urination. Indicated in gouty forms of Sycosis; great heaviness and weariness of feet; gouty nodosities on toes; rheumatic pains in joints, especially hip joints. Indicated in pale, gouty, delicate women who are cold all the time; pains aggravated by heat of bed; pains ascend upward. Venous stases, puffy, mottled appearance during menses; gout of feet relieved by cold bathing.

LEPTANDRA

Leucorrhœa in shreds of mucus, with ulceration of os; general languor and prostration; urine red or orange color; sore, lame feeling in small of back; chronic congestion and disorders of the liver; stool often black, tarry or clay colored. "Dull aching in the liver with a weak sinking sensation in pit of stomach". (Hering's Guiding Symptoms).

LILIUM TIGRINUM

Leucorrhœa very copious, thin, and brownish with bearing-down sensation in pelvic organs, feeling as if the organs would push out through the vagina, > by supporting vulva with hand. Leucorrhœa stains the linen brown (Nit. acid), or it is bright-yellow and excoriating after a scanty menstruation. As soon as the profuse, acrid leucorrhœa begins, menses cease; the bearing down is worse standing (Sulphur), better sitting or lying down; sensation as if heart were grasped in a vice (Cactus); often indicated in any displacement or relaxation of uterus; palpitation with fluttering of the heart; low-spirited, apprehensive, burning and pressure, with dragging down sensation in all the pelvic organs, even in rectum, with desire to stool (Nux vom., Aloe, Sepia). Reddish sediment; great nervous irritation, always in a hurry, indicated in light-haired, blue or grey eyed people with florid complexions, vivacious and inclined to be fleshy, with lax muscular system; uterine complaints from child bearing. It is syco-psoric.

LYCOPODIUM

Rose-colored leucorrhœa < before the full of the moon, or it may be milky or bloody; pain and rumbling in left hypochondria; much distension and flatulence of abdomen; acid digestion, often indicated in the uric acid diathesis; following Sycosis in tertiary stage the leucorrhœa is often acrid and corrosive; dryness in vagina; gas escapes from the vagina; gnawing, itching, burning in vulva after menstruation (Kreosotum), indicated from the gastric symptoms more often than anything else. It is a deep acting remedy; acts on every tissue and on all the miasms; face is sallow, pale, or sickly; aggravated by heat of bed, > by eating dry food; low-spirited, moody; dreads solitude; great discomfort and bloating after eating.

MAGNESIA CARBONICA

Leucorrhœa white mucus, often acrid after menses, then watery, scanty, with pinching pain about the umbilicus; tongue coated white; mouth full of white mucus; leucorrhœa smells sour; stool like clay, hard, dry, crumbling. Face pale, waxy, sallow; she always feels tired and relaxed in the morning. Menses dark, acrid, pitch-like, with cutting colic, sour belching and desire for meat.

MAGNESIA MURIATICA

Leucorrhœa with great nervous excitement, often with uterine spasms; stool hard and knotty like sheep dung (Sepia). Leucorrhœa < after exercise and after stool. Leucorrhœa alternating with uterine cramps or with flow of menses. Pain in small of back as if burned; uterine diseases in nervous, hysterical women. Indicated in scirrhus of uterus ; aggravated by salt, sea-bathing, warm room ; < in open air (like Pulsatilla) ; loss of power in bladder, little power to expel urine. Backache relieved by hard pressure (Kali carb.). Eructations taste like rotten eggs ; takes cold easily, sensitive to cold and chilly, yet feels > when walking in open air.

MAGNESIA PHOSPHORICA

Another remedy having spasmodic pains in uterus during menses or spasmodic colic, also < from damp, cold weather, cold bathing ; ameliorated by hard pressure, and from heat ; often indicated in school girls (Cal. phos.), who suffer from mental emotion, study ; occipital headaches with flushed face or supra-orbital neuralgia ; menses are dark and stringy ; she is subject to chorea and spasmodic symptoms. Pains < on right side, from the least draft of cold air or cold bathing. Leucorrhœa stringy, membranous, the same as menses. Lightning-like ovarian and neuralgic pains.

MAGNESIA SULPHURICA

Leucorrhœa bloody between the menses ; bruised pain in small of back and groin. Discharge thick, white, profuse like the menses. Leucorrhœa causes burning when walking. Great heaviness in the head during menses ; greenish colored urine ; dry cough, with burning at pit of stomach ; pyrosis, water rising in the mouth ; taste bitter ; mentally of a sad and weeping mood.

MANGANUM

Indicated in waxy, chlorotic, pallid, sickly, tubercular women who have great anxiety and fear as if something were going to happen; sad, low-spirited, silent also. Leucorrhœa in chlorosis or pernicious anæmia (Ferrum, Ars.,); menses very scanty, lasting but a day or so. Discharge, greenish-yellow, tubercular pus.

MERCURIUS SOL

Leucorrhœa either acrid or bland; it may be whitish, greenish, bloody or sweet smelling; when it is purulent it produces burning, rawness, pimples, and pustules on the labia; the itching and burning is relieved by washing in cold water, also < in the evening and at night. There is much viscid cottony saliva in the mouth; the tongue is usually large and flabby, taking the imprint of the teeth; taste metallic or bitter, putrid; gums are soft, spongy, recede from teeth and bleed easily. Not infrequently the discharge is muco-purulent, thin, acrid, lumpy, there is milk in the breasts during menses. Burning and throbbing in the vagina, aphthæ; patches on labia; weakness and weariness in lower limbs; skin sallow; jaundiced looking.

MERCURIUS CORROSIVUS

Leucorrhœa pale, yellow, sweet smelling, tinged with blood, or composed of mucus and thin water; it is very acrid, causing intense heat and burning of genitals, pimples, nodules, even ulcers. Gonorrhœal leucorrhœa greenish with vesical tenesmus, with burning in the orifice; bloody urine passes in drops, with much pain and tenesmus.

MERCURIUS DULCIS

Leucorrhœa greenish-yellow; moist, burning condylomata about the external genitals; perineum and anus discharging a greenish, watery, offensive secretion; foul smell from mouth with salivation and mercurial symptoms in general. Syphilitic symptoms or syco-syphilitic symptoms (Thuja, Nit. acid, Cinnabaris).

MERCURIUS IODATUS FLAVUS

Leucorrhœa copious, muco-purulent, comes from the os uteri. Leucorrhœa in young girls or children with a syphilitic history; great weariness and weight in lower extremities, often cramp-like pains, < at night, from warmth, during summer or spring-time.

MUREX PURPUREA

Leucorrhœa watery, greenish during the day only. Leucorrhœa bloody and excoriating, feeling of great heaviness in the vagina or sensation of constriction in the uterus. Study its eruptive diseases. It is a remedy like

Sulphur which is greatly aggravated by washing and >
from warmth of bed.

MEDORRHINUM

Anti-sycotic. Gonorrhœal leucorrhœa usually profuse ; whitish or yellow ; corrosive, producing biting and pruritus of the vulva and vagina ; cannot retain urine long ; stains napkin dirty brown ; leucorrhœa opaque, white mucus ; stains linen yellow ; soreness and burning when urinating. Leucorrhœa like dirty water, thin, offensive, corrosive, producing pruritus ; odor like stale fish, musty, and pungent. Breasts sensitive and sore ; vagina and cervix mottled, with alternate bluish or pinkish spots. Sensation as if something were pulling down in left ovary ; ovary sensitive ; leucorrhœa suppressed by medicated douches. She has great difficulty in telling symptoms ; stops and begins over again ; mind weak and forgetful ; cannot remember names ; gonorrhœa of rectum or nose with thin, scanty, watery oozing. Pruritus vulvæ which is < while thinking about it.

MURIATIC ACID

Leucorrhœa, with much backache ; great soreness in anus, either from hemorrhoids or fissures. Uterine ulceration with putrid discharges, accompanied with a sense of great weakness. She is sad, ill-humored, anxious, apprehensive, disposed to be angry ; gums scorbutic; slow emission of urine from great weakness of the bladder; external genitals very sensitive to touch; heaviness of the anus; weariness of the lower extremities. Hemorrhoids protruding, dark-purple with burning in anus, > from hot bathing. Pressing sensation in the genitals as if the menses would appear; leucorrhœa with backache, pressing in genitals, soreness in anus, often indicated in low febrile states and exhausting diseases. Suitable to dark-haired, dark-eyed women. Aggravation from 9 a.m. to 1 p. m.

NATRUM CARBONICUM

The discharge of this remedy is thick, heavy, white, or yellowish mucus, pus-like, more copious during urination; the leucorrhœa like the menses is often accompanied with pressure in the hypogastrium, extending towards the genitals, as if everything would issue from the abdomen (Lil., Bell., Sepia). As a catarrhal remedy Natrum carbonicum is worthy of careful study. The thick, yellow or greenish discharge shows its sycotic curative qualities; as with all the Natrums the patient is sad, despondent, trembles from exertion, is weak minded, has a peculiar aversion to men and to society in general. She is very sleepy during the day, awakens in the morning unrefreshed. These patients cannot digest starches, therefore suffer from flatulence caused by indigestion of starchy food. They suffer with nervous hunger (like Psor., Ign., Sepia, Sulp.); they are always tired and have cold knees and cold extremities ; are nervous, dyspeptic and catarrhal. The leucorrhœas are often like the nasal catarrh, thick, greenish and copious, and comes out of the vagina in gushes ; aggravation during full moon, and during a thunder-storm, and from 5 to 11 a.m.

NATRUM MURIATICUM

Leucorrhœa thick, white or transparent, profuse, acrid, with smarting in the vulva. We often have a bearing-down or pressure-like sensation as if the menses were coming, or a cutting pain in the urethra after urinating. Leucorrhœa greenish, especially when walking ; aversion to sexual intercourse, very irritable afterwards. Melancholy, sad, despondent, dejected, and made < by consolation ; extremely sad during menstruation; she has headache every morning as if it would burst. Sensation as if sand were in the eyes or fiery zigzag flashes before the eyes. The skin is pale, waxy, greasy, often dropsical and she is subject to goose-flesh when she becomes chilled. She drops things from her hands because of a nervous weakness ; gets into a passion about trifles ; the tongue is often mapped, and she suffers with herpes about the chin and mouth during the menstrual period, or urticaria ; aggravation from 10 to 11 a.m.

NITRIC ACID

Leucorrhœa after menses, greenish mucus, or flow is watery (Lil.), flesh-colored or cherry-colored ; leucorrhœa acrid, offensive, brownish water (Sycosis) ; it is occasionally stringy (Kali bich., Hydras.) ; head aches as if head were tightly bound ; stitches in vagina ; soreness of vulva with itching. Taking cold greatly aggravates the leucorrhœa and pruritus ; bearing down in lower abdomen is quite a constant symptom. Face pale, sallow or brownish (Sepia, Lyc.) ; ulceration in corners of mouth ; aversion to meat and bread ; likes salt fish, herring, chalk, and lime (Kali carb.). Urine brownish, strong smelling, fetid (Benzoic acid), indicated frequently in tall, dark, lean women, with black eyes and hair ; she is generally < at night and > from riding in a carriage or car ; adapted to diseases coming from secondary or tertiary syphilis or syco-syphilis. The ulcers, warts, and abnormal growths bleed easily or ooze a thin yellowish-green or dirty-water secretion. It is suitable also to hemorrhages due to a syphilitic taint ; as Phosphorus is to the tubercular, so it is to the syco-syphilitic.

NUX MOSCHATA

Indicated in very hysterical women who are subject to fainting fits, and have a sort of vicarious leucorrhœa in place of the menses. Mouth and tongue become so dry they are unbearable, almost adhere to the roof of the mouth. Menses scanty, dark and suppressed, followed by profuse leucorrhœa. Great dryness of the eyes ; great inclination to laugh when out of doors (hysteria.) Great distension of the abdomen with flatulence of a nervous origin ; vanishing of thought. Pain in the back as of a piece of wood lying across it ; slimy, leucorrhœal discharge when the menses should appear ; palpitation of the heart with attacks of fainting.

PETROLEUM

Pseudo-psoric. Leucorrhœa like albumen, copious with burning in the genitals. Desire beer ; aversion to meat and fats ; itching herpes in the perinium ; soreness and moisture in the genitals ; fetid sweat in axilla ; itching and burning in different parts of the body ; skin diseases and eruptions about the genitals of both sexes ; cracks and fissures behind the ears, hands and feet ; burning and itching with redness of the skin ; chilblains.

PHYTOLACCA DECANDRA

Anti-sycotic. Uterine leucorrhœa ; cervical ulceration ; scirrhus or cancer of the cervix (Conium) ; discharge profuse, yellow, thick and often tenacious and irritating. Saliva tenacious, yellow, ropy, metallic-tasting ; pain at the root of tongue when swallowing ; inflammation, swelling and induration of the mammæ.

PHOSPHORUS

Pseudo-psoric. Leucorrhœa from chlorosis in tubercular individuals in advanced stages of the disease. In tall, thin people with narrow, pigeon-shaped and contracted chests. It sometimes takes the place of the menses, and it may be either bland or acrid ; typically, however, it is acrid, corrosive, smarting and blistering the parts passed over. Leucorrhœa milky or watery with a sense of great weakness across the abdomen ; with heat and burning in the back ; night or evening cough, < from lying down ; occasionally the leucorrhœa is pinkish or reddish, with a weak empty feeling in the abdomen and great burning of the hands and feet, which is < at night. Before the menses, a weeping (like Puls.) with bleeding from the gums and nose ; leucorrhœa with hæmoptysis in place of the menses, or spitting of blood in place of the menses ; petechia, spots on the skin. Aggravations: Evening, thundertorms, and when lying on the left side.

PHOSPHORIC ACID

Acrid leucorrhœa, profuse, bloody or yellowish with much itching, coming on a few days after menses. Leucorrhœa after exhausting fevers or diseases like pneumonia. Pale, sickly complexion with great indifference and apathy ; disinclination to talk and low-spirited ; longs for juicy, acid fruits ; stools thin and whitish or thin and yellow. Great bodily weakness, emaciation, dull, listless and apathetic, especially in the a.m. Leucorrhœa with a severe backache in young girl students (Cal. carb., Cal. phos., and Nat. mur.). Leucorrhœa after onanism ; urine clear, watery ; nervous or milky urine.

PLATINA

Leucorrhœa with constipation and great sensitiveness of the external genitals. Albuminous leucorrhœa only in the daytime, with pinching pains in abdomen and pressing down in the groins; voluptuous tingling in the pudenda.

PSORINUM

Leucorrhœa in large lumps with an unbearable odor. It leaves a yellow stain on the linen; leucorrhœa with a constant increasing debility and loss of strength; great sensitiveness to cold or sudden change of weather; leucorrhœa thin, corrosive and exceedingly offensive; perspiration sour and offensive; skin sallow, dingy, pimply, unwashed appearing, scaly, rough, moist; eczema behind the ears and corners of the mouth sore; body has a filthy smell, even after a bath; tired, weary and desire to lie down.

RANUNCULUS BULBOSUS

Psoric and pseudo-psoric in its action; leucorrhœa bland at first but in a day or two it becomes very acrid and corrosive in its character. The patients suffers with pressure and tightness across the chest, or with stitching pains across the chest; intercostal neuralgia.

RHODODENDRON

Leucorrhœa of a bloody character; gonorhœa of ovaries and tubes; cysts of ovaries. It produces itching and soreness of genitals and thighs. Choleraic symptoms arising from gonorrhœal rheumatism either hereditary or acquired. It has much burning in the uterine region, acute inflammation of joints and general rheumatism, which is brought on by damp weather or getting wet; < before a storm, especially a thunder-storm. Laboring women, strong constitutions, suffering from sycotic rheumatism. She has much fear and dread of storms. Rheumatism and all her complaints are aggravated by electrical storms. Aggravated by wet, windy, or stormy weather (Rhus tox).

ROBINIA

Leucorrhœa whitish or greenish with a bruised feeling in the womb. Leucorrhœa thick, yellow and acrid, with a very fetid smell; womb hard, firm and swollen; between the menstrual periods discharges of blood followed by an acrid, thick, purulent leucorrhœa, great acidity of the stomach. Indicated more frequently in dark-eyed and dark-complexioned people.

RHUS TOX

Rheumatic dysmenorrhœa, secondary or tertiary Sycosis; leucorrhœa like dirty water, coming on from lift ing, over-straining or getting wet. It is often acrid and excoriating and not infrequently produces herpes or vesicles on external genitals, with intense itching, smarting and burning. Extra exertion brings on menses again. Suppression of menses from getting wet and leucorrhœa follows, which is very acrid ; rheumatic pains in muscles and tendons ; stiffness, lameness, soreness all over the body which is < on beginning to move, yet > when in motion, until the muscles become tired. Aggravation, rest, quiet, afternoon, and cold. > from motion, warmth, warm and dry weather, rubbing the affected part. Sycosis in its manifestations on the muscular system, tendons and skin. It is a true anti-sycotic.

SABINA

Anti-sycotic. Leucorrhœa thin, milky, fetid ; suppression of the menses, with a milky discharge, *or with a copious and starch-like discharge with drawing pains in the small of the back through to the pubes*. Sycotic or gouty leucorrhœa, yellowish, ichorous, producing severe itching, suitable to plethoric women ; bloody leucorrhœa coming on every two weeks, offensive, smelling ; weariness and bad feeling in the lumbar region, dragging from back forwards. *Leucorrhoea after abortion or miscarriage about the third month of pregnancy*. Fig warts with itching and burning ; > in cool fresh air, music intolerable.

SANGUINARIA

This remedy is said to be especially good for leucorrhœa following the cessation of the menses, at the menopause. The discharge is fetid and corrosive. In tubercular patients with a cough, uterine polypi, cancer or ulceration of the os. It has flatulence from the vagina (Lyc.). There is pain in the loins extending down through the hypogastric region and uterus to thighs. Climactric difficulties with acrid leucorrhœa accompanied with severe burning of the hands and feet (like Phos., Sulp.). Throws the bed-coverings off (like Lach., Sulp.).

SARRACENIA PURPUREA

Anti-sycotic and pseudo-psoric. Leucorrhœa milky, thick, foul smelling, with spasmodic pains in the uterus; leucorrhœa produces an irritating eruption on the external genitals, urging to urinate with a feeling that the bladder is very full (Caladium). Great commotion in abdominal regions while lying down (Lyc.); taste very oily and bitter. Stools dark, hard, covered with mucus (Alum).

SARSAPARILLA

Anti-sycotic. Menses retarded, scanty, acrid and burning on the inside of thighs. Leucorrhœa slimy, mucous, scanty; < when walking or riding; severe pain at the close of urination. Urinary deposit like gray sand;

urine reddish, turbid, containing flakes of mucus. The patient has an old look. Indicated after suppressedgonorrhœa where the suppression manifests itself upon the urinary tract and bladder. Often the urine dribbles while sitting ; renal colic with passage of sand or gravel from the kidneys ; often indicated in sycotic children in bladder or urinary difficulties (Benzoic acid, Nit. acid).

SECALE CORNUTUM

An anti-psoric remedy, but it acts in all the miasms, even in Syphilis. Leucorrhœa is brownish and offensive or it is jelly-like, alternating with menorrhagia ; not infrequently it is dark, sanious, putrid as found in malignancies. In uterine ulcer or cancer, the discharge is dark, putrid, bloody, burning pains in uterus ; leucorrhœa that looks like coffee grounds or disorganized blood (Ars., Con., Pyro). General coldness, although heat aggravates her. Indicated in feeble, cachetic, thin, scrawny women who are full of fear, and who are very despondent and melancholy. Skin cold to touch ; < from warm covering and > in the cold air.

SEPIA

Syco-psoric. The leucorrhœa of this wonderful remedy is varied and changeable, but I have found it to be either milky and white or thick and yellow, staining the linen. Occasionally it is yellowish-green in gonorrhœa ; it is sometimes lumpy and of a fetid odor. In the latter case it is often accompanied by stitches in the cervix and is quite acrid, causing soreness of the pudenda ; in most forms there is a sensation of a downward pressure, and in displacements and malpositions, this is very marked ; crossing the limbs relieves the downward pressure; dirty-yellow or moth spots on the face are commonly present. Sepia is suited to physically feeble women, dark eyed ; skin fine with rigid fiber, but mild and gentle disposition. General weakness of the sexual sphere. Aggravation, forenoon and evening ; > from severe exercise. Sensation as of a ball in inner parts, causing the genitals to feel as though distended and as if everything were coming out through the vagina. This gives us a good picture of Sepia in pelvic difficulties.

SILICA

Pseudo-psoric but acts in tertiary stages of all the miasms. Leucorrhœa milky, watery and sometimes brownish or she has bloody discharges between the periods. Discharges of whitish water from the vagina between the menstrual periods, < after eating sour things. Leucorrhœa with severe itching and smarting of the pudenda. Again in Silica we have milky leucorrhœa or a copious, yellow leucorrhœa that is corrosive and excoriates. Aggravation in open air, cold, new moon ; amelioration by warmth, and wearing warm clothing. Adapted to light-haired, lax-muscled, pale-faced and thin blooded people ; also dry-skinned women of an irritable, nervous and tubercular taint.

STANNUM

Pseudo-psoric. Leucorrhœa with prolapsus uteri, great debility, and a sensation in the uterus as if menses would appear; weakness about the chest and throat; voice husky, deep, hollow, and weak. Leucorrhœa whitish, albuminous, transparent, mucous, or thin and watery with great debility. Pain in the malar bone during the menses. Dry cough in the evening until midnight, expectoration greenish or greenish-yellow, tastes sweet and smells musty; limbs give out easily; desire to sit or lie down constantly.

SULPHUR

Anti-psoric. Leucorrhœa with cutting and pinching pains about the navel; *scanty, acrid, inducing soreness, itching, smarting and burning of the vulva.* Leucorrhœa thick, yellow, smarting like salt and itching < at night, when she becomes warm in bed. Burning in the soles of the feet, with much heat and restlessness with desire for cool air, throwing the clothing off. Old chronic cases of leucorrhœa with a marked psoric or sulphur diathesis.

VERATUM ALBUM

Menses too early and too profuse, with cerebral congestion and choleraic symptoms; great mental disturbances ; exhaustion with cold perspiration especially on the forehead ; cold sensation on vertex with constriction of the heart ; vomiting, rice water discharges from the bowels ; general collapse ; great thirst for cold water ; lemonade or acids ; but wants everything cold ; aversion to warm things ; sudden sinking of strength like Arsenicum, adapted to lean, choleric, melancholy young women with light brown hair and lax muscles.

ZINCUM METALLICUM

Pseudo-psoric. Leucorrhœa thick, < before menses and after stool, with stinging and biting in the pudenda ; < when walking, as the result of masturbation in young girls ; great nervous exhaustion and restlessness of feet and lower extremities. Leucorrhœa preceded by cutting pain in bowels, and distension of the abdomen. Sexual mania from pruritus vulva in young girls ; pricking and twitching with soreness in the spine ; hysterical symptoms; mind acts slowly; patient weary, tired and forgetful. Indicated in spinal irritation in feeble minded girls.

REPERTORY

THERAPEUTICS OF GONORRHOEA

Aconite 165
Agaricus 166
Agustura 170
Alumina 166
Ammonium Carb 168
Ammonium Muriaticum 168
Anantherum 170
Apis 167
Argentum Nitricum 169,236
Arsenicum Album..168,169
Asparagus 167,168

Balsam of Peru 172,173
Benzoic Acid 171,204
Berberis,..........171,172
Bondonnean, ...173
Borax 170,171
Bryonia, ...172,241,246

Caladium 178
Calcaria Carb 173,174
Cannabis Indica 175
Cannabis Sativa 175,176,252
Cantharis 174,240
Capsicum 174
Carbolic Acid 176
Causticum 252

Chimaphila Umbel 178
Clematis..........176,177
Colchicum 261
Copaiba 177
Colocynthis 261
Cubeba 177,178

Digitalis 179
Doryphora 179, 180

Epigæa Repens 181
Erechthites 181
Erigeron Can......181,182
Eryngium Aquat 180
Eupatorium Pur.......180
Euphorbia Pil. 182

Fagopyrum Escu 182
Fluoric Acid 182

Gelsemium 183
Graphites 236
Gnaphalium 183,184

Hydrastis 184

Kali Bichromicum
          185,186,232

Kali Iodatum 185	Petroselinum 194,195
Kali Mur 184,185	Piper Nig. 195,196
Kali Sulph. 186,187	Prunus Spinosa........196
	Psorinum 250
Lac Can 187,188	Pulsatilla,........ 196,197
Lachesis, ...188,261	
Lycopodium, ...188,189	Saccharum Lac. 197
	Sanicula 197
Medorrhinum	Sarsaparilla 199,252
189,190,191,240,241, 261	Senecio 197,198
Mercurius Sol.........189	Senega 198
	Sepia 198,199, 204, 206, 261
Natrum Mur. 193,216	Silica 200, 216, 253
Natrum Sulph. 261	Stillingia 200
Nitrate of Uranium ..194	Staphisagria 199,200
Nitric Acid 193,194,204,248	Sulphur............. ....
Nux Vomica	....216, 236, 249, 250,251
.... 191,192,193,240	
	Terebinthinum........202
Palladium, ...195	Thuja 201

THERAPEUTICS OF THE URINARY TRACT

Aconite 202,203	Baryta Carb. 216,232
Agaricus..........203,204	Berberis 213,213
Alumina 205	Benzoic Acid 210, 211,212
Ammonium Carb. 206,207	
Ammonium Mur. 204	Cannabis Ind. 219
Antimonium Crude ..206	Cannabis Sativa ..213,214
Anthrokokali 209	Capsicum 214, 215, 216, 217
Argentum Met. 207,208,209	Carbo Veg. 218,219
Arsenicum 246,248	Causticum 221,222
Arundo 205,206	Chamomilla 217,261
Asparagus Off. 204	Chimaphila 221

Cinnabaris 219,220
Coffea 249
Cyclamen 241

Dulcamara ....
.....222,223,224,225,246

Euphrasia 225,226,227
Fluoric Acid 227,228

Gambogia 218
Gelsemium 228

Kali Nit. 229,230

Lachesis 230,231
Lac Caninum..233,234,235
LacDefloratum 231,232,233

Manganum 235,236
NuxVomica236,237,238,239

Papaya Vul 239
Pareira Brava 239,240
Petroselinum 240
Phosphorus 236,240
Pulsatilla, 240,241,242,243

Ratanhia 245
Rhus Tox ....
..243,244,245,241,246,261

Sarsaparilla 245,246
Sepia 246,247
Staphisagria 247,248
Stramonium 248,249
Sulphur 249,250,261
Syphilinum 248

Tabacum 253,254
Thuja 251,252,253

THERAPEUTICS OF DYSMENORRHOEA

Absinthium 278,180
Aconite 263,296
Acetic Acid 272,273
Actea Rac. ....
.....264,265,266,331,336
Aesculus Hip......280,281
Agaricus.........281,182
Agnus Castus ....274,275'
Aletris Far 267,268
Aloe 283,284,331,336
Alumina 269,270,316
Ammonium Carb. 278,279

Ammonium Mur. 278
Anacardium 266,267
Anatherum 273,274
Angustura 285,286
Ambra Gris 277,278
Antimonium Crude ..268
Antimonium Tart..268,269
Apis Mel. 282,283
Apocynum 285
Aralia Racemosa 270
Argentum Nit. 284,285,310
Arnica Montana 273

REPERTORY.

Arsenicum Album ......
..270,271,272,282,296,297
Arsenicum Iodide 270
Aurum Met 263,264
Arundo 274
Asafoetida 275,276,297
Asarum Europ 276,277

Baryta Carb. 286
Belladona 286,287,266,267,
  298,317,326,331,332,
  333,336,346,352.
Benzoic Acid.......... 296
Berberis 290,291
Borax 288,289
Bovista.... 289,290,296,331
Bromium 293
Bryonia .. 292,293,355,356
Bufo 293,352
Bursa Pastoris 291,292

Calcarea Carb. 311,321,325
Calcarea Phos. 311,312,313
Carbo Anamalis .. 309,310
Carbo Veg 308,309,302,310
Causticum 311
Chamomilla 308
Chimaphila 307,308
Cicuta Vir 303,304
Cinchona 302,310,313
Cinnabaris 294
Cinnamomun 296,297
Coca 306,307
Cocculus Ind., ... 300,301
Coccus Cacti 304,305

Coffea 310,311,308
Colchicum 303
Colocynthis 294,295,301,333
Conium Mac. 305,306,300
Crocus Sativus 301,302,357
Crotalus 299,300
Croton Tig. 299
Cubeba 298,299
Cuprum Met. 295,296,299
Cyclamen 305,341

Eupionum............ 313

Ferrum Met 314,315
Ferrum Phos. 317

Gelsemium ....
.... 317,318,296,330,340.
Glonoinum 315,267
Gossypium 315,316
Graphites 316,317,315
Gratiola Off 318

Hamamelis Vir .. 320,321
Helleborus 267
Helonias.......... 319,320
Hepar Sulph. 304
Hydrastus 297
Hyoscyamus 318,319,302,
  323

Ignatia .. 322,323,352,346
Iodine 321,322,341
Ipecacuanha .. 324,355,357

Kali Bich 323

Kali Carb. 324,325
Kali Iod. 323, 324,352
Kreosotum............325,326

Lac Caninum...326,327,300
Lac Defloratum 330,331,355
Lachesis 325,
267, 298, 300, 304, 319, 326
Lilium Tig. 331,332,336,340
Lithium Carb. 304
Lobelia......327, 328, 355
Lycopodium......328, 329
......266,301,310, 347,352

Magnesium Carb. 332,333,
.......................293
Magnesium Phos......333
Medorrhinum 352
Mercurius Cor.........335
Mercurius Sol. 334,
................335,303,347
Mezereum 337,338
Millefolium 333,334
Moschus..........336,337
Murex..335, 336, 334, 340
Muriatic Acid 338

Natrum Carb. 339,340
Natrum Mur. 340,
341, 342,311, 332,352,355
Natrum Sulph. 340
Niccolum 342
Nux Vomica ....
..338, 339, 296,331,347,355

Oleum Animale ..343,344
Oleum Cajeputi 344
Oleum Jec. 344,345

Opium 345,346
Origanum 342,343

Palladium 349,350
Phosphorus 348,304,340,353
Platinum..304,338,266, 336
Podophyllum......348,349
Prunus Spinosa ..347, 348
Pulsatilla, 346,347, 329,265,
277, 291, 296, 333, 340, 341

Rhus Tox 351,265,282, 293,
.........313, 317, 319, 342

Sabadilla 267
Sabina 267
Sepia ..265, 296, 304, 320,
........331, 332, 336, 343
Silicea 355,340
Stannum 353
Staphisagria ..353,354,355
Stramonium 298
Sulphur 316,352
Syphilinum 351,352

Tabacum 355,356
Terebinthina 356,357
Thuja 301
Tuberculinum 341,348

Ustilago 357

Veratrum Alba 299,355
Veratum Vir. 326
Xanthoxylum 357,358

Zinc 326,350

THERAPEUTICS OF LEUCORRHOEA

Aconite 365	Calendula 377,378
Actea Race 365	Capsicum 383
Aesculus......... 365,366	Cargo Veg. 378,379
Agaricus 366	Carbolic Acid 385,386
Agnus Castus 366	Castoreum 379
Aletris 366,367	Caulophyllum 379
Allium Sativum 367	Causticum 379,380
Aloe 367	Chamomilla 380
Alumina......... 367,368	Cina 380,381
Ambra Grisea...... 368	Cinchona, ... 381
Ammonium Carb... 368,369	Cocculus Ind. 381
Ammonium Mur. 369,373	Coccus Cacti 382
Anacardium 369	Coffea 382,383
Anantherum 369	Colchicum 383
Antimonium Crude 369,370	Collinsonia 383
Apis Mel 370	Conium 383,384
Aralia Race 370,371	Copaiba 386
Argentum Nit. 372,379,382	Crocus Sat. 384
Arnica 371	Crotalus Hor. 384,385
Arsenicum 371,372	Croton Tig. 385
Asafoetida 372	Cubeba 385
Asarum Europ. .. 372,373	Curare 385
	Cyclamen 386
Baryta Carb...... 373,374	Daphne Mezereum 387
Belladona 374	Dulcamara 386,387
Berberis 375,376	Dictamnus 387
Borax 374,375	
Bovista 375	Erigeron......... 387,388
Bufo 376	Eupion 387,388
	Ferrum Met. 388
Caladium 378	
Calcarea Carb 376,377	Gelsemium 388,389
Calcarea Phos 377	Graphites 389

Hamamelis Vir. ..389,390
Helonias 399
Hepar Sulph 399,400
Hydrastis 391
Hypericum 391,392

Ignatia 392
Iodine 392

Kali Bich 392,393
Kali Carb 393
Kali Fer 393,394
Kali Hydro 394
Kali Mur 395
Kali Phos 395
Kreosotum........394,395

Lac Canium 397
Lac Defloratum....395,396
Lac Felinum 397
Lachesis 396
Lapsis Albus 396
Laurocerasus......396,397
Ledum 398
Lilium Tig 399
Leptandra 398,399
Lycopodium 399,400
Lyssin 397,398

Magnesia Carb........400
Magnesia Mur 400,401
Magnesia Phos 401
Magnesia Sulph ..401,402
Manganum 402
Medorrhinum 404

Mercurius Cor 402,403
Mercurius Dul 403
Mercurius Iod. Flav ..403
Mercurius Sol. 402,372
Murex 403,404
Muriatic Acid 404,405

Natrum Carb 405,406
Natrum Mur 375
Nitric Acid........406,407
Nux Moschata 407,408

Petroleum 408
Phosphorus 408,409
Phosphoric Acid 409
Phytolacca 408
Platina 410
Psorinum 410

Ranunculus Bul 410
Rhododendron 411
Robinia..............411
Rhus Tox 411

Sabina 412
Sanguinaria 413
Sarracenia Par 413
Sarsaparilla 413
Secale Cor 414
Sepia 414,415
Silicea 415
Stannum 416
Sulphur 416

Veratum Vir 416,417

Zincum Met. 417